THE SKIN AND INFECTION

A Color Atlas and Text

THE SKIN AND INFECTION

A Color Atlas and Text

EDITORS

CHARLES V. SANDERS, M.D.

Edgar Hull Professor and Chairman
Department of Medicine
Louisiana State University School of Medicine
New Orleans, Louisiana

LEE T. NESBITT, JR., M.D.

Chairman
Department of Dermatology
Louisiana State University School of Medicine
New Orleans, Louisiana

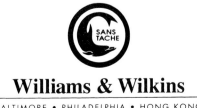

Williams & Wilkins

BALTIMORE • PHILADELPHIA • HONG KONG
LONDON • MUNICH • SYDNEY • TOKYO

A WAVERLY COMPANY

Editor: Jonathan W. Pine, Jr.
Managing Editor: Molly L. Mullen
Copy Editor: Harriet Felscher
Designer: Norman Och
Illustration Planner: Ray Lowman
Production Coordinator: Kimberly S. Nawrozki

Accurate indications, adverse reactions, and dosage schedules for drugs are provided in this
book, but it is possible that they may change. The reader is urged to review the package
information data of the manufacturers of the medications mentioned.

Printed in United States of America

Library of Congress Cataloging-in-Publication Data

The skin and infection : a color atlas and text / editors, Charles V. Sanders, Lee T. Nesbitt, Jr.
  p.   cm.
  Includes index.
  ISBN 0-683-07539-X
  1. Skin—Infections. 2. Skin—Infections—Atlases. I. Sanders, Charles V. II. Nesbitt, Lee
T.
    [DNLM: 1. Skin Diseases—diagnosis—atlases. WR 17 S628 1995]
    RL201.S55 1995
  616.5—dc20
  DNLM/DLC
  for Library of Congress   94-26490
                                                                 CIP

                                 94 95 96 97 98
              1   2   3   4   5   6   7   8   9   10

Reprints of chapters may be purchased from Williams & Wilkins in quantities of 100 or
more. Call Isabella Wise in the Special Sales Department, (800) 358-3538.

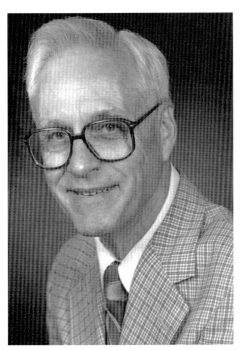

Dedicated to

Henry W. Jolly, Jr., M.D.,

a wonderful teacher and friend, who will always be a role model and source of inspiration for me. His enthusiasm, sense of humor, and zest for life contribute to the respect and admiration he has earned from all of those who know him!

Lee T. Nesbitt, Jr., M.D.

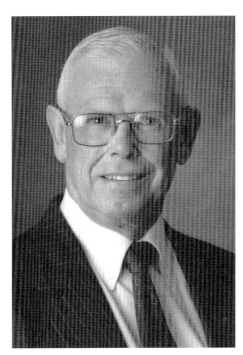

Dedicated to

Jay P. Sanford, M.D.,

my early mentor and a continual source of inspiration. His zeal for the field of infectious diseases fueled my own fascination with the subject, and his untiring committment to medical education helped build the foundation for my career.

Charles V. Sanders, M.D.

FOREWORD

The skin is the largest organ system of the body and the one with the greatest surface area. By virtue of its exterior location it is subject to contact with a variety of infectious agents that may colonize its surface or, following trauma, penetrate into the deeper epidermis, dermis, or subcutaneous tissues. Such invasion can produce a variety of well-defined primary bacterial pyodermas, such as impetigo, folliculitis, furunculosis, erysipelas, cellulitis, or necrotizing fasciitis, to mention but a few. Similarly, distinctive lesions occur with various infections that are viral (e.g., herpes simplex, molluscum contagiosum, human papillomavirus), mycotic (e.g., sporotrichosis), spirochaetal (e.g., syphilitic chancre, erythema migrans of Lyme disease), and mycobacterial (e.g., primary inoculation tuberculosis) as well. Not only is the skin the site of primary cutaneous infections, but it may also serve to mirror systemic infections (e.g., infective endocarditis, dermatitis-arthritis syndrome of disseminated gonococcal infection, meningo-coccemia, rose spots of typhoid fever, mucocutaneous lesions of secondary syphilis).

Definition of the specific microbial etiology of (1) a primary skin infection, (2) a secondarily infected noninfectious process (e.g., viral infection of underlying atopic dermatitis, (3) toxin-induced changes in the skin due to infection elsewhere in the body (e.g., scalded skin syndrome, toxic shock syndrome), or (4) bacteremia (e.g., infective endocarditis) is essential in selecting appropriate antimicrobial therapy. To make such an initial determination of the likely etiologic agent, the physician needs to employ all the tools of clinical diagnosis: detailed history with emphasis on epidemiologic evidence, careful physical examination, and laboratory testing.

The morphology of skin lesions can offer useful clues as to the underlying process and the likely infecting agent. Despite the advances in laboratory tests (e.g., fluorescent antibody staining of tissue biopsy specimens, polymerase chain reaction in the identification of specific microbial DNA sequences), and radiologic procedures (radionuclide and magnetic resonance imaging of soft tissue infections), physical examination unquestionably provides the most valuable preliminary information as to the likely etiology. It initiates the thinking about differential diagnosis by establishing the category of cutaneous lesions that should be considered. Thus, the lesions of nodular lymphangitis ("sporotrichoid syndrome"), gangrenous cellulitis, purpura, generalized maculopapular eruption, and chancriform ulceration will each bring to the fore specific etiologic considerations. Since infections in the skin may evolve over hours (e.g., change from macular to petechial lesions in Rocky Mountain spotted fever; from papules to vesicles in varicella), repeated evaluations of the character of the lesions provide further insight into etiology.

The status of the immune system in a given patient can alter the appearance of specific microbial infections of the skin and/or affect the spectrum of potential invasive microorganisms. Thus, in immunocompromised patients such as those with HIV infection, the grouped vesicles of genital herpes may recur more frequently and have a more prolonged course. Deep, rapidly progressive ulcers may occur or the lesions may appear gangrenous with overlying eschars. Similarly, molluscum contagiosum viral infection may have extremely widespread lesions. Opportunistic pathogens such as *Cryptococcus neoformans* or *Candida* spp. may produce, in patients with altered cell-mediated immunity, lesions with an appearance similar to cellulitis caused by various streptococci and *Staphylococcus aureus*. Novel opportunistic pathogens, such as the *Rochalimaea* species *R. henselae* and *R. quintana*, have produced distinctive violaceous, papular, hemangioma-like cutaneous lesions in immunocompromised patients with AIDS.

The clinician's initial evaluation of cutaneous lesions in a febrile patient, or of lesions of likely infectious nature even though present in a patient without fever, leans heavily on their gross appearance. Although well-chosen words can serve to describe the wide range of types of skin lesions or their arrangement and distribution, there is no substitute for direct observation of the lesions themselves to help in their identification.

The great value of an extensive collection of hundreds of illustrations, as in this volume, lies in the ability to convey a useful picture of the identifying features and overall gestalt of these cutaneous manifestations of infection. Carefully selected photographs and slides, such as are included in this color atlas, can provide a "visual memory" for the physician who may not often encounter some of these lesions among his patients. The presentation of the pictorial material under clinically relevant rubrics provides a convenient framework for the approach to the patient and for differential diagnosis. Such rubrics include chapters on necrotizing and gangrenous soft tissue infection, infections in the immunocompromised host, diagnosis of the patient with fever and a rash, and cutaneous signs of septicemia.

The value in presenting representative images of cutaneous lesions is enhanced by the inclusion herein of a listing of causes of similar lesions to be considered in the differential diagnosis. Emphasis is appropriately placed on the use of simple diagnostic tests, such as Gram-stained smears of exudates, Ziehl-Neelsen-stained smears, dark-field microscopy, fluorescence under Wood's lamp, Tzanck preparations of scrapings from vesicular lesions, and histologic examination of biopsy specimens.

In compiling this extensive color atlas of skin lesions in local and systemic infections, the editors and authors have made available a remarkably comprehensive collection of excellent photographs of characteristic skin lesions. By accompanying these visual images with a descriptive text that includes commentary on epidemiologic aspects, clinical course, diagnostic tests, differential diagnoses, and treatment they have provided a comprehensive presentation of "the skin and infection." This collective effort provides a sharply focused and extremely well-illustrated volume that will be of continuing value to practicing clinicians, infectious disease specialists, dermatologists, teachers of medicine, and medical students.

Morton N. Swartz, M.D.
Professor of Medicine
Harvard Medical School

PREFACE

Students provide the primary stimulus for teachers. This is certainly the case in the stimulus for this color atlas and text. Over the years, many residents and medical students have inspired our dedication to providing instruction in a subject in which we all have a vital interest—the skin and infection.

In fact, the impetus for this atlas began almost 15 years ago with one medical student in particular, when B. Eugene Beyt, Jr. approached Dr. Sanders with an idea. A talented photographer, he was interested in developing a text on infectious diseases and the skin that would feature extensive color plates of the clinical and pathologic manifestations. He believed, as we do, that good photographic documentation of skin lesions is important in both medical education and in following the disease course of individual patients.

Dr. Beyt went on to train in infectious diseases, and, although he eventually moved in a different direction, he helped formulate the book's contents during meetings with Doctors Sanders, David S. Feingold from Tufts, and Arnold Weinberg of the Massachusetts Institute of Technology. While Dr. Weinberg left to pursue other commitments, Dr. Feingold remained involved to become a chapter contributor. These initial meetings gave the book its shape.

In 1990, the new Head of Dermatology at Louisiana State University, Dr. Lee T. Nesbitt, Jr.,was enlisted as co-editor, lending a meticulous perspective to the effort. Finally, a new coordinating editor, Ms. Caroline Helwick, solidified the team in 1993 and provided invaluable assistance in bringing this volume to completion.

The result is *The Skin and Infection: A Color Atlas and Text*. Certainly, other infectious disease texts are available to students and residents, academicians and clinicians; indeed, many of them are excellent resources. However, a number of such publications rely more heavily on illustrations than on written material to convey information. This atlas, on the other hand, combines both approaches in a more balanced, practical format: almost 500 color illustrations accompany 22 chapters to provide extensive coverage of the cutaneous manifestations of infection. Contributors include nearly 30 leading dermatologists, infectious disease specialists, pathologists, and microbiologists from throughout the United States. Their chapters comprehensively cover a gamut of critical topics in the field.

We begin with a summary of general considerations in evaluating patients who present with skin infections as well as a review of histological skin patterns seen most commonly in infection. Subsequent chapters are devoted to staphylococcal and streptococcal infections, septicemia, necrotizing and gangrenous soft tissue infections, infectious zoonoses, and a range of sexually transmitted diseases.

Lyme disease, the rickettsioses, and tuberculous and nontuberculous mycobacteria are examined, as are superficial and systemic fungal infections. Separate chapters deal with skin manifestations in the immunocompromised host—those stemming from HIV and AIDS and those that are nonHIV-related. Leprosy, viral exanthems and other viral infections, and protozoan and helminth infections are surveyed at length, and a separate chapter is devoted to bites, stings, and infestations. We conclude with an overview of fever and rash.

We hope this extensive collection will prove invaluable to students, trainees, and clinicians alike, both as a detailed introduction to the challenging array of cutaneous manifestations in infection and as a trusted standard reference.

Charles V. Sanders, M.D.
Lee T. Nesbitt, Jr., M.D.

NOTICE: In light of the ever-changing nature of the field of medicine, the editors and publisher of this text encourage the reader to confirm information contained herein, especially regarding the administration of medications. Indications, contraindications, dosages, and side effects should, in particular, be validated with current product information inserts, since these features change as research and clinical experience broaden the knowledge base. While we have made every effort to produce a text of the highest academic quality, checking with sources we believe to be reliable, no party involved in the publication of this work warrants that the information contained herein is complete in every aspect and instance.

ACKNOWLEDGMENTS

No labor of this type would be possible without the support of many persons. Our deepest gratitude goes first to our wives, Julia Sanders and Yvette Nesbitt, for the many years they have been part of our lives and work. Their unflagging support and their understanding of our love for the field of medicine—as well as the latitude they have generously extended to us in demanding careers—have made this book and other achievements possible. Over the years, they have been willing and supportive participants in many discussions of this project, particularly on those occasions when it seemed the book would never materialize. Special thanks are due, as well, to our children—Laura, Jonathan, and Benjamin Sanders, who pulled reprints so long ago they may no longer remember it, and Julye and Terrell Nesbitt, who were an inspiration and joy when efforts on this work seemed insurmountable.

Contemporaries in the practice of infectious diseases and dermatology as well as the residents that we have each taught have contributed greatly to our knowledge, have shared interesting cases that add to the scope of this volume, and have voiced their own enthusiasm for this project. Particularly, we want to thank Eugene Beyt, M.D., who as a medical student first approached one of us (C.V.S.) about doing an atlas and who, with that idea in mind, photographed a number of patients.

Contributors for each chapter are to be cited for their outstanding expertise and their continued devotion to this project. They have made the book possible.

Finally, co-workers in our departments have made some of the toil on this project a pleasure because of their cooperative spirit, sense of humor, and special talents. We thank Donald L. Greer, Ph.D., for his helpful reviews of chapters dealing with mycoses and acid-fast infections. Chuck Chapman, then editor at Louisiana State University School of Medicine, coordinated initial efforts to launch the book and helped lay the groundwork. Caroline Helwick later assumed the role of coordinating editor, and we thank her for her astute editorial advice and her tireless committment to seeing this to press. Holly Tietjen's able handling of manuscript preparation and her skill in devising chart and table configurations were invaluable. Zack Wilson and Jim Lilly, Jr. made countless trips to the library to track down essential references, and Marsha Brock and Linda Munoz demonstrated unwavering professionalism and patience during their many years as our administrative secretaries. In the late stages of the project, Anne Compliment provided additional editorial support. Each contributed mightily to the final product.

Charles V. Sanders, M.D.
Lee T. Nesbitt, Jr., M.D.

CONTRIBUTORS

Jack L. Arbiser, M.D., Ph.D.
Fellow in Dermatology, Harvard Medical School and Howard Hughes Medical Institute, Boston, Massachusetts

Kenneth A. Arndt, M.D.
Professor of Dermatology, Harvard Medical School, Boston, Massachusetts

Marc Avram, M.D.
Resident in Dermatology, Harvard Medical School, Boston, Massachusetts

Bernard W. Berger, M.D.
Clinical Assistant Professor of Dermatology, State University of New York at Stonybrook, Southampton, New York

Edward Chan, M.D.
Intern in Medicine, Harvard Medical School, Boston, Massachusetts

Bruce H. Clements, M.D.
Chief, Clinical Branch, Gillis W. Long Hansen's Disease Center, Carville, Louisiana

William E. Dismukes, M.D.
Professor and Vice Chairman for Educational Programs, Director, Medical Housestaff, University of Alabama School of Medicine, Birmingham, Alabama

Mervyn L. Elgart, M.D.
Professor and Chairman of Dermatology, The George Washington University Medical Center, Washington, D.C.

Carmen G. Espinoza, M.D.
Professor of Pathology, Louisiana State University School of Medicine, New Orleans, Louisiana

Douglas P. Fine, M.D.
Professor and Vice Chairman of Medicine, Chief, Medical Services, V.A. Medical Center, Chief, Infectious Diseases, University of Oklahoma Health Sciences Center, Oklahoma City, Oklahoma

Jo-David Fine, M.D.
Professor of Dermatology, Adjunct Professor of Epidemiology, University of North Carolina Schools of Medicine, and Public Health, Chapel Hill, North Carolina

David S. Feingold, M.D.
Professor and Chairman of Dermatology, Professor of Medicine, Tufts University School of Medicine, Boston, Massachusetts

Wesley King Galen, M.D.
Clinical Associate Professor of Dermatology, Louisiana State University School of Medicine and Tulane University School of Medicine, New Orleans, Louisiana

Leonard E. Gately, III, M.D.
Clinical Assistant Professor of Dermatology, Louisiana State University School of Medicine, New Orleans, Louisiana

Stephen E. Gellis, M.D.
Assistant Professor of Dermatology (Pediatrics)
Harvard Medical School, Director, Dermatology Program
Children's Hospital, Boston, Massachusetts

Donald L. Greer, Ph.D.
Professor of Clinical Mycology, Departments of Dermatology, Pathology, and Microbiology, Louisiana State University School of Medicine, New Orleans, Louisiana

Michael K. Hill, M.D.
Assistant Clinical Professor of Medicine, Section of Infectious Diseases, Louisiana State University School of Medicine, New Orleans, Louisiana

Jan V. Hirschmann, M.D.
Professor of Medicine, University of Washington School of Medicine, Assistant Chief, Medical Service, Seattle V.A. Medical Center, Seattle, Washington

Joy D. Jester, M.D.
Assistant Professor of Dermatology, Louisiana State University School of Medicine, New Orleans, Louisiana

Richard Allen Johnson, M.D.
Instructor in Dermatology, Harvard Medical School, Boston, Massachusetts

Debra Chester Kalter, M.D. (deceased)
Silver Spring, Maryland

W. A. Krotoski, M.D., Ph.D., M.P.H.
Research Physician, Laboratory Research Branch, Gillis W. Long Hansen's Disease Center, Carville, Louisiana, Clinical Associate Professor of Infectious Diseases, International and Tropical Medicine, and Parasitology, Louisiana State University School of Medicine, New Orleans, Louisiana

Brian D. Lee, M.D.
Clinical Associate Professor of Dermatology, Louisiana State University School of Medicine, New Orleans, Louisiana

James L. Leyden, M.D.
Professor of Dermatology, University of Pennsylvania School of Medicine, Philadelphia, Pennsylvania

David H. Martin, M.D.
Harry E. Dascomb, M.D. Professor of Medicine, Professor of Microbiology, Chief, Section of Infectious Diseases, Louisiana State University School of Medicine, New Orleans, Louisiana

Tomasz F. Mroczkowski, M.D.
Research Professor of Dermatology and Venereology, Section of Infectious Diseases, Department of Medicine, Louisiana State University School of Medicine, New Orleans, Louisiana

Daniel M. Musher, M.D.
Professor of Medicine, Microbiology, and Immunology, Baylor College of Medicine, Chief, Infectious Disease Section, Veteran's Administration Medical Center, Houston, Texas

Lee T. Nesbitt, Jr., M.D.
Professor and Chairman of Dermatology, Louisiana State University School of Medicine, New Orleans, Louisiana

Robert H. Rubin, M.D.
Chief of Transplantation Infectious Disease, Massachusetts General Hospital, Director, Center for Experimental Pharmacology and Therapeutics, Harvard-M.I.T. Division of Health Sciences and Technology, Boston, Massachusetts

Andrew H. Rudolph, M.D.
Clinical Professor of Dermatology, Baylor College of Medicine, Houston, Texas

Rolando E. Saenz, M.D.
Associate Professor of Medicine, Louisiana State University School of Medicine, New Orleans, Louisiana, Chief of Infectious Diseases, University Medical Center, Lafayette, Louisiana

Charles V. Sanders, M.D.
Edgar Hull Professor and Chairman, Department of Medicine, Louisiana State University School of Medicine, New Orleans, Louisiana

Edward J. Septimus, M.D.
Clinical Professor of Internal Medicine, University of Texas Health Sciences Center, Director, Infectious Diseases Program, Memorial Healthcare System, Houston, Texas

Alan M. Stamm, M.D.
Associate Professor of Medicine, University of Alabama School of Medicine, Birmingham, Alabama

CONTENTS

CHAPTER 1

Evaluating the Patient with a Skin Infection—General Considerations

LEE T. NESBITT, JR.

In medical practice, the nature of the patient's chief complaint commonly directs the physician in pursuing much of the pertinent history and physical examination. This is certainly true when the presenting complaint involves the skin and an infection is suspected.

In the diagnosis of many skin disorders, taking an initial detailed history before the physical examination is not as mandatory as with certain other medical problems. The rationale for this occurrence is that many skin lesions are almost immediately visible to the physician, with physical diagnosis beginning early in the patient interview and orienting the physician to important questions to be asked later in the history. In fact, dermatologists often prefer to look at skin lesions before obtaining a detailed history or review of systems so that there will be no bias in the history to eliminate any of the complete differential diagnostic considerations. In many other disciplines as well, skilled clinicians often obtain much of the history during the physical examination of the patient.

The experienced and astute clinician will know the proper amounts of general medical and cutaneous histories to obtain in each case and will be able to direct the patient with the proper questions for the greatest detection of essential and significant information. In patients who present with skin eruptions that may be related to a systemic infection, it is extremely important to consider the patient as a whole and perform a detailed complete medical history and physical examination.

Patient History

A good history must always be obtained at some point during the patient visit for the absolute best clinical impression to be made. Initially, the age, sex, and race of the patient must be considered, since certain infections are more prevalent depending upon these factors.

For example, primary syphilis is diagnosed much more frequently during years of greatest sexual activity in males, as primary chancres may commonly go undetected on mucosal surfaces in females due to lack of pain. Disseminated gonococ-

cal disease with skin lesions, in contrast, almost always occurs in females due to the organism gaining access to hematogenous dissemination during menses.

Besides the routine history of present illness, past medical history, social and family history, and review of systems, several key pieces of information are necessary in the proper evaluation of skin lesions, especially those believed to be related to infection. The following considerations should always be obtained in evaluating a patient of this type.

TIME OF ONSET OF SKIN LESIONS

The approximate times of onset of the lesions is one of the most important pieces of information and should be determined as accurately as possible. Exacerbations, remissions, and recurrences of the skin eruption should also be determined. Chronic meningococcal or gonococcal sepsis, for example, will show skin lesions during periods of fever and bacteremia, with the timing and association of these recurrent symptoms of utmost diagnostic importance.

SITE OF ONSET

The initial area of the body involved by the lesions is extremely important and can often be a key in diagnosis. The pattern of spread or dissemination to other parts of the body is also vital information to obtain. A classic example is that of erythema infectiosum, which begins with bright erythema of the cheeks followed in a few days by reticulated erythema of the extremities, providing a diagnostic clinical picture.

CHANGE OF LESIONS

The patient should be asked to attempt to describe the original lesions and how they may have evolved since the onset of the eruption. Lesions present at one particular examination or point in time may be quite different from the lesions that initially appeared. Lymphopathia venereum, for example, will show a very transient genital lesion that heals, followed in a few weeks by significant inguinal lymphadenopathy. The time of examination will vary greatly in physical findings.

CUTANEOUS SYMPTOMS

The presence or absence of itching, burning, other types of discomfort, or any other symptomatology is extremely important in affording the most educated differential diagnostic considerations. For example, the symptoms of neural pain followed by typical skin lesions of herpes zoster makes diagnosis of that disorder almost unquestioned.

PROVOKING FACTORS

The patient should be asked if any known factors precipitated the lesions. It is also important to ascertain if any other illness occurred prior to or at the time of onset of the skin lesions, as this could possibly be associated. An example of a common clinical association is that of herpes simplex infection preceding the development of skin lesions of erythema multiforme.

PREVIOUS TREATMENT

A very important piece of information is whether there has been any self-treatment or previous treatment by physicians that affected the skin lesions in either a positive or negative way. Any infectious process, for example, may be greatly affected by the use of topical or systemic corticosteroid therapy, causing a pronounced change in the clinical lesions and often making diagnosis more confusing. Tinea infections are common processes in which the appearance is often changed by glucocorticoid therapy.

OCCUPATION AND HOBBIES

These are very important subjects in determining various types of exposure the patient may have had in regard to specific infections. Persons whose occupation or hobby is gardening would be much more prone to develop sporotrichosis, whereas those persons with occupations or hobbies related to water could more likely develop *Mycobacterium marinum* infections.

GEOGRAPHIC FACTORS

Where the patients have lived and where they have traveled prior to the onset of lesions can be useful information, especially in infections that are seen most commonly in certain geographic locations. In the United States, coccidioidomycosis is usually contracted in the southwestern states, whereas blastomycosis and histoplasmosis are seen with much higher frequency in the Mississippi and Ohio River valley areas.

CONSTITUTIONAL AND PRODROMAL SYMPTOMS

In evaluating a possible systemic infection, acute symptoms such as fever, sweats, sore throat, and gastrointestinal upset are of immense importance as are symptoms of chronic illness, such as fatigue, malaise, and weight loss.

PATIENT OPINION

The patient's own opinion should never be disregarded. Although patients may be incorrect, their opinions in many instances may help the physician arrive at the correct diagnosis.

Individual Lesions

Every field of medicine has a certain language of its own. This is as true for the study of skin diseases as for any other medical discipline. Dermatologists essentially speak this language each day of their professional lives, but nondermatologist physicians have less familiarity with the words necessary to communicate fully in regard to skin disorders. This discussion is meant as a basic introduction to the language of skin lesions so that the rest of this text and atlas will offer the greatest possible value to all physicians.

Basic terminology has not always been standardized in describing skin lesions. A glossary of basic lesions has been produced by the International League of Dermatologic Societies to alleviate this problem. This discussion will utilize those standardized terms.

MACULES

A macule is a circumscribed, flat lesion that differs from surrounding skin by color (Fig. 1.1). It may have any size or shape, with very large macular lesions often called "patches." Macules can show an erythematous color through capillary dilatation or can manifest various other colors, including hyperpigmentation and hypopigmentation.

Certain specialized lesions are commonly macular. These include telangiectasia and purpura. Telangiectasia represent persistent capillary dilatations, most types of which blanch on pressure. Purpuric lesions represent discolorations of skin caused by extravasation of red blood cells (Fig. 1.2), and they are commonly divided into two categories: ecchymoses, which are large, bruise-like purpuric lesions, and petechiae, which are small, pin-point purpuric lesions.

A technique that is often utilized to distinguish between purpura and certain other lesions, including telangiectasia and erythema, is diascopy. This is a technique whereby a magnifying lens or a glass slide is applied to the surface of a reddish skin lesion. If the redness remains under the pressure of the lens or slide, the lesion may represent purpura. Alternatively, erythema or telangiectasia produced by capillary dilatation usually will blanch under pressure.

PAPULES

A papule is a circumscribed, solid, elevated skin lesion that is palpable and usually smaller than 0.5 cm in diameter (Fig. 1.3). Papules may have varying shapes and may be dome-surfaced, flat-topped, or verrucoid. When papules have scaling at the surface, these lesions are usually referred to as papulosquamous lesions (Fig. 1.4). Papules may be of any color, may sometimes conform to openings in the skin (as in folliculitis), or may coalesce into larger lesions called plaques.

In some instances, both telangiectasia and purpura can be elevated and are therefore papular. Papular areas of purpura are often called palpable purpura and can distinguish certain types of cutaneous vasculitis from other causes of purpura.

The term maculopapular eruption is often used for a skin eruption consisting of both macules and papules (Figs. 1.5, 1.6).

To appreciate very slight papular elevations of the skin, it may be necessary to direct light onto the lesions from a source located at an oblique angle to the lesions.

PLAQUES

A plaque is a large, solid, elevated skin lesion that is palpable (Fig. 1.7). Plaques are larger than papules, but sometimes may be formed by coalescence of smaller papules.

WHEALS

A wheal is a specialized plaque or papule that contains edema and is characteristically transient, usually lasting less than a day. Wheals can occur as an allergic or non-allergic response to innumerable agents, including insect bites and various infections. Angioedema represents a giant, deep wheal that is seen clinically as a large area of swelling in the skin due to edema.

LICHENIFICATION

Lichenification refers to a plaque or patch that has become thickened due to chronic scratching or rubbing. This cutaneous lesion is essentially always indicative of chronic pruritus.

NODULES

A nodule is a circumscribed, solid, palpable skin lesion with depth as well as elevation (Figs. 1.8, 1.9). Depth of involvement and/or greater palpability differentiate nodules from papules and plaques. Nodules may sometimes involve the epidermis as well as the dermis and subcutaneous tissue. They may be round, ellipsoid, or irregular in shape. It is usually clinically beneficial to determine if a nodule is hard or soft, firm or fleshy, fixed or movable, painful or painless, and if the nodule is warm to the touch. Physicians also use tumor as a general term for a large nodule or for any mass produced by a growth of a particular cell type, be it benign or malignant.

VESICLES AND BULLAE

Vesicles and bullae are circumscribed, elevated lesions of the skin containing fluid. Vesicles are lesions smaller than 0.5 cm in diameter (Figs. 1.10, 1.11), and bullae may be any size greater than 0.5 cm in diameter. These lesions may form at any level within the epidermis, at the epidermal-dermal junction, or in the upper dermis. Those vesicles and bullae that are in the uppermost portions of the epidermis are more fragile and have a greater tendency for easy rupture. When a vesiculobullous lesion does rupture, the area of denuded skin left is known as an erosion, which is a moist area that may be slightly depressed in relation to surrounding skin. Usually, erosions quickly develop crusts, consisting of dried serum and other exudates, on their surfaces.

PUSTULES

A pustule is a circumscribed, raised lesion containing pus (Fig. 1.12). This purulent material, containing leukocytes with or without other debris, may contain microorganisms or may be sterile. Pustules may have varying sizes and shapes and may be various colors, including white, yellow, or green.

Variations of pustules include furuncles, carbuncles, and abscesses (Fig. 1.13). A furuncle is a deep form of folliculitis, containing pus, with necrosis of the follicle and surrounding connective tissue. Several furuncles may coalesce to form a larger lesion, called a carbuncle. An abscess is a broad term encompassing both furuncles and carbuncles in which the accumulation of purulent material is very deep and in which pus is usually not visible at the skin surface. Collectively, pustules and other related lesions are often called pyodermas, which relates to any purulent skin process. Any purulent or pyodermatous process may also produce crusts when there is rupture of pus at the skin surface.

Sometimes a purulent skin disorder may develop a tract leading to the skin surface, which is called a sinus. Sinus tracts can be seen in actinomycosis, scrofuloderma, botryomycosis, mycetoma, and gummas of syphilis.

CYSTS

A cyst is a circumscribed, closed cavity or sac containing a liquid or semisolid material (Fig. 1.14). On palpation, a cyst usually has a similar feeling to that which occurs with pressure over the eyeball.

ULCERS

An ulcer is a depressed defect of the skin in which the epidermis and at least the upper (papillary) dermis has been lost (Figs. 1.15, 1.16). Ulcers can have various shapes, borders, bases, and discharge. All of these features are of importance in a clinical attempt to determine the ulcer etiology. Location on the body is also very important in determining what is suspected clinically as causing the ulcer.

Ulceration can result from tissue infarction due to vascular compromise, from rapid tissue growth (as in malignancy), from severe inflammatory processes, and from excoriations or other types of trauma. Ulcers are more common on areas of pressure, over bony prominences, and in body folds. Nodules adjacent to ulcerations may suggest a granulomatous (Fig. 1.17) or neoplastic process.

SCARS

A scar is an area of skin in which one type of tissue that has been destroyed by injury or disease is replaced by fibrous tissue. In many instances, an ulceration or infectious process has taken place previously and the pattern of healing results in a scar (Fig. 1.18). Scars may be hypertrophic when the skin is elevated with excessive fibrous tissue, atrophic when the skin is thin and wrinkled, or cribriform, in which the scar tissue is perforated with multiple small pits. Sometimes, increased amounts of connective tissue result in sclerosis, a term often used for diffuse hardening or induration of the skin.

SCALES

A scale represents a flake of stratum corneum that is shed from the skin surface (Fig. 1.19). These are among the most common individual lesions of the skin and often occur on a background of macules, papules, plaques, or other primary lesions. Scales may be light or dark, and may vary in thickness from very thin (branny) to heaped-up (ostraceous) with all gradations between. Collarettes of scale at the edges of lesions are seen classically in pityriasis rosea (which is likely related to some unidentified microorganism), but can also be seen in superficial mycoses and secondary syphilis. When scales desquamate in large sheets or to a severe degree, this type of desquamation is often called exfoliation.

CRUSTS

A crust is a hardened deposit at the skin surface resulting from serum, pus, or blood drying on the skin surface (Figs. 1.20, 1.21). Crusts may be various colors depending on the type of exudate and are often said to be honey-colored in impetigo. They may be extremely thick in conditions such as ecthyma, when they involve the entire thickness of the epidermis, or in favus-type superficial fungal infections of the scalp.

OTHER LESIONS

Certain other dermatologic terms should also be recognized. Excoriations are superficial epidermal excavations produced by scratching that may be linear or sharply circumscribed. They usually indicate significant pruritus, as seen in infestations, and may lead to scarring. Fissures are linear splits in the skin related to inflammation (Fig. 1.22), and they may be painful. They may be seen in body folds and can sometimes be caused by dermatophytes or *Candida* organisms. Burrows are small tunnels in the skin caused by a parasite, such as is seen in scabies. Gangrene represents death of tissue from a severe necrotizing and sloughing process. It can result from arterial occlusion or an infectious process with marked tissue destruction. Finally, atrophy is a diminution in size of a particular portion of the skin. It can refer to a decrease in epidermal, dermal, or subcutaneous thickness, or a combination thereof. With epidermal atrophy, one can usually easily see underlying superficial dermal blood vessels, whereas atrophy of deeper tissues is usually characterized by depressed areas of the affected skin.

Shape and Arrangement of Lesions

After the types of lesions are identified, their individual shape and arrangement on the skin are the next important considerations and can be major keys to diagnosis. Some terms can be used to apply to the shape of a single lesion or the arrangement of multiple lesions. For example, a single lesion may have a linear quality, or multiple lesions may be arranged in a linear pattern. Another example is that of a single lesion that may be annular, or multiple lesions that may be arranged in an annular pattern (Fig. 1.23).

The shape of individual lesions may be round, annular (ring-shaped), arciform, iris, oval, polygonal, polycyclic, linear, serpiginous (snake-like), or umbilicated (Fig. 1.24).

Annular lesions are not identical to round lesions. Annular lesions have borders that contrast with their centers; round ones do not, being completely uniform throughout the lesion. A spe-

cial type of annular lesion is the iris (target) lesion characterized by rings of varying degrees of erythema, sometimes surmounted by a central vesicle or bulla. A round or annular lesion can sometimes be explained by a relationship to the vascular supply from an individual arteriole, or from the centrifugal extension of an infection from the point of inoculation. An arciform lesion relates to a partial ring-like lesion. Polycyclic lesions have variable annular, arciform, oval, or other unusual ring-like shapes.

A linear lesion can be an important feature that may indicate an exogenous cause or inoculation of an infectious process. The isomorphic (Koebner) phenomenon occurs in certain disorders when trauma plays a role in the induction of a lesion, or lesions. This may be linear, for example, with trauma such as that produced by scratches. Serpiginous lesions, in contrast, take very unusual shapes and often indicate a parasitic infestation.

Papules or vesicles may have a surface that is umbilicated, which means that there is a central depression on the surface of the lesion. This finding is often indicative of certain viral infections, such as papules of molluscum contagiosum or vesicles of the now world-eradicated viral infection, variola (smallpox).

Arrangement of lesions on the skin is defined by how the lesions are related to one another. There are three major arrangement patterns of lesions: linear, annular, and grouped.

LINEARITY

As in a single linear lesion, a linear arrangement of lesions may also indicate an exogenous cause or inoculation of an infectious process. The isomorphic phenomenon may be operative. Papules, vesicles, and pustules are lesions that most often can be arranged in a linear pattern. Nodules, however, may also occur in a linear pattern, such as sporotrichosis nodules along the course of lymphatic channels. The term sporotrichoid pattern is sometimes used in this clinical situation, since sporotrichosis is a prototype disease for its spread along lymphatic channels. Many other infections may also have a similar spread, including atypical mycobacterial infections. Macular lesions may also sometimes be linear, as in the linear erythema produced by lymphangitis from an infectious process.

ANNULARITY

As in a single lesion, multiple lesions may also occur in an annular, arciform, or polycyclic pattern. Certain infections tend to spread in this type of pattern. The individual nodules of lupus vulgaris or gummatous syphilis, for example, may exhibit these patterns. In many instances, however, lesions of these diseases are arranged in incomplete or broken ring-like patterns. Secondary syphilis, dermatophyte infections, and Lyme borreliosis may also produce annular maculopapular lesions in the skin.

GROUPING

Vesicles, papules, wheals, or nodules may occur in groups in certain disorders. Groups of vesicles clustered together are so characteristic of herpes simplex and herpes zoster infections that this type of grouping is commonly termed herpetiform (Fig.

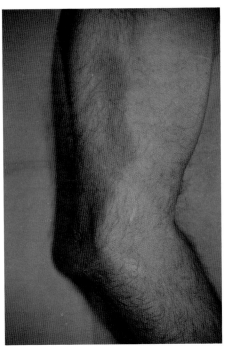

Figure 1.1.   Streptococcal lymphangitis. A linear, macular erythematous lesion. (Courtesy of Dr. Charles V. Sanders)

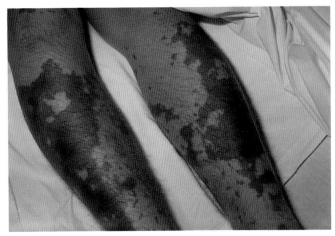

Figure 1.2.   Meningococcemia. Purpuric lesions showing large ecchymoses and small satellite petechiae.

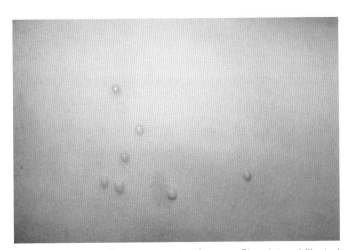

Figure 1.3.   Molluscum contagiosum. Pinpoint umbilicated papules in close proximity to each other.

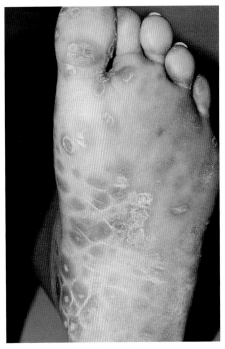

Figure 1.4.   Secondary syphilis. Reddish-brown papulosquamous lesions on the sole of the foot.

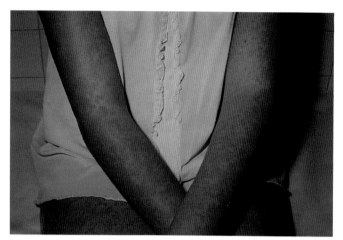

Figure 1.5. **Infectious mononucleosis.** Generalized maculopapular eruption in a patient who took ampicillin.

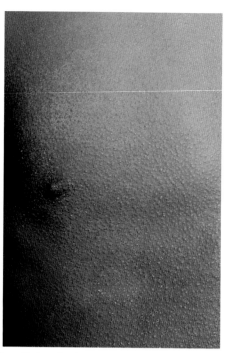

Figure 1.6. **Rubeola.** Generalized fine maculopapular eruption.

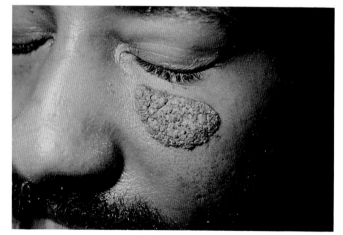

Figure 1.7. **Blastomycosis.** Large verrucoid plaque of the left cheek.

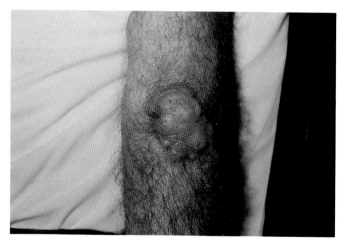

Figure 1.8. *Mycobacterium marinum* **infection.** Large nodular lesion of the elbow related to an injury in a fisherman.

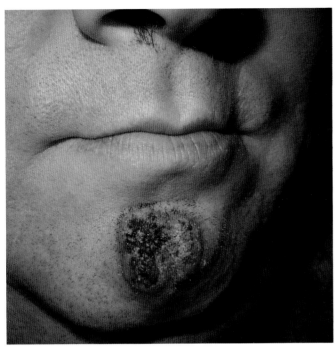

Figure 1.9.   Blastomycosis. Ulcerated, crusted nodule of the chin.

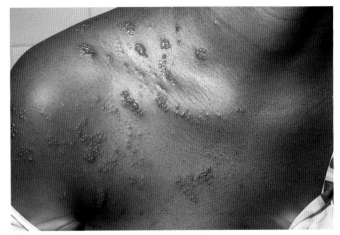

Figure 1.10.   Herpes zoster. Grouped vesicular lesions of the anterior chest and shoulder that are unilateral, stopping at the midline.

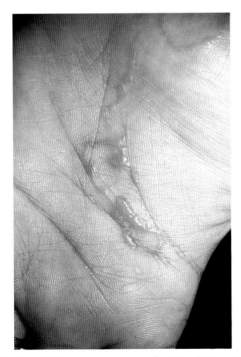

Figure 1.11.   Cutaneous larva migrans. Linear serpiginous papulovesicular to bullous lesions of the palm.

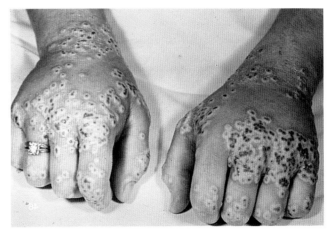

Figure 1.12.   Vaccinia. Large numbers of umbilicated pustules in a patient vaccinated for prevention of smallpox prior to its total world eradication.

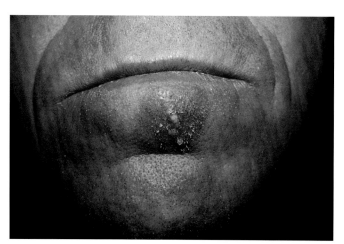

Figure 1.13.   Tinea barbae. Furuncular lesion of the chin with overlying follicular pustules, due to *Trichophyton rubrum.*

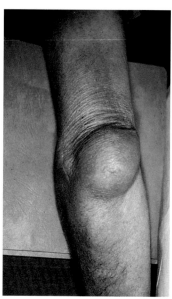

Figure 1.14.   Atypical mycobacterial infection. Large cystic lesion due to *Mycobacterium marinum* involving bursa of the elbow. The lesion contained large amounts of fluid as well as granulomatous inflammation. (Courtesy of Dr. Charles V. Sanders)

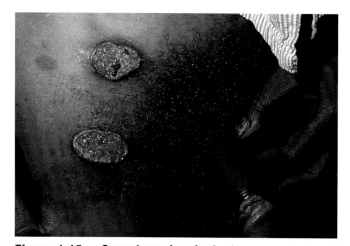

Figure 1.15.   Granuloma inguinale. Large granular-based ulcers on the penis and inguinal area with sharply defined, overhanging edges.

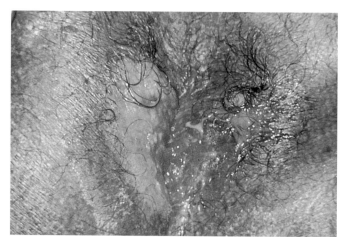

Figure 1.16.   Orificial tuberculosis. Irregular ulcerative and eroded lesion of the perianal area in a patient with active tuberculosis.

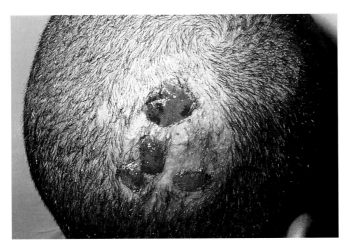

Figure 1.17.   Tinea capitis. Nodular ulcerations of the scalp in a child with granulation tissue response in resolving kerion.

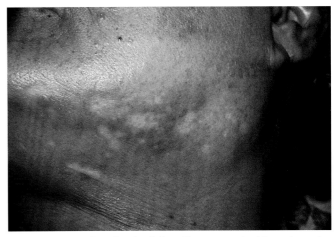

Figure 1.18.   Cervicofacial actinomycosis. Linear hypopigmented and atrophic scars in a patient with "lumpy jaw."

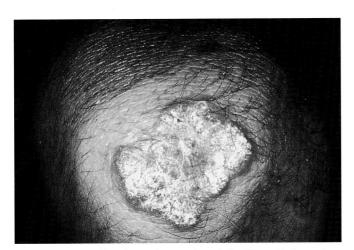

Figure 1.19.   *Mycobacterium marinum* **infection.** Erythematous plaque with silvery scale of the elbow due to trauma. The lesion resembled psoriasis.

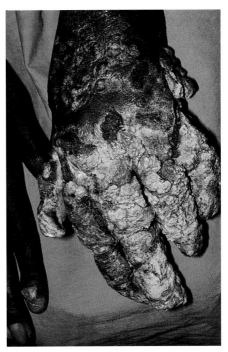

Figure 1.20.   Chronic mucocutaneous candidiasis. Heavy, verrucoid crusts of the hands in a patient with specific immunodeficiency to *Candida*.

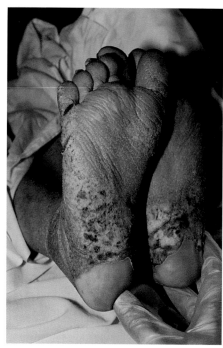

Figure 1.21.   Norwegian scabies. Thick crusts with scaling and fissures of the soles in an institutionalized patient.

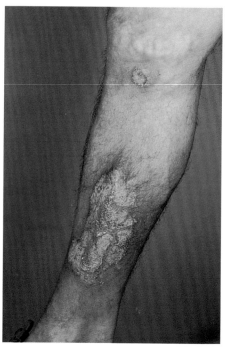

Figure 1.22. Chromomycosis. Large verrucoid and scaly plaques of the leg showing fissures within the larger lesion.

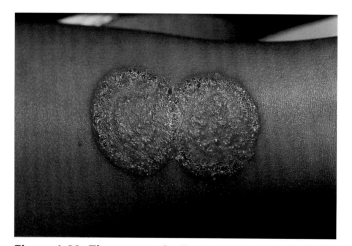

Figure 1.23. Tinea corporis. Two coalescing annular plaques showing raised, active borders contrasting with scaly, less-active centers.

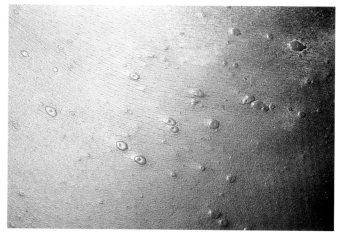

Figure 1.24.   Varicella-zoster infection. Generalized umbilicated vesicular eruption in a patient with zoster who had chronic leukemia for 8 years.

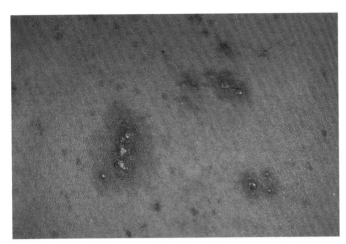

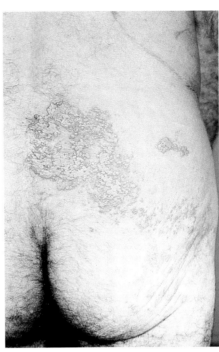

Figure 1.25.   Herpes zoster. Herpetiform, grouped vesicles on erythematous bases.

Figure 1.26.   Herpes zoster. Zosteriform, dermatomal grouping of vesicular lesions on erythematous bases of the lower back, stopping at the midline.

CHAPTER 2

Histopathology and Pathophysiology

CARMEN G. ESPINOZA

Histological examination of skin specimens removed at biopsy is useful in deciphering the nature of infectious diseases. Combining morphological identification of organisms with known tissue reaction to them gives strong support to clinical findings.

The number of cell types and the pattern of responses in the skin are limited, as are the mediating mechanisms directing these responses. Only a few pathogens, such as the molluscum contagiosum virus, may cause a unique or pathognomonic histological skin pattern. Most organisms can cause two to three different histological patterns that are shared not only with other pathogens but also with noninfectious processes. For example, *Candida* causes a spongiform pustule reaction; however, dermatophytes and psoriasis vulgaris may cause a similar pattern. *Candida* may also cause a suppurative granulomatous reaction, one similar to that with many pathogens, including blastomycosis. In addition, in immunosuppressed hosts having disseminated candidiasis, the organisms may be found growing in the dermis with no inflammatory cells.

Discussed in this chapter are the histological skin patterns most commonly seen in infection; the infectious agents most likely to cause such patterns; and, briefly, the mechanisms of lesion production.

Histological Patterns and Pathophysiology

MINIMAL OR NO INFLAMMATORY REACTION (TABLE 2.1)

The intraepithelial organisms listed in Table 2.1 have in common their tendency to multiply at the site of entry and shed directly to the exterior. Although the stratum corneum is the ideal place to escape immunological surveillance (Figs. 2.1–2.3), it meets the nutritional requirements of only a few organisms. The epidermis lacks blood vessels needed for pro-

Table 2.1. Minimal or No Inflammatory Reaction

Location of Lesion	Disease	Usual Pathogen	Site of Organism
I. Intraepithelial			
A. Nonproliferative	Erythrasma	*Corynebacterium minutissimum*	Stratum corneum
	Pitted keratolysis	*Corynebacterium* species	Stratum corneum
	Pitted keratolysis	*Micrococcus sedentaris*	Stratum corneum
	Tinea nigra	*Cladosporium werneckii*	Stratum corneum
	Tinea versicolor	*Malassezia furfur*	Stratum corneum
B. Cytoproliferative	Verruca vulgaris	Human papillomavirus	Epidermis above basal-cell layer
	Condyloma acuminatum	Human papillomavirus	Epidermis above basal-cell layer
	Molluscum contagiosum	Poxvirus	Epidermis above basal-cell layer
II. Intradermal	Cryptococcosis	*Cryptococcus neoformans*	Upper dermis

ducing an inflammatory response; however, it has Langerhans' cells in the stratum epinosum, and those cells usually process antigens for stimulation of T lymphocytes.

Papilloma and molluscum contagiosum viruses do not invade the basal-cell layer and have a decreased number of Langerhans' cells (Fig. 2.4). To explain the paucity of Langerhans' cells in the epidermis of these lesions, investigators have postulated the production of substances toxic to the Langerhans' cells, which block their reproduction. Another theory is that the cells have migrated to carry a signal to lymphocytes. As a rule, although the cells infected with these viruses produce a small amount of interferons, the viruses are resistant to their action. Thus, in the control of these infections, cell-mediated immunity plays an important role. Lesions showing dermal inflammatory infiltrate have lymphocytes and many Langerhans' cells in this infiltrate.

The response to infection by an organism is determined essentially by both the organism's characteristics and the host's response. *Cryptococcus* appears in tissue as a single budding yeast covered with a thick, poorly antigenic, mucinous capsule. As a rule, it causes a space-occupying lesion in the dermis but no inflammatory infiltrate; however, occasionally, it may produce a granulomatous response. Because opportunistic fungal infections in immunosuppressed hosts lack cellular inflammatory infiltrate but usually cause thrombosis of blood vessels, these infections are discussed below under the heading "Vascular Patterns."

Table 2.2. Acute Inflammatory Reaction

Location of Lesion	Disease	Usual Pathogen	Site of Organism
I. Epidermis			
A. Intracorneal pustule	Staphylococcal scalded skin syndrome (SSSS)	*Staphylococcus* toxin exfoliatin	Absent in lesion
	Impetigo	*Staphylococcus aureus* *Streptococcus pyogenes*	Pustule
B. Subcorneal pustule	Impetigo	*Staphylococcus aureus* *Streptococcus pyogenes*	Stratum corneum
	Candidiasis	*Candida* species	Pustule
C. Intraspinous pustule	Dermatophytosis	Dermatophytes	Stratum corneum
	Candidiasis	*Candida* species	Pustule
	Secondary syphilis	*Treponema pallidum*	Epidermis and blood vessels
II. Dermis	Erysipelas	*Streptococcus pyogenes*	Deep dermis
	Erysipeloid	*Erysipelothrix rhusiopathiae*	Deep dermis
	Abscess	*Staphylococcus aureus* *Nocardia* species Anaerobes	Abscess
III. Dermis & subcutaneous tissue	Cellulitis	*Streptococcus pyogenes* *Staphylococcus aureus* *Haemophilus influenzae*	Deepest portion of dermis or fat
IV. Follicles	Superficial folliculitis	*Staphylococcus aureus* *Pseudomonas aeruginosa*	Pustule in infundibulum
	Deep folliculitis		
	1. Furuncle	*Staphylococcus aureus* *Pseudomonas* species	Pus
	2. Carbuncle	*Staphylococcus aureus* *Pseudomonas aeruginosa* Aerobes	Pus
V. Nail	Paronychia	*Pseudomonas aeruginosa* Aerobes	Nail and skin

ACUTE INFLAMMATORY REACTION (TABLE 2.2)

The organisms causing this type of response are usually small, rapidly dividing bacteria in an extracellular location. They elicit all stages seen in an acute inflammatory response with migration of leukocytes, particularly neutrophils. Pus is formed when great numbers of neutrophils are present. Because of the potential to produce pus, many of these bacteria are called "pyogenic." As the acute response subsides, chronic inflammation appears, or healing and repair take place.

Staphylococcal scalded skin syndrome appears in young children and persons with impaired renal function. The lesion is produced by exfoliatin, an epidermolytic toxin caused by staphylococci, phage group II. The skin is the target, although the organism is always present elsewhere in the body. The early lesion contains no inflammatory cells and is characterized by splitting of the epidermis and acantholysis just below the granular layer. The detached epidermis becomes necrotic and produces chemotactic factors for neutrophils.

Candida is a yeast-like saprophyte of the epidermis and mucosa. It is recognized as a pathogen by the presence of pseudohyphae. When pseudohyphae are formed, the organism produces chemotactic factors for neutrophils. The epidermis acts as a semipermeable membrane, and, because the organisms are close to the stratum corneum, the pustule is usually formed at this level. A similar mechanism is suspected in dermatophytes.

Folliculitis in the dermis is associated with a perifollicular inflammatory infiltrate. If the follicle ruptures, the normal elements of the follicle and its contents will elicit a granulomatous reaction regardless of the size of the organisms.

VESICULAR REACTION (TABLE 2.3)

Bullous impetigo and staphylococcal scalded skin syndrome (SSSS) are caused by phage group II *Staphylococcus*. In bullous impetigo, a superficial local infection, the organisms are present in clear subcorneal blisters that later become pustules. SSSS is caused by the toxin produced by the *Staphylococcus.*

The spongiotic vesicles caused by infectious agents and by noninfectious agents are similar. First, multiple foci of spongiosis with exocytosis arise in the epidermis and become confluent, usually forming a multiloculated blister. The cells identified in early spongiotic vesicles usually are T lymphocytes and Langerhans' cells.

Some viruses characteristically cause blisters to form by the mechanism of ballooning degeneration of the epidermis (Fig. 2.5). The infected epidermal cells undergo considerable swelling with loss of intercellular bridges, resulting in acantholysis. The severe swelling causes the cells to burst, and bullae arise in which the residual cell walls form septae. The process is called reticular degeneration of the epidermis because of the bullae's appearance.

CHRONIC INFLAMMATORY REACTION (TABLE 2.4)

Succeeding the acute inflammatory cell infiltrate is the chronic infiltrate in viral and spirochetal infections; however, a chronic inflammatory cell infiltrate tends to be present early in the course of the infection.

In the viral exanthems, the infiltrate is mainly lymphocytic. In rubella, the rash most likely is caused by the damaging effect of an antibody counteracting the virus, because a correlation exists between the onset of the rash and the presence of antibodies in blood. In rubeola, the virus is present within the epidermis, causing multinucleated cells. In the exanthem caused by human immunodeficiency virus, the putative mechanism is primary infection of epidermal Langerhans' cells.

Lesions resulting from syphilis and other spirochetal infections have many plasma cells (Figs. 2.6, 2.7). Erythema chronicum migrans in Lyme disease may have variable histological features. Usually a chronic inflammatory infiltrate is evident—with vary-

Table 2.3. Vesicular Reaction

Location of Lesion	Disease	Usual Pathogen	Site of Organism
I. Subcorneal	Staphylococcal scalded skin syndrome (SSSS)	*Staphylococcus* toxin exfoliatin Phage group II	Not in lesion
	Bullous impetigo	*Staphylococcus*	Blister
II. Spinous layer			
A. Spongiotic	Dermatophytosis	Dermatophytes	Stratum corneum
	Gianotti-Crosti syndrome Id reaction	Hepatitis B virus Dermatophytes	Not in lesion
B. Ballooning degeneration	Herpes/varicella Smallpox Vaccinia Hand, foot, and mouth disease Ecthyma contagiosum (Orf) Milker's nodule	Herpesvirus Poxvirus variola Poxvirus vaccinia Coxsackievirus Parapoxvirus Pseudocowpox	Blister

Table 2.4. Chronic Inflammatory Reaction

Location in Dermis	Disease	Usual Pathogen	Site of Organism
I. Superficial	Viral exanthem:		
	1. Fifth disease	Parvovirus	Not in lesion
	2. Rubella	Rubella virus	Not in lesion
	3. Rubeola	Rubeola virus	Epidermis
	4. Acquired immunodeficiency syndrome	HIV virus	Langerhans' cells
	5. Dermatomyositis-like eruption	*Toxoplasma*	Not in lesion
		Borrelia	Dermis
	6. Superficial fungal infection	*Malassezia furfur*	Horny layer
		Dermatophytes	Horny layer
II. Superficial and deep perivascular	Secondary syphilis	*Treponema pallidum*	Near blood vessels
	Borderline leprosy	*Mycobacterium leprae*	Histiocyte
	Erythema chronicum migrans	*Borrelia burgdorferi*	Dermis

Table 2.5. Suppurative Granulomatous Reaction

Type of Lesion	Disease	Usual Pathogen	Site of Organism
I. Draining sinuses	Actinomycosis	*Actinomyces israelii*	Sulfur granule
	Mycetoma		
	1. Actinomycetoma	*Actinomyces* species *Streptomyces madurae* *Nocardia brasiliensis* *Nocardia asteroides*	Grain
	2. Eumycetoma	*Allescheria boydii* *Madurella grisea* *Madurella mycetomatis* *Phialophora jeanselmei*	Grain
	Botryomycosis	*Staphylococcus aureus* *Pseudomonas aeruginosa*	Grain
II. Pseudoepitheliomatous hyperplasia and epidermal microabscesses	Blastomycosis	*Blastomyces dermatitidis*	Lesion
	Paracoccidioidomycosis	*Paracoccidioides brasiliensis*	Lesion
	Chromomycosis	*Fonsecaea pedrosoi* *Fonsecaea compacta* *Cladosporium carrionii* *Phialophora verrucosa*	Lesion
	Blastomycosis-like pyoderma	*Staphylococcus aureus* *Wangiella dermatitidis*	Lesion
III. Dermal	Mycobacteriosis	Atypical mycobacteria	Lesion
	Deep folliculitis	Bacteria Fungi Herpesvirus	Hair follicle, rarely perifollicular

ing numbers of lymphocytes, eosinophils, histiocytes, and plasma cells (mainly perivascular) throughout the dermis. Sometimes an acute inflammatory infiltrate is also present, especially near the tick bite in primary lesions. Chronic lesions of erythema chronicum migrans may resemble scleroderma.

SUPPURATIVE GRANULOMATOUS REACTION (TABLE 2.5)

In this type of reaction, neutrophils are present as is a chronic inflammatory cell infiltrate containing histiocytes and multinucleated giant cells (Fig. 2.8). Neutrophils and macrophages work to ingest, kill, and digest microorganisms. Multinucleated

Table 2.6. Granulomatous Inflammatory Reaction

Type of Granulomatous Reaction	Disease	Usual Pathogen	Site of Organism
I. Diffuse histiocytic	Lepromatous leprosy	*Mycobacterium leprae*	Histiocytes Schwann cells
	Leishmaniasis	*Leishmania* species	Histiocytes
	Malacoplakia	*Pseudomonas aeruginosa* *Escherichia coli* *Staphylococcus aureus*	
	Disseminated histoplasmosis	*Histoplasma capsulatum*	
	Rhinoscleroma	*Klebsiella rhinoscleromatis*	
II. Discrete granulomas			
A. Noncaseating	Tuberculosis	*Mycobacterium tuberculosis*	Histiocytes
	Leishmaniasis	*Leishmania* species	Histiocytes
	Tuberculoid leprosy	*Mycobacterium leprae*	Schwann cells
	Brucellosis	*Brucella* species	Histiocytes usually
	Late secondary syphilis	*Treponema pallidum*	absent in lesion
B. Caseating	Tuberculosis	*Mycobacterium tuberculosis*	Histiocytes, caseous
	Tertiary syphilis	*Treponema pallidum*	Absent in lesion
	Histoplasmosis	*Histoplasma capsulatum*	Center of lesion
	Mycobacteriosis	Mycobacteria other than M. tuberculosis	Histiocytes, extracellular
C. Necrobiotic (Stellate abscess)	Lymphogranuloma venereum	*Chlamydia trachomatis*	Not identified in tissue
	Tularemia	*Francisella tularensis*	Not identified in tissue
	Cat-scratch disease	Gram-negative bacillus	Rarely seen in tissue

cells are formed by the fusion of histiocytes when the organism's large size precludes management by a single macrophage.

The first group listed in Table 2.5 is characterized clinically by intermittent discharge of pus containing grains (Fig. 2.9). The grains in actinomycosis and mycetoma represent microcolonies, whereas the grains of botryomycosis represent bacteria trapped in proteinaceous material.

Because of the chronicity of the lesion, pseudoepitheliomatous hyperplasia with epidermal microabscesses and dermal fibrosis may also be present. When pseudoepitheliomatous hyperplasia and epidermal microabscesses are histologically present, the lesions have a verrucous appearance (Fig. 2.10). The organism may be found in the dermis or undergoing transepidermal elimination.

GRANULOMATOUS INFLAMMATION (TABLE 2.6)

Granulomatous inflammation is characterized by histiocytes and multinucleated cells having varying numbers of lymphocytes and plasma cells. The organisms that cause this type of reaction can multiply within the histiocyte. A diffuse histiocytic pattern is associated with decreased cell-mediated immunity in the host. Discrete granulomas are seen in immunocompetent hosts. The organisms are more abundant in diffuse histiocytic reactions than in discrete granulomas. Granulomas with caseous necrosis may have organisms at the center. Stellate abscesses do not contain organisms identifiable in tissue sections.

In lepromatous leprosy, investigators have postulated a spe-

cific deficiency of T lymphocytes in recognizing the bacterial antigen, whereby the inadequately instructed macrophage fails to destroy the phagocytized *Mycobacterium leprae*, thus allowing its proliferation (Fig. 2.11). Malacoplakia is believed to result from an acquired defect of the macrophage in the lysosomal enzymes, which prevents it from digesting the phagocytized bacteria.

Early granulomas in tuberculosis do not undergo caseous necrosis. The organism multiplies within the macrophage and destroys it. If viable organisms are present when the histiocytes disintegrate, these organisms will infect other macrophages and perpetuate infection. Multinucleated giant cells in these granulomas most likely interact with antigens rather than bacteria. In tuberculoid leprosy (Fig. 2.12), the bacilli may be seen in Schwann cells. Macrophages then digest the infected cells and destroy the bacilli and the Schwann cells of the nerves.

ULCERATIVE PATTERN (TABLE 2.7)

Complete or partial loss of the epidermis is called an erosion, whereas the term "ulcer" includes loss of epidermis and at least some of the superficial dermis. Erosions and ulcerations allow the infected material to be shed to the environment; however, such environmental contamination is not essential for the spread of these infections.

Uncomplicated syphilitic chancre and the primary lesion of granuloma inguinale are histological erosions. *Corynebacterium diphtheriae* produces an exotoxin that inhibits cell protein syn-

Table 2.7. Ulcerative Pattern

Type of Lesion	Disease	Usual Pathogen	Site of Organism
I. Erosion	Syphilis (Primary chancre)	*Treponema pallidum*	Lesion
	Granuloma inguinale	*Calymmatobacterium granulomatis*	Lesion
II. Ulceration	Diphtheria	*Corynebacterium diphtheriae*	Ulcer bed
	Chancroid	*Haemophilus ducreyi*	Ulcer bed
	Lymphogranuloma venereum	*Chlamydia trachomatis*	Ulcer bed
	Tularemia	*Francisella tularensis*	Lesion, but not visible
	Ecthyma	*Streptococcus pyogenes*	Ulcer bed
	Buruli ulcer	*Mycobacterium ulcerans*	Necrotic tissue
	Swimming pool granuloma	*Mycobacterium marinum*	Ulcer bed
	Leishmaniasis	*Leishmania braziliensis*	Ulcer bed
		Leishmania mexicana	Ulcer bed

Table 2.8. Vascular Pattern

Type of Lesion	Disease	Usual Pathogen	Site of Organism
Organism present			
1. Angioinvasive			
A. Vasculitis and thrombosis	Rocky Mountain spotted fever	*Rickettsia rickettsii*	Endothelium
	Typhus	*Rickettsia prowazekii`*	Endothelium
	Progressive ulcerative ulcer	Herpesvirus	Endothelium
B. Necrotizing vasculitis	Cellulitis due to vibrio	*Vibrio vulnificus*	Scattered in dermis and subcutaneous tissue
	Ecthyma gangrenosum	*Pseudomonas aeruginosa*	Capillary wall
		Aeromonas species	Capillary wall
		Candida species	Capillary wall
C. Thrombosis, vasculitis and pustules	Chronic gonococcemia	*Neisseria gonorrhoeae*	Pus, around vessels
	Acute meningococcemia	*Neisseria meningitidis*	Thrombus, vessel wall
	Subacute bacterial endocarditis	Cocci, bacilli	Thrombus
	Staphylococcal septicemia	*Staphylococcus aureus*	Thrombus
D. Thrombosis and infarcts	Aspergillosis	*Aspergillus*	Thrombus and dermis
	Zygomycosis	Zygomycetes	Thrombus and dermis
	Opportunistic infections	*Fusarium* species	Thrombus and dermis
2. Angioproliferative	Bacillary epithelioid angiomatosis	*Rochalimaea henselae*	Macrophages, dermis
	Bartonellosis	*Bartonella bacilliformis*	Macrophages, endothelial cells
Organism absent			
A. Vasculitis	Leukocytoclastic vasculitis	Antigen-antibody complex	Not in lesion
		Streptococcus pyogenes	Not in lesion
		Mycobacterium tuberculosis	Not in lesion
		Haemophilus influenzae	Not in lesion
B. Thrombosis	Disseminated intravascular coagulation	*Streptococcus pyogenes*	Not in lesion
		Varicella-zoster virus	Not in lesion
		Neisseria meningitidis	Not in lesion
		Rubella	Not in lesion

Table 2.9. Panniculitis and Diffuse Cellulitis

Location of Lesion	Disease	Usual Pathogen	Site of Organism
Septal panniculitis	Erythema nodosum	*Coccidioides immitis* *Streptococcus pyogenes* Many other organisms	Not in lesion
Lobular panniculitis	Erythema induratum Subcutaneous abscess	*Mycobacterium tuberculosis* *Mycobacterium* other than *M. tuberculosis* *Nocardia* species Deep fungi	Not in lesion Lesion Lesion Lesion
Diffuse cellulitis with crepitis and gas	Clostridial anaerobic cellulitis Nonclostridial anaerobic cellulitis	*Clostridium perfringens* *Clostridium septicum* *Bacteroides* species	Devitalized tissue Devitalized tissue Lesion

Diffuse cellulitis with deeper infection	Synergistic necrotizing cellulitis
	
	Draining sinuses
	
	Gangrenous cellulitis
	
	Acute infectious cellulitis
		Mixed bacterial infections:
		    anaerobes and enteric Gram-
		    negative organisms
		Bacteroides
		Fusobacterium species
		Mixed bacterial infections:
		    microaerophilic anaerobes, cocci
		Aspergillus species
		Zygomycetes
		Pseudomonas aeruginosa
		Vibrio vulnificus
		Streptococcus B
		Haemophilus influenzae
		Pneumococcus
			Lesion

thesis and causes epithelial necrosis. Most of the granulomatous inflammation associated with caseous necrosis or other types of necrosis can result in an ulcer when the necrotic material is eliminated to the surface.

VASCULAR PATTERN (TABLE 2.8)

Angioinvasive lesions are classified according to the primary site of vascular involvement by the organism and the most salient histological features (Figs. 2.13, 2.14). The fungi listed in Table 2.8 are opportunistic, and no cellular inflammatory response may occur, despite the presence of many organisms in the thrombus, blood vessel wall, and dermis (Fig. 2.15).

In the angioproliferative infectious diseases, production of an angiogenic factor by the organisms has been postulated.

Leukocytoclastic vasculitis is an immune complex disorder. The immune complexes are deposited within the wall of the postcapillary venules and lead to complement activation and production of C5a, which is chemotactic for neutrophils. Leukocytoclasis and the coincident release of lysosomal enzymes cause the vascular damage and extravasation of erythrocytes. Thrombosis and epidermal necrosis may also be present.

Disseminated intravascular coagulation is characterized histologically by widespread noninflammatory thrombosis of small blood vessels. The extreme manifestation, called purpura fulminans, is associated with infarction and hemorrhagic necrosis.

Thrombosis causes a consumption of platelets, fibrinogen, prothrombin, and plasminogen. In purpura fulminans, protein C, which is needed for its anticoagulant and profibrinolytic activities, is severely deficient.

PANNICULITIS AND DIFFUSE CELLULITIS (TABLE 2.9)

Erythema nodosum involves predominantly the subcutaneous septae, while other types of panniculitis predominantly affect the lobules of the subcutaneous fat (Fig. 2.16). Bacteria and fungi are by far the most common agents identified in infectious panniculitis. Diffuse cellulitis tends to have variable amounts of necrosis.

Morphology of Infectious Agents in Tissue Sections

Correlation between the histological pattern and morphology of the organisms is vital for accurate histological diagnosis (Table 2.10). Most organisms can be identified in hematoxylin-and-eosin-stained sections; however, special stains ease the search. The larger the organism, the easier the recognition by light microscopy. Current light microscopic techniques, such as immunoperoxidase staining and in situ hybridization with DNA probes, are becoming popular. The latter is so sensitive that the presence of an infectious antigen may be detected when no morphological tissue change is evident.

Table 2.10. Morphology of Infectious Agents in Histological Sections of Skin

Pathogen	Characteristics
I. Virus	In routine H&E sections, can sometimes be recognized by the cytopathic changes in the infected cell.
A. Herpesvirus	Ground-glass appearance of nuclei. Multinucleated cell with nuclear molding. Cowdry type A of intranuclear inclusions. Affects keratinocytes and endothelial cells.
B. Measles virus	Multinucleated epidermal cells.
C. Pseudocowpox virus	Eosinophilic intracytoplasmic inclusion bodies in keratinocytes.
D. Molluscum contagiosum virus	Large eosinophilic intracytoplasmic inclusion bodies.
E. Poxvirus variolae	Eosinophilic intracytoplasmic inclusion bodies (Guarnier bodies).
F. Poxvirus vaccinia	Eosinophilic intracytoplasmic inclusion bodies.
G. Papillomavirus	Koilocytes or changes in the keratohyline granules in the epidermal granular layer.
II. Bacteria	
A. Rickettsia	Small size (0.3 x 1 μm) requires special stain. Direct immunofluorescence with antibodies against rickettsia is the preferred method of visualization.
B. Eubacteria	
1. *Streptococcus*	Cocci. Gram-positive, small, round organisms.
2. *Corynebacterium minutissimum*	Delicate filamentous forms, 1 μm or less in diameter.
3. *Pseudomonas*	Gram-negative rods.
4. *Klebsiella rhinoscleromatis*	Small, round or ovoid bodies within large histiocytes, better seen with *rhinoscleromatis* PAS or silver stains.
5. *Bacillus anthracis*	Gram-positive rods.
6. *Neisseria gonorrhoeae*	Gram-negative diplococci. Fluoresceinated antibodies against gonococcus are very effective in demonstrating gonococcus.
7. *Vibrio vulnificus*	Gram-negative rods.
C. Mycobacteria	Not visualized in H&E, requires special stain for acid-fast bacilli. Fite is preferred for *M. leprae* and Kinyon or Auramine-Rhodamine for the others.
D. Spirochetes	Visualized with silver stains. *Treponema* is slender and has more coils than *Borrelia*.
E. Actinomycetes	*Nocardia* is better seen with silver stain as branching filaments 1 μm in diameter.

Table 2.10. *cont.*

Pathogen	Characteristics
III. Fungi	Most seen in H&E, however, periodic acid-Schiff and Gomori chromic methenamine silver are used for better visualization. The diameters of the fungal elements are listed.
A. Superficial mycosis	
1. *Cladosporium wernekii*	Septated, pigmented hyphae 1.5–3 µm
2. *Malassezia furfur*	2.5–4.0 µm. Hyphae and spores (spaghetti and meatballs).
3. Dermatophytes	Hyphae and spores 3–15 µm.
B. Subcutaneous mycosis	
1. *Sporotrichum schenckii*	3–5 µm budding yeast, some cigar-shaped.
2. Zygomycetes	10–30 µm. Broad, nonseptated, or rarely septated hyphae.
3. *Dematiaceous fungi* (Chromomycosis)	Pigmented fungal elements and sclerotic bodies of 6–12 µm in diameter.
4. *Eumycotic* organisms	0.5–2.0 mm grains containing hyphae and spores.
C. Systemic mycosis	
1. *Candida* species	Yeast, 2.5–4.0 µm; pseudohyphae.
2. *Cryptococcus neoformans*	Budding yeast 5–20 µm with thick, gelatinous capsule. Capsule stains positive with mucicarmine.
3. *Histoplasma capsulatum*	Single, oval, budding yeast, 1–5 µm.
4. *Blastomyces dermatitidis*	Single budding yeast, 5–15 µm, with thick wall.
5. *Coccidioides*	Round sporangia, 20–60 µm, with 2- 5-µm endospores.
6. *Paracoccidioides braziliensis*	10–60 µm yeast with multiple buds.
7. *Aspergillus* species	Slender, septated hyphae with acute angle branching 2–4 µm in diameter.

ANNOTATED BIBLIOGRAPHY

Abele DC, Anders KH. The many faces and phases of borreliosis I. Lyme disease. J Am Acad Dermatol 1990;23:167.
Comprehensive review of Lyme disease with a brief description of histopathological findings.

Abele DC, Anders KH. The many faces and phases of borreliosis II. J Am Acad Dermatol 1990;23:401.
Review of the manifestations of different diseases definitely linked to *Borrelia,* with an excellent discussion of histological features.

Ayers LW, Koneman EW, Merrick TA. Surgical pathology of infectious diseases. In: Principles and practice of surgical pathology. 2nd ed. Silverberg SG, ed. New York: Churchill Livingstone, 1990.
Up-to-date review of tissue diagnosis of infectious diseases, including current histological methods for visualization of microorganisms.

Drijkoningen M, De Wolf-Peeters C, Degreef H, Desmet V. Epidermal Langerhans' cells, dermal dendritic cells, and keratinocytes in viral lesions of skin and mucous membranes: An immunohistochemical study. Arch Dermatol Res 1988;280:220.
Findings from a study of 68 biopsies, which included warts, condylomata acuminata, molluscum contagiosum, and herpesvirus infection.

Feingold DS, Hirschmann JV, Leyden JJ. Bacterial infections of the skin. J Am Acad Dermatol 1989;20:469.
A synopsis of current literature on the subject, evaluating the references and highlighting their key points.

Friedman-Kien AE. Color atlas of AIDS. Philadelphia: WB Saunders, 1989.
An atlas focusing on the cutaneous manifestations of AIDS, including opportunistic infections seen in this disease.

Hulsebosch HJ, et al. Human immunodeficiency virus exanthem. J Am Acad Dermatol 1990;23:483.
Report of three patients with acute HIV infection characterized by a cutaneous exanthem, fever, and malaise. Includes photomicrograph of the skin biopsy specimen.

Reyes-Flores 0. Granulomas induced by living agents. Int J Dermatol 1986;25:158.
Review of infections causing granulomas or granulomatous reactions.

Slater LN, Welch DF, Min KW. *Rochalimaea henselae* causes bacillary angiomatosis and peliosis hepatica. Arch Intern Med 1992;152:602.
The authors cultivated the organism from patients with pathological changes of these processes.

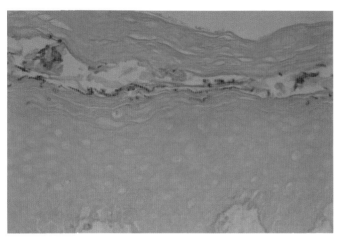

Figure 2.1.   Dermatophytosis. Hyphae and neutrophils in the most superficial layer of the epidermis are readily seen with periodic acid-Schiff stain (PAS 160X).

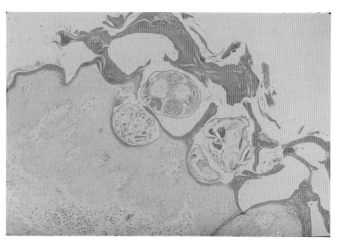

Figure 2.2.   Biopsy of a patient with scabies. Note multiple intertwining tunnels filled with scabies organisms. (Dermatol Clin 8: 253, 1990. Courtesy of Dr. Mervyn Elgart)

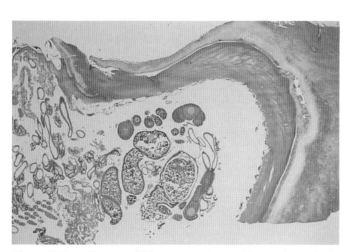

Figure 2.3.   Biopsy of *Tunga penetrans.* Biopsy shows flea in relationship to keratin of the sole. (Courtesy of Dr. Mervyn Elgart and Dr. George Elgart)

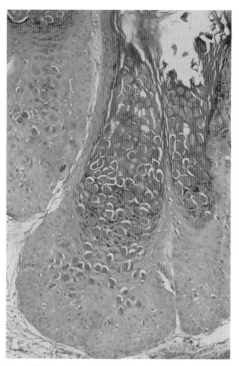

Figure 2.4.   Molluscum contagiosum. Sparing of the epidermal basal cell layer and progressive differentiation of the molluscum bodies toward the surface in hemotoxylin and eosin stain (H&E 40X).

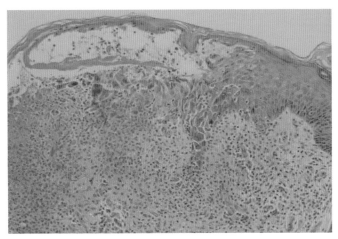

Figure 2.5.   Herpesvirus infection. Intraepidermal vesicle with ballooning degeneration and formation of multinucleated cells. Herpes simplex and herpes zoster/varicella have similar histological features (H&E 40X).

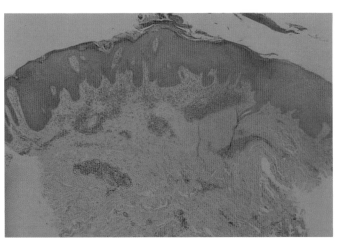

Figure 2.6.   Secondary syphilis. Biopsy from a patient suspected clinically of having systemic lupus erythematosus. Acanthosis and a dense perivascular inflammatory infiltrate are present. The lesions and symptoms resolved with antibiotic therapy (H&E 10X).

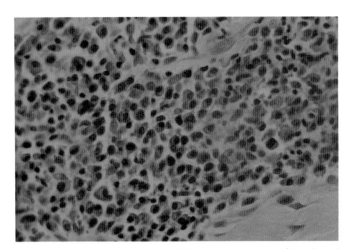

Figure 2.7.   Secondary syphilis. High-power view of the dermal infiltrate shown in Figures 2.2–2.4. The inflammatory cell infiltrate is largely composed of plasma cells, some of them binucleated (H&E 160X).

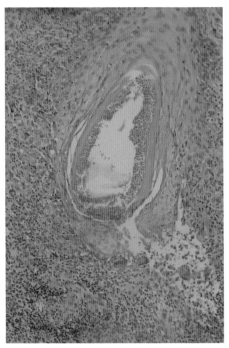

Figure 2.8.   Deep folliculitis. Fungal elements are present around and within the hair shaft. The suppurative granulomatous inflammation is mainly perifollicular (H&E 40X).

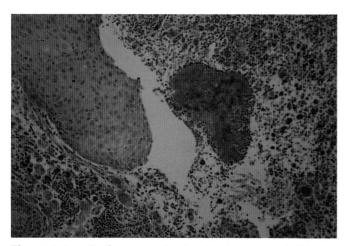

Figure 2.9.   Actinomycosis. Acanthosis and a typical "sulfur granule" amid acute and chronic inflammatory infiltrate with some multinucleated giant cells (H&E 100X).

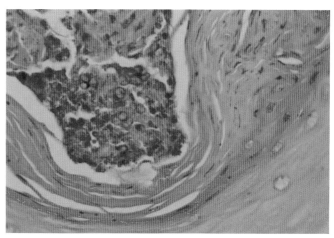

Figure 2.10.   Chromomycosis. Intraepidermal microabscesses containing pigmented fungal elements. The organism in this verrucous skin lesion was identified by culture as *Cladosporium* (H&E 160X).

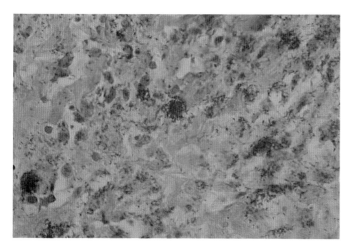

Figure 2.11.   Lepromatous leprosy. Dermis with many intracellular acid-fast bacilli treated with Fite stain (100X). (Courtesy of Dr. Lee T. Nesbitt, Jr.)

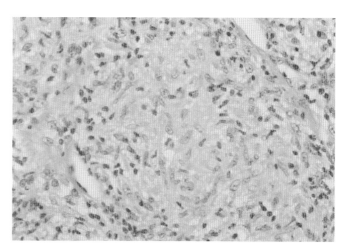

Figure 2.12.   Tuberculoid leprosy. Discrete granulomas in dermis. No organisms were identified with Fite stain (H&E 252X).

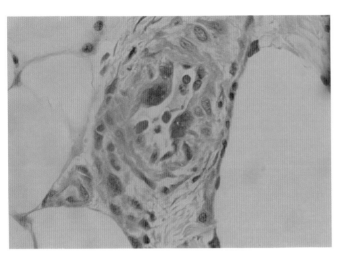

Figure 2.13.   Herpesvirus vasculitis, early stage. Cytopathic changes are present in the endothelium of a blood vessel in the subcutaneous tissue. The biopsy specimen was taken from a progressively expanding ulcer in the buttocks of an immunosuppressed patient (160X).

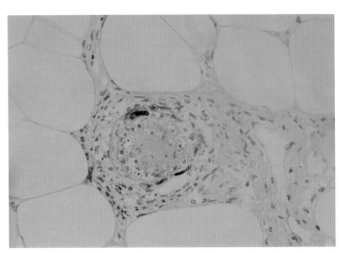

Figure 2.14. Herpesvirus vasculitis, fully developed. Photomicrograph from the same biopsy of Figure 2.13. Blood vessel with thrombosis and inflammation of the wall. Brown staining identified herpesvirus antigen in endothelial cells. Areas of infarcted epidermis did not contain a virus. Immunoperoxidase stain with antibody against herpes simplex (100X).

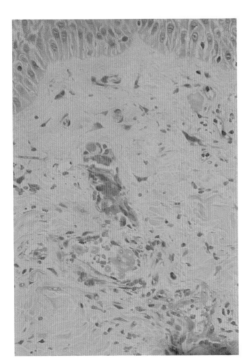

Figure 2.15.   *Curvularia*. Biopsy specimen from a localized forearm lesion in a bone marrow transplant patient. Notice the paucity of inflammatory cell infiltrate. Numerous hyphae are seen in dermis and in vascular fibrin thrombi (H&E 100X).

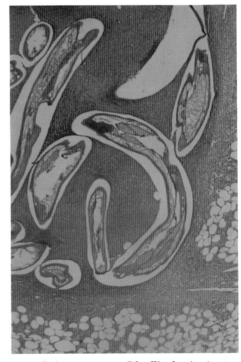

Figure 2.16.   Subcutaneous *Dirofilaria*. A migratory urticarial lesion associated with a burning sensation developed after a mosquito bite. Sections of the parasite are surrounded by intense neutrophilic inflammatory infiltrate (10X).

CHAPTER 3

Staphylococcal and Streptococcal Infections

JAMES J. LEYDEN and LEONARD E. GATELY, III

Bacterial infections are among the most common of skin disorders. *Staphylococcus aureus* and *Streptococcus pyogenes* are very frequent causative organisms, occurring singly or as "mixed infections" when *Staphylococcus aureus* colonizes the exudative crust of a lesion initially produced by *Streptococcus pyogenes*. Although the clinical-bacteriologic correlates of such cutaneous infections were once unclear, clinical morphological characteristics are now established for infections caused by *Staphylococcus aureus* and *Streptococcus pyogenes*, which should enable the physician to distinguish these infections with confidence.

Staphylococcal Infections

Skin infections caused by staphylococcal bacteria invariably arise from strains of *Staphylococcus aureus*. While it is frequently recovered from normal intact skin, *S. aureus* is rarely a true member of the resident bacterial flora, except in the perineum of 10% to 15% of persons living in tropical environments. Other staphylococcal species, such as *S. epidermidis, S. saprophyticus*, and other members of the Micrococcaceae family, clearly can induce serious systemic infection, particularly in the immunocompromised host. They have not, however, proved causative in cutaneous infection.

• PATHOGENESIS •

Staphylococcus aureus strains are classified into major groups by their susceptibility to various bacteriophages: strains for groups I, II, and III are responsible for cutaneous infections. *Staphylococcus aureus* strains vary considerably in the capacity to produce toxins and other noxious materials that contribute to their virulence. Certain toxins are particularly virulent and produce specific syndromes. They include (*a*) exfoliating toxins A and B, which produce bullous impetigo lesions and the staphylococcal scalded skin syndrome (SSSS), (*b*) the enterotoxins A, B, C1, C2, C3, D, and E, which are responsible for food poisoning, and (*c*) those toxins responsible for the toxic shock syndromes. Most other strains of *S. aureus* produce less virulent toxins.

Specific clinical lesions occur with infections caused by strains producing the toxin exfoliatin. Infections caused by other strains produce lesions that represent an interplay between the host response (primarily an influx of polymorphonuclear leukocytes) and the ability of the particular strain of *S. aureus* to produce toxic substances that penetrate these host defense mechanisms. This host-parasite interaction can cause various typical lesions, which range from superficial, relatively noninflammatory pustules and furuncles to rapidly spreading, inflammatory pustules or deep, highly inflammatory dermal abscesses.

Streptococci, particularly group A streptococci, are now known to produce toxins that are similar in structure to the enterotoxins causing toxic shock syndrome produced by *S. aureus*. These streptococcal toxins can produce syndromes characterized by fever, shock, and erythematous rash. More interestingly, these toxins bind to human and mouse major histocompatibility proteins, and the complex ligand has specificity for T-cell receptors. The interaction of the toxin-major histocompatibility complex can then activate T cells. Staphylococcal enterotoxins can behave similarly, activating up to 40% of T cells in mice and causing symptoms due to massive T-cell stimulation and the release of lymphokines, such as interleukin-2 or tumor necrosis factor. Furthermore, the binding of these toxins to major histocompatibility molecules could activate macrophages and mast cells with release of their various mediators of inflammation. On the other hand, exfoliating toxins A and B bind weakly or not at all to major histocompatibility molecules; therefore, the fever and systemic toxicity associated with SSSS are less dependent on the release of mediators from cells activated through interaction of toxins with major histocompatibility molecules.

Kawasaki syndrome, long thought to have an infectious cause, has recently been shown to have an association with *S. aureus*-produced toxic shock syndrome toxin in many patients and streptococcal pyogenic exotoxins in a few, thereby also linking this childhood disorder to bacterial toxins (1).

Infection with *S. aureus* usually begins with colonization of the skin surface. While this occurs most easily when the integrity of the skin is broken, experimental evidence indicates that the skin does not have to be damaged for infection to occur. The resident flora appears to be a first line of defense against infection with *S. aureus*, according to two lines of evidence. First, the newborn does not immediately acquire a resident flora and is clearly more vulnerable to infections with *S. aureus* during the first few days of life. Secondly, experimental infections in human volunteers are more easily produced by degerming the skin surface before inoculation of *S. aureus*. One possible mechanism by which the resident flora may protect against *S. aureus* infection is through the production of antibiotic substances known as bacteriocins.

As is apparent from clinical observations as well as from experimentally induced infections, *S. aureus* infection frequently results from invasion of the skin via hair follicles. Superficial follicular pustules (lesions of folliculitis) are among the hallmark lesions of *S. aureus* infection. Virulent strains are capable of penetrating to the dermis, resulting in a dermal abscess or furuncle. If the particular strain of *S. aureus* is extremely virulent or the host response is inadequate, rapidly enlarging carbuncle lesions or cellulitis can develop.

Rapidly progressing, highly inflammatory abscesses and/or cellulitis are often caused by strains of *S. aureus* that are susceptible to semisynthetic ß-lactamase-resistant penicillins (such as oxacillin or nafcillin) but resistant to penicillin G and related drugs, such as ampicillin. Methicillin-resistant strains are those that can produce life-threatening infections. Culture for antibiotic sensitivity, therefore, should be done on all rapidly spreading *S. aureus* infections. Furthermore, since infections caused by these virulent strains are often contagious, the physician should inquire about infections among family members.

S. aureus infections with strains capable of producing the toxin known as exfoliatin are usually caused by group II phage type 71 strains, which produce toxic changes in the skin as opposed to invading the skin and eliciting a host response of an influx of polymorphonuclear leukocytes. Colonization of the skin surface is followed by elaboration of a toxin that produces superficial necrosis of the skin, resulting in a lesion equivalent to a superficial burn. This toxin has been shown to be mediated by both plasmids and chromosomal alterations in *S. aureus* DNA. The host response to this process is that of an antitoxin antibody. Skin infections or colonization of the nasopharynx and conjunctivae in infants or in immunosuppressed adults who either lack antibodies to this toxin or do not produce an efficient antibody response can lead to syndromes of widespread scarlatina-like erythema or the widespread erythema associated with sloughing or desquamation, known as SSSS. This process can be life-threatening because of secondary sepsis or because of loss of fluid and electrolytes. Patients with impaired renal function are at increased risk for prolonged, severe SSSS because the causative toxin is excreted by the kidney.

Staphylococcus aureus infection of dermatitic skin is common. By poorly understood mechanisms, various types of dermatitis, especially atopic dermatitis, somehow favors colonization by *S. aureus*, which can then proliferate to the point of frank secondary infection.

• CLINICAL FEATURES •

The primary lesion of *S. aureus* infection is a follicular pustule, called folliculitis (Fig. 3.1). Virulent strains usually produce many rapidly spreading lesions with intense perifollicular erythema (Fig. 3.2). Dermal abscesses (Figs. 3.3, 3.4) develop when *S. aureus* is introduced directly to the dermis if the integrity of the skin is impaired or when virulent, toxin-producing strains overwhelm the host reaction.

Strains of *S. aureus* that produce the toxin known as exfoliatin induce a superficial, flaccid bulla, called bullous impetigo, as the primary lesion (Figs. 3.5, 3.6). This blister is clear at first, then pustular. After rupture, it forms a crusted lesion similar to that seen in streptococcal nonbullous impetigo (Fig. 3.7). Patients often have multiple lesions that can include follicular pustules, superficial flaccid bullae, and localized areas of "scalded skin." Extensive production of the toxin results in either a scarlatina-like rash or a generalized erythematous eruption with splitting in the outer epidermal layers, the staphylococcal scalded skin syndrome or SSSS (Fig. 3.8).

Toxic shock syndrome, caused in most cases by *S. aureus*, is characterized clinically by acute onset, fever, and a widespread macular erythematous eruption (Fig. 3.9). Mucous membrane erythema (Fig. 3.10), especially of the conjunctivae where there may also be hemorrhage (Fig. 3.11), is prominent. Certain mucosal surfaces may ulcerate. Desquamation of the skin is highly characteristic, occurring 10 days to 3 weeks after disease onset, and especially involving the fingertips and palmoplantar surfaces. Vomiting and diarrhea are common early symptoms, and circulatory shock is the most severe complication, producing a mortality rate of about 7%.

Kawasaki disease, also called mucocutaneous lymph node syndrome, has many clinical similarities to toxic shock syndrome, but predominantly affects preschool-age children and was initially reported in Japan. Acute onset, fever, conjunctival injection, strawberry tongue (Fig. 3.12), and an erythematous eruption that especially affects palms and soles, producing desquamation of the skin of the digits, are characteristic findings. Cervical lymphadenopathy is seen in the majority of patients, and cardiac involvement is the most serious late sequela. Kawasaki disease is the most common cause of acquired heart disease in children and has an overall mortality of about 1%.

Staphylococcus aureus secondary infections in dermatitic skin produce follicular pustules and serosanguineous exudate with crusting. They rarely progress to deeper infections, such as furuncles or cellulitis.

The most common pyoderma among HIV-infected persons is due to *S. aureus*. This stems from colonization of the nares with the organism and subsequent ease of cutaneous infection due to lack of normal immune defenses, and also from the frequency of eczematous dermatoses and of indwelling catheters in these patients. Lesions of staphylococcal pyoderma in HIV-infected patients may appear as vesiculobullous lesions or erythema and superficial crusting, but the most common presentation is folliculitis on the upper trunk and/or face.

Seborrheic dermatitis of the face and scalp may also become secondarily infected with *S. aureus*.

Blastomycosis-like pyoderma (Fig. 3.13) and botryomycosis are chronic granulomatous reactions to bacterial infection, with the latter containing granules resembling the sulfur granules of actinomycosis. The organism involved in most cases is *S. aureus*, and a variety of underlying or predisposing factors have been described. Very extensive skin forms have been reported with a high percentage of these in association with diabetes. In AIDS, different forms have been reported ranging from disseminated cutaneous papules to extensive perianal sinus formation. A history of abrasion is common, stressing the importance of foreign substances in wounds as well as infection. The size of bacterial inoculation may be crucial.

A resemblance to actinomycosis can also occur uncommonly. Most lesions of this type are on the limbs but other sites, including the perianal region and the face, can be affected. In the primary cutaneous form, single or multiple abscesses of skin and subcutaneous tissues break down to discharge serous fluid through multiple sinuses. These heal after a course of many months to leave atrophic scars. Patients may present with smaller painful papules without sinus formation.

• DIAGNOSIS AND DIFFERENTIAL DIAGNOSIS •

The diagnosis of *S. aureus* infections is usually apparent from clinical inspection alone, but one must consider other possibilities. Follicular pustules can be caused by *Candida albicans*, although these pustules are usually not follicular; by *Propionibacterium acnes* in sebaceous areas in persons with acne vulgaris; and by noninfectious causes, such as erythema toxicum and pustular melanosis in the newborn, iodides and other drugs producing acne-like lesions in the adult, and cutting oils or other irritants in occupational exposure. In immunocompromised persons, numerous organisms can produce pustular skin lesions.

Spreading pustules can be caused by herpes simplex infections in the immunocompromised and especially in the newborn. Abscess or furuncle lesions can occur on an inflammatory basis in acne, hidradenitis suppurativa, and noninfectious disorders, such as panniculitis. In the immunocompromised patient, and occasionally in the intact host, unusual organisms such as *Nocardia*, *Cryptococcus*, and atypical mycobacteria can produce furunculoid lesions.

Differentiation of *Staphylococcus aureus* scalded skin syndrome from the drug-induced reaction known as toxic epidermal necrolysis is important. Frozen section of the sloughing skin shows full-thickness necrosis in the drug-induced process, whereas only superficial necrosis is found in SSSS produced by *S. aureus* toxin.

Infections caused by other organisms can be ruled out by performing smears with Gram's stain, Giemsa stain (to identify multinucleated giant cells in herpes simplex and zoster), and KOH (potassium hydroxide) test (to identify the pseudohyphae and yeast cells of *Candida albicans*), and by culturing for bacteria, viruses, and fungi.

• TREATMENT AND CLINICAL COURSE •

Superficial pustular lesions and superficial secondary infection of dermatitic skin can be successfully treated in many patients with topical antibiotics, although systemic antibiotics are needed if more than a few lesions are present. Topical 2% mupirocin ointment is very effective in the treatment of impetigo. Deeper lesions, such as furuncles, require systemic antibiotic therapy. The majority of strains are resistant to penicillin G and related drugs, but many are sensitive to erythromycin and most are responsive to penicillinase-resistant penicillins. For recurrent furunculosis, the addition of topical mupirocin will help eradicate reservoir populations of *Staphylococcus aureus* from the anterior nares or the perineum. In the case of bullous impetigo, systemic antibiotic therapy with penicillinase-resistant penicillins or erythromycin is usually indicated because lesions may develop rapidly over multiple body sites.

SSSS is a potentially fatal condition and usually requires hospitalization for fluid and electrolyte management as well as intravenous antibiotic therapy. Intravenous γ-globulin has recently been demonstrated to reduce systemic inflammation and the prevalence of coronary artery aneurysms in patients with Kawasaki disease. The treatment, however, is effective only if administered early in the illness. Hence, prompt and accurate diagnosis is essential.

Streptococcal Infections

Cutaneous infections caused by *Streptococcus pyogenes* are among the most common skin diseases in the world, particularly in tropical climates among populations living in crowded, unsanitary conditions.

Streptococcus pyogenes strains are classified into various groups by the presence of cell-wall polysaccharides and subclassified by the presence of specific cell-wall proteins, called M & T proteins. The strains that produce cutaneous infections differ from those responsible for pharyngitis. The host immunological response to strains causing pharyngitis and cutaneous infections also differs in significant ways. The hallmark of infection associated with pharyngitis is the antistreptolysin O (ASO) titer, whereas strains causing skin infection are associated with a feeble ASO titer and a brisk rise in anti-DNAse and antihyaluronidase titers. Cutaneous infection is now recognized to be a potential complication of an immune complex-mediated, postinfection glomerulonephritis.

• PATHOGENESIS •

The pathogenesis of infection with *S. pyogenes* differs from that of *Staphylococcus aureus*, which will not survive for prolonged periods on intact normal skin. Unlike *S. aureus*, the resident flora apparently is not an important first line of defense, because degerming the skin surface does not increase the survival of *Streptococcus pyogenes* on intact skin. Skin lipids, on the other hand, particularly certain fatty acids, do inhibit the survival of *S. pyogenes* and seem to be the major factor limiting the growth of this organism on the skin surface. Colonization of the skin and subsequent infections develop quickly if the stratum corneum barrier is disrupted. For example, inoculation of *S. pyogenes* onto superficially scarified skin results in infection, whereas the same inoculum applied to intact skin dies off quickly. The serum that is present in abraded skin seems to provide sufficient nutrients for growth of *S. pyogenes* and subsequent infection. Once the outer stratum corneum has been breached, rapid spread is facilitated by the production of various toxins and other substances. The ability of *S. pyogenes* to produce hyaluronidase, also referred to as the "spreading factor," facilitates penetration into the dermis. Because *S. pyogenes* can penetrate the dermis and make its way into lymphatics and dermal vessels, systemic signs such as fever and regional lymphadenopathy often develop early in the course of infection, even with only a single lesion.

Streptococcus pyogenes most commonly infects the lower extremities, sites of more frequent trauma. Lesions from these organisms are more common in children than adults, probably reflecting more minor cuts and abrasions coupled with close contact with playmates. *Streptococcus pyogenes* can also produce syndromes similar to those seen with the toxic shock syndrome toxin and the enterotoxins of *Staphylococcus aureus*. Although rare, the possibility of a streptococcal infection should be remembered when one encounters a patient with fever, shock, and rash.

There is also concern that group A streptococci, which in recent decades have caused less serious infection in the United States, may be acquiring greater virulence. In one series of 20 patients, necrotizing fasciitis was seen in 11, shock in 19, and renal impairment in 16; the mortality rate was 30% (2). Exotoxin A or scarlet fever toxin A was produced by 80% of strains. This scarlet fever toxin has rarely been isolated in recent years and was more common in strains recovered from patients with scarlet fever prior to 1940. Host factors did not appear to explain the high mortality in this series, since most patients were under age 50, did not have other underlying disease or immunocompromise, and frequently did not have obvious portals of entry. The role of other toxins such as streptolysin O and pyrogenic exotoxin A is unclear, but their toxicity in animals suggests the possibility of additional effects.

• CLINICAL FEATURES •

The initial single lesion of infection with *Streptococcus pyogenes* is usually not seen because the process evolves so quickly. The earliest lesion of impetigo is a vesiculopustular lesion on an erythematous base that rapidly progresses to a yellow-brown, serosanguineous crust (Fig. 3.14). Deeper penetration of the dermis produces a crater-like ulceration referred to as ecthyma (Figs. 3.15, 3.16). As the host reaction intensifies, more serosanguineous exudate and a thicker crust develop. Further penetration into lymphatics may occur (Fig. 3.17). Lateral spread in the dermis results in a localized cellulitis (Figs. 3.18, 3.19), which can progress to a more extensive cellulitis (Figs. 3.20, 3.21). More superficial involvement with rapid spread of erythema is best called erysipelas (Fig. 3.22). In the presence of

devitalized tissue and/or a hematoma producing a more anaerobic environment, a rapidly progressive infection can evolve, with extensive toxin production (Fig. 3.23), with tissue damage associated with high fever, and with hypotension as the infection extends through the skin into muscle (Figs. 3.24, 3.25). Extensive debridement and intravenous antibiotic therapy are required in such cases. *Staphylococcus aureus* colonization can occur in up to 50% of streptococcal pyodermas.

As mentioned above under the heading "Pathogenesis," streptococcal exotoxin A produces a febrile disorder with bright erythema of the skin, i.e., scarlet fever. Associated mucocutaneous findings are strawberry tongue, Pastia's sign of body folds (Fig. 3.26), and desquamation of the fingertips, palms, and soles (Fig. 3.27). The same toxin may also produce streptococcal toxic shock syndrome, a recently recognized disorder that has the same clinical features as staphylococcal toxic shock syndrome (3).

• DIAGNOSIS AND DIFFERENTIAL DIAGNOSIS •

Diagnosis and differentiation from staphylococcal infections are usually apparent on clinical inspection. When necessary, cultures confirm the diagnosis if proper swabs are used. Since many cotton-tipped swabs contain fatty acids that can inhibit *S. aureus*, calcium alginate swabs are preferable.

• TREATMENT AND CLINICAL COURSE •

Early streptococcal infections can be successfully treated with topical antibiotics, particularly with the introduction of mupirocin. Multiple superficial and deeper lesions, including cellulitis, require systemic antibiotic therapy. Patients with even deeper infections, such as necrotizing fasciitis, may need surgical debridement, intravenous antibiotic therapy, and fluid and electrolyte management.

REFERENCES

1. Leung DY, et al. Toxic shock syndrome toxin-secreting *Staphylococcus aureus* in Kawasaki syndrome. Lancet 1993;342 (8884):1385.
2. Stevens DL, et al. Severe group A streptococcal infections associated with a toxic shock-like syndrome and scarlet fever. N Engl J Med 1989;321:1.
3. Hoge CW, et al. The changing epidemiology of invasive group A streptococcal infections and the emergence of streptococcal toxic shock-like syndrome. JAMA 1993;269(13):1638.

ANNOTATED BIBLIOGRAPHY

Barnett BO, Frieden IJ. Streptococcal skin diseases in children. Semin Dermatol 1992;11(1):3.
   Reviews direct infection, toxin-mediated infection, and immunologically-mediated disease produced by streptococci with emphasis on the changing bacteriology of impetigo and streptococcal toxic shock-like syndrome.
Cone LA, Woodard DR, Schlievert PM, Tomory G. Clinical and bacteriologic observations of a toxic shock-like syndrome due to *Streptococcus pyogenes*. New Engl J Med 1987;317:146.
   Toxic shock syndrome in two patients due to group A streptococci producing pyrogenic toxin A.
Dajani AS, Ferrieri P, Wannamaker LW. Natural history of impetigo. II. Etiologic agents and bacterial interactions. J Clin Invest 1972;1:2863.

Excellent review from the group who delineated many of the clinical, microbiological, and epidemiological factors involved in streptococcal infection. Excellent description and photographs distinguishing streptococcal and staphylococcal infections.

Dillon HC. Impetigo contagiosa: suppurative and non-suppurative complications. Am J Dis Child 1968;115:530.

Classic description of staphylococcal and streptococcal infections delineating the clinical differences.

Grossman KL, Rasmussen JE. Recent advances in pediatric infectious diseases and their impact on dermatology. J Am Acad Dermatol 1991;24(3):379.

Discusses recent advances in pediatric infectious disease with emphasis on the changing etiology of impetigo associated with *Staphylococcus aureus*.

Isaphani P, Donald FE, Aveline AJD. *Streptococcus pyogenes* bacteremia: An old enemy subdued, but not defeated. J Infect Dis 1988;16:37.

Reviews 40 cases with a 35% mortality demonstrating the potential virulence of group A streptococcal infection even in previously healthy persons.

Leung DYM, et al. Toxic shock syndrome toxin-secreting *Staphylococcus aureus* in Kawasaki syndrome. Lancet 1993;342:1385.

Discusses 16 patients with Kawasaki syndrome. Isolation of a new strain of toxic shock syndrome toxin produced by *Staphylococcus aureus* occurred in 11 patients and streptococcal pyrogenic exotoxin B and C was isolated in 2 patients.

Leyden JJ. Mupirocin—A new topical antibiotic. J Am Acad Dermatol 1990;22:879.

Review of the role of this new antibiotic in the treatment of impetigo and secondarily infected dermatoses.

Leyden JJ, Nordstrom KM, McGinley KJ. Cutaneous Microbiology. In Biochemistry and Physiology of the Skin. 2nd ed. Goldsmith LA, ed. New York: Oxford University Press, 1991:1403.

Summarizes the classification of cutaneous microorganisms, factors influencing cutaneous flora in different body areas, and the role of various organisms in a variety of skin diseases.

Marrack P, Krappler J. The staphylococcal enterotoxins and their relatives. Science 1990;248:705.

Reviews the emerging story of the similarity between staphylococcal and streptococcal toxins and how their interaction with the immune system helps explain their pathogenesis.

Resnick SD. Staphylococcal toxin-mediated syndromes in childhood. Semin Dermatol 1992;Mar 11(1):11.

Reviews the effects of toxins produced by staphylococci that are etiologically related to toxic shock syndrome and staphylococcal scalded skin syndrome in children.

Stevens DL, et al. Severe group A streptococcal infections associated with a toxic shock-like syndrome and scarlet fever toxin A. N Engl J Med 1989;321:1.

Reviews 20 cases of life-threatening infection due to toxin-producing strains of group A streptococci.

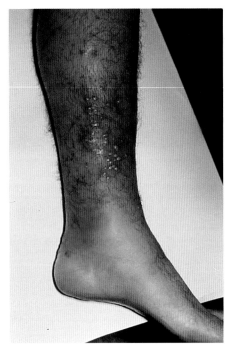

Figure 3.1.   Staphylococci. Folliculitis of the leg. (Courtesy of Dr. Lee T. Nesbitt, Jr.)

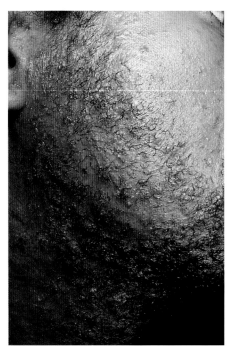

Figure 3.2.   Staphylococci. Folliculitis of the beard in a 21-year-old male. (Courtesy of Dr. Lee T. Nesbitt, Jr.)

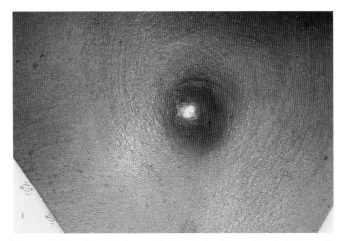

Figure 3.3.   Staphylococci. Infected epidermal cyst of the medi-al thigh secondary to *Staphylococcus aureus*.

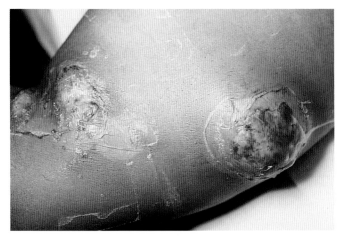

Figure 3.4.   Staphylococci. Multiple abscesses of the arm occur-ring after a mastectomy.

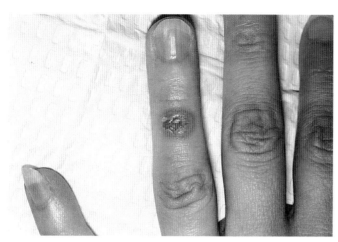

Figure 3.5.   Staphylococci. Bullous pyoderma of the finger. (Courtesy of Dr. Lee T. Nesbitt, Jr.)

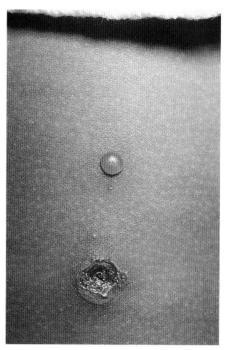

Figure 3.6.   Staphylococci. Bullous impetigo, with an early vesicle and later lesion showing crust formation. (Courtesy of Dr. Lee T. Nesbitt, Jr.)

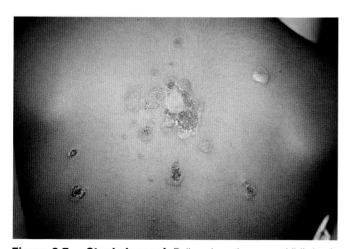

Figure 3.7.   Staphylococci. Bullous impetigo on a child's back. (Courtesy of Dr. Lee T. Nesbitt, Jr.)

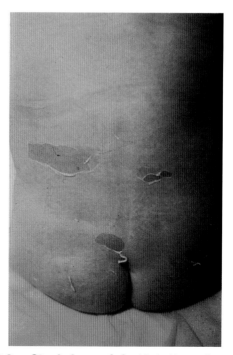

Figure 3.8.   Staphylococci. Scalded skin syndrome showing superficial desquamating lesions in a child. (Courtesy of Dr. Gene Beyt)

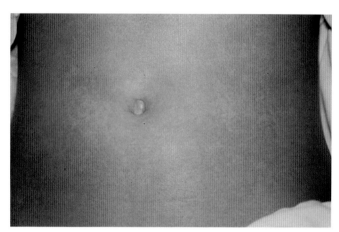

Figure 3.9.   Staphylococcal toxic shock syndrome.
Erythematous maculopapular eruption on the abdomen. (Courtesy of
Dr. Charles V. Sanders)

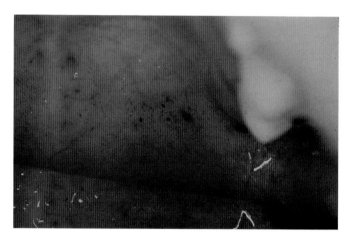

Figure 3.10.   Staphylococcal toxic shock syndrome.
Petechial hemorrhages on the oral mucosa. (Courtesy of Dr. Charles V.
Sanders)

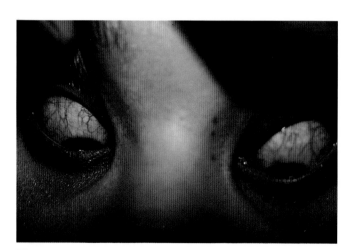

Figure 3.11.   Staphylococcal toxic shock syndrome.
Conjunctival suffusion. (Courtesy of Dr. Charles V. Sanders)

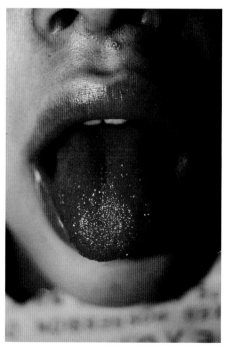

Figure 3.12.   Kawasaki disease. Strawberry tongue. (Courtesy
of Dr. Charles V. Sanders)

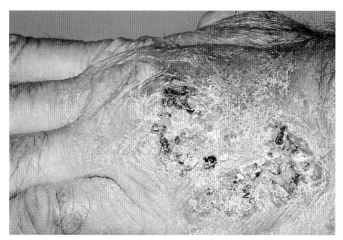

Figure 3.13.   Staphylococci. Blastomycosis-like pyoderma of the back of the hand.

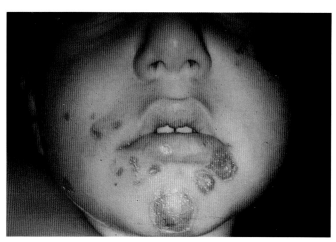

Figure 3.14.   Streptococcal impetigo. Honey-colored crusts of the face.

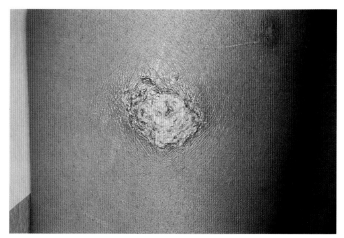

Figure 3.15.   Streptococci. Ecthyma, showing thick crust with surrounding erythema of the leg. (Courtesy of Dr. Lee T. Nesbitt, Jr.)

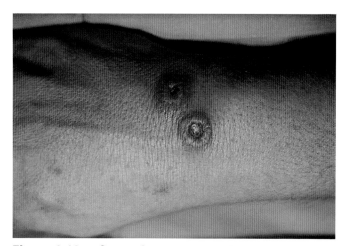

Figure 3.16.   Group A streptococcal ecthyma. Annular lesions, one showing central pustulation and the other showing central ulceration. (Courtesy of Dr. Charles V. Sanders)

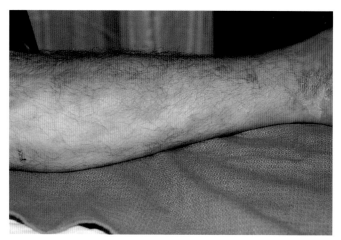

Figure 3.17.   Streptococci. Lymphangitis with erythema conforming to lymphatic drainage.

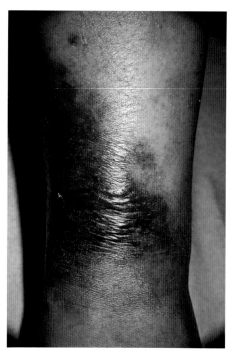

Figure 3.18.   Streptococci. Early cellulitis on an adult's leg. Note the hemorrhagic nature of the lesion. (Courtesy of Dr. Lee T. Nesbitt, Jr.)

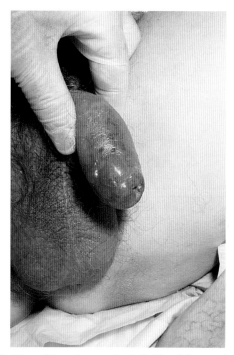

Figure 3.19.   Streptococci. Cellulitis of the penis following catheterization. (Courtesy of Dr. Lee T. Nesbitt, Jr.)

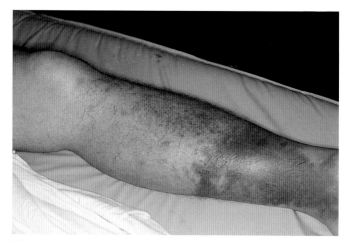

Figure 3.20.   Streptococci. Cellulitis of the leg with hemorrhage and erythematous border.

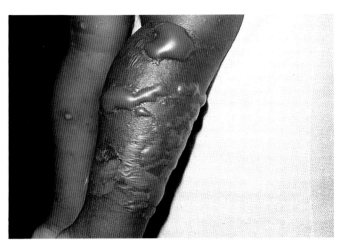

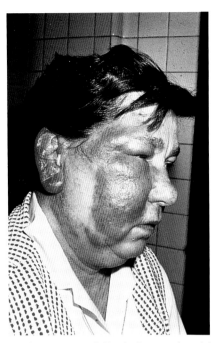

Figure 3.21.   Streptococci. Cellulitis with bullous lesions on the leg of a child. (Courtesy of Dr. Lee T. Nesbitt, Jr.)

Figure 3.22.   Streptococci. Erysipelas on a female's face.

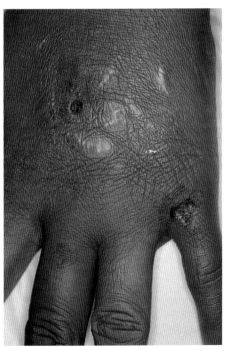

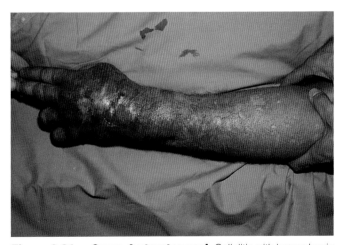

Figure 3.23.   Group A streptococcal toxic shock syndrome. Hemorrhagic necrotic lesions on erythematous bases. (Courtesy of Dr. Deborah Hoadley)

Figure 3.24.   Group A streptococci. Cellulitis with hemorrhagic induration, bullae formation, and erosions of the hand and arm. (Courtesy of Dr. Charles Genovese)

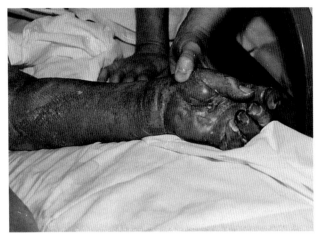

Figure 3.25.   Group A streptococci. Severe infection with peripheral gangrene and swelling of the hand and arm. (Courtesy of Dr. Charles Genovese)

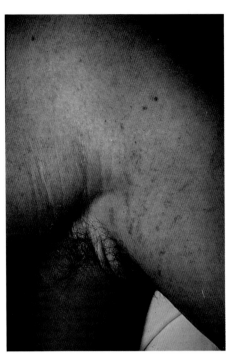

Figure 3.26.   Scarlet fever. Pastia's sign of the axillary area. (Courtesy of Dr. Charles V. Sanders)

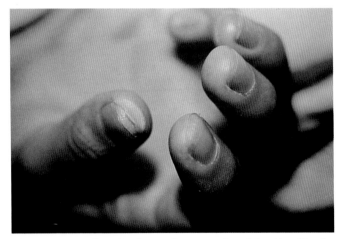

Figure 3.27.   Scarlet fever. Desquamation of the skin of the fingertips. (Courtesy of Dr. Charles V. Sanders)

CHAPTER 4

Cutaneous Signs of Septicemia

JAN V. HIRSCHMANN

Although skin lesions are not the rule in most systemic bacterial infections, when they are present, they may be important clues for identifying the infecting organism. Accurate recognition of these cutaneous abnormalities may allow a rapid presumptive diagnosis and prompt institution of appropriate therapy before results of cultures are available. Occasionally, a skin biopsy provides the earliest or the only histologic or microbiologic information that confirms the cause of an infection.

The mechanisms responsible for the skin lesions in systemic bacterial infections are often unclear, but four pathogenic sequences produce most cutaneous abnormalities:

1. Bacteria-induced vascular damage: Circulating bacteria can cause vascular or perivascular injury when they reach the small cutaneous vessels where they may provoke acute or chronic inflammation or other vascular changes. Cultures or aspirates of these skin lesions are usually positive, and organisms are often visible on stains.

2. Immune-mediated vascular injury: Damage to cutaneous vessels may result from a local immunological response to bacterial antigens or from circulating immune complexes deposited in the vasculature. Because the antigen does not consist of viable organisms, cultures and bacterial stains of material obtained from the skin lesions are usually negative. Immunofluorescent techniques, however, may confirm the presence of the antigen or the immune complexes.

3. Production of circulating toxin: Bacteria present in the bloodstream or at another site may elaborate circulating toxins that cause widespread skin damage. Because bacteria, bacterial antigens, and immune complexes are not present in the skin, cultures and stains of lesions, including immunofluorescent techniques, are negative.

4. Altered hemostasis: Some bacterial infections can produce isolated thrombocytopenia or initiate disseminated intravascular coagulation, either of which can result in cutaneous hemorrhage. Because bacteria are usually not present in the skin lesions, stains and cultures of cutaneous biopsies or aspirates are typically negative.

Some organisms can produce skin lesions by more than one of these mechanisms. Several types of skin lesions, for example, may occur with bacteremia due to *Staphylococcus aureus*. When endocarditis is present, the cutaneous manifestations mentioned below—petechiae, splinter hemorrhages, Osler's nodes, and Janeway lesions—may develop. Gram's stain of these lesions usually reveals Gram-positive cocci in clusters, and cultures are positive for the organism. Pustules, without petechiae, and subcutaneous abscesses may occur in staphylococcal bacteremia whether or not endocarditis is present. Gram's stain and culture of pus from these lesions are almost always positive. Bacteria from *S. aureus* may also provoke disseminated intravascular coagulation, producing purpuric skin lesions discussed more completely below under "Sepsis-Induced Hemostatic Disorders." Finally, when staphylococci elaborate certain toxins, either the toxic shock syndrome or the staphylococcal scalded skin syndrome, described in Chapter 3, may occur.

In this chapter, most forms of bacterial septicemia are discussed. Miscellaneous Gram-negative organisms, including *Vibrio* species, are also discussed in Chapter 5 due to the expertise of the contributing author.

Bacterial Endocarditis

• PATHOGENESIS •

Bacterial endocarditis, an infection of the cardiac valves, is most commonly caused by various streptococci and staphylococci. Most patients have a heart murmur, fever, and other manifestations of a systemic infection such as anorexia, malaise, weight loss, arthralgias, and anemia. Emboli to other organs are also common: with right-sided endocarditis, they are typically septic emboli to the pulmonary arteries; with left-sided disease, they are usually evident as stroke or ischemic renal infarcts.

Four kinds of cutaneous lesions occur: petechiae, splinter hemorrhages, Osler's nodes, and Janeway lesions. Whether these abnormalities are caused by emboli from vegetations breaking off the valve surface or are manifestations of immune-complex vasculitis is debated. Most of the evidence, however, indicates that they result from septic emboli. In several cases of Osler's nodes and Janeway lesions, skin biopsies have shown emboli, and bacteria have grown on culture.

• CLINICAL FEATURES •

The most common lesions seen in bacterial endocarditis are nonpalpable petechiae. Cutaneous petechiae develop most frequently on the distal extremities (Fig. 4.1), but they may also appear on the upper chest. Palpable purpuric lesions can also be present occasionally (Fig. 4.2). Mucous membrane petechiae, like those on the skin, develop in about 10% to 20% of cases of endocarditis. They occur primarily on the palate and on the palpebral conjunctivae under both the lower and upper lids (Fig. 4.3), important areas to examine in suspected cases.

Splinter hemorrhages are red, brown, or black linear discolorations beneath the nail plate (Fig. 4.4). These nonblanching lesions, usually present beneath the distal third of the nail, develop in about 20% of cases of endocarditis. Nail trauma, however, is a much more common cause of splinter hemorrhages, which are seen frequently in the general population. Only if fresh splinter hemorrhages develop in the absence of injury is their presence diagnostically significant in patients with suspected endocarditis.

Osler's nodes are painful, red-to-purplish nodules on the pads of the fingers and toes (Fig. 4.5). Present in about 10% of cases of endocarditis, they last from several hours to several days. Janeway lesions, occurring in about 5% of cases, are probably pathogenetically identical to Osler's nodes and differ clinically only in being nontender, usually macular, erythematous lesions on the palms and soles (Fig. 4.6). Another abnormality discernible on cutaneous examination is nail clubbing of recent onset, present in about 5% of cases. Its pathogenesis is unknown.

• DIAGNOSIS AND DIFFERENTIAL DIAGNOSIS •

The skin lesions, while suggestive of endocarditis, are not pathognomonic. Petechiae are clinically indistinguishable from those resulting from thrombocytopenia or other causes. Palpable purpuric lesions are morphologically and histologically identical to other types of leukocytoclastic vasculitis. Atherosclerotic emboli to the fingers and toes and various types of vasculitis can resemble Osler's nodes and Janeway lesions.

Blood cultures are mandatory to identify the causative organism. Because the bacteremia of endocarditis is continuous but low-grade, three blood culture specimens, each removing at least 10 ml, should be obtained from separate venipunctures within the first 24 hours of evaluation. Unless the patient has received recent antimicrobial therapy or the infecting organism is very unusual, one or more of the blood cultures will almost always grow the responsible bacteria within a few days.

Skin biopsies are not usually helpful in the diagnosis. The findings present in petechial lesions are endothelial proliferation, hemorrhage, and variable inflammatory cell infiltration consistent with cutaneous vasculitis. Biopsies of some Osler's nodes have demonstrated microemboli in dermal arterioles, microabscesses in the dermis, and organisms on some occasions. Others have shown endothelial swelling, neutrophilic vascular and perivascular inflammation, and dermal microabscesses without organisms on stain or culture. Splinter hem-

orrhages consist of masses of blood cells embedded in a layer of squamous cells adherent to the undersurface of the nail.

• TREATMENT AND CLINICAL COURSE •

Endocarditis due to penicillin-sensitive *Streptococcus viridans* is curable with 2 weeks of penicillin and streptomycin therapy. Less sensitive *S. viridans* is usually treated with 4 weeks administration of these agents. In either case, vancomycin therapy for 4 weeks is appropriate for penicillin-allergic patients. Enterococcal endocarditis usually requires 4 to 6 weeks of therapy with a penicillin (penicillin G or ampicillin) plus an aminoglycoside (streptomycin or gentamicin). Penicillin-allergic patients can receive vancomycin plus an aminoglycoside. *Staphylococcus aureus* endocarditis is usually treated with 4 weeks administration of a penicillinase-resistant penicillin such as nafcillin or oxacillin. When the patient is penicillin-allergic or the organism is resistant to these agents, vancomycin is used. *Staphylococcus epidermidis* endocarditis, common in prosthetic valves, is treated with 6 weeks of vancomycin, plus either gentamicin or oral rifampin.

Meningococcal Infections

ACUTE MENINGOCOCCEMIA

• PATHOGENESIS •

Humans are the only reservoir for *Neisseria meningitidis*, of which there are 13 serogroups that differ in their polysaccharide capsules. Groups A, B, and C usually account for more than 90% of meningococcal disease. Ordinarily, meningococci are present in the oropharynx and nasopharynx of 2% to 10% of the population, but the colonization rate can exceed 80% in certain epidemic conditions. Such carriage usually lasts from days to months, with person-to-person spread occurring via airborne droplets or possibly by inanimate objects contaminated by the secretions of a carrier.

Disease develops when meningococci from the upper airway invade the bloodstream to cause meningitis, meningococcal bacteremia without meningitis, or, less commonly, infections in other sites, such as the pericardium or joints. Such invasive disease usually occurs shortly after exposure to the meningococcus; disease is uncommon in chronic carriers. The skin lesions of acute meningococcemia are produced by both bacteremia-induced vasculitis and disseminated intravascular coagulation.

Protection against this organism depends on serogroup-specific bacteriocidal antibodies that require complement for immune bacteriolysis. At special risk for meningococcal disease are those persons without previous exposure to the organism, especially in situations where overcrowding introduces them to immunologically unfamiliar strains. Meningococcal disease is most common in children younger than 5 years old, but it also occurs in military recruits during the first weeks of service, in patients with complement deficiency, and in those in poor general health, especially alcoholics.

• CLINICAL FEATURES •

Acute upper respiratory tract symptoms, such as sore throat and rhinorrhea, often antedate the abrupt onset of fever, rigors, weakness, nausea, vomiting, arthralgias, and moderate headache. With meningitis there may be confusion, neck stiffness, and coma.

Skin lesions occur in about half of patients with meningitis and nearly all with acute meningococcemia. Early, they may be inconspicuous, red macules that blanch or have central petechiae; later, petechiae and purpuric lesions occur, typically 1 to 15 mm in diameter (Fig. 4.7). Larger lesions may become plaque-like or tender (Fig. 4.8). The rash may evolve from sparse lesions to numerous generalized purpuric lesions within a few hours (Fig. 4.9). Sometimes, crops of macular lesions appear and disappear as the temperature rises and falls. The purpuric lesions may transform into hemorrhagic bullae or coalesce into large ecchymotic areas that can become ulcerated or gangrenous (Fig. 4.10). The syndrome of disseminated intravascular coagulation, most commonly associated with acute meningococcemia, is discussed later in this chapter.

• DIAGNOSIS AND DIFFERENTIAL DIAGNOSIS •

Blood cultures are positive in nearly all cases of acute meningococcemia without meningitis and in about one-third of patients with meningococcal meningitis. Stains of aspirates from skin lesions reveal organisms in as many as 80% of the cases. Wright's stains or methylene blue stains may be easier to interpret than Gram's stains.

Skin biopsies demonstrate dilated vessels, swollen endothelial cells, neutrophilic inflammation and necrosis of the vessel walls, and vascular thrombi consisting of platelets, fibrin, and red blood cells. Organisms are often visible. Perivascular hemorrhages and inflammation occur from extravasation of erythrocytes and neutrophils.

Both acute meningococcemia and Rocky Mountain spotted fever cause fever and petechial eruptions that usually begin as blanching macules. With Rocky Mountain spotted fever, the eruption typically starts on the wrists and ankles, involves the palms and soles, and, only after 6 to 12 hours, extends centripetally to affect the axillae, buttocks, trunk, neck, and face. The lesions commonly become petechial after several days. In contrast, the eruption of acute meningococcemia commonly begins on the trunk, does not affect the palms and soles, and becomes petechial over several hours. Nevertheless, the two diseases occasionally may be very difficult to distinguish in an individual patient. Other bacteremias and vasculitides may also be included in the differential diagnosis of acute meningococcemia.

• TREATMENT AND CLINICAL COURSE •

Intravenous penicillin G or ceftriaxone are drugs of choice. Chloramphenicol is a reasonable alternative in patients with life-threatening penicillin allergies. The mortality is about 5% for meningococcal meningitis and about 20% to 30% for acute meningococcemia without meningitis. Patients with large pur-

puric or ecchymotic lesions have a higher fatality rate than those with macular, papular, or petechial eruptions. The course of acute meningococcemia may be fulminant, with fatal hypotension occurring a few hours after onset. For those who survive, the petechial and purpuric lesions resolve in days to weeks, leaving a residual light-brown pigmentation. Areas of cutaneous necrosis tend to heal slowly, sometimes requiring skin grafts, and amputation may be necessary for gangrene of the fingers and toes.

CHRONIC MENINGOCOCCEMIA

• PATHOGENESIS •

Chronic meningococcemia, a rare disease, seems to develop when a patient has incomplete immunity to the infecting organism. Invasion into the bloodstream occurs, but a partial immune response prevents or delays the development of hypotension, meningitis, and other suppurative foci of infection. Some of the manifestations may originate from circulating immune complexes. Most reported patients have been between the ages of 10 and 40 years.

• CLINICAL FEATURES •

Usually, a relapsing fever occurring every 2 to 10 days is accompanied by throbbing headache, migrating arthralgias without frank arthritis, and a skin eruption. The patient feels relatively well between episodes. In a minority of patients, the fever occurs daily, with the cutaneous eruption appearing as crops of lesions when the temperature rises. The rash is most extensive on the trunk and extremities, especially the extensor surfaces, but nearly always spares the palms and soles. The lesions are macular or papular in about 50% of patients (Fig. 4.11), petechial in 10%, nodular in 15%, and polymorphous in 25%. Ecchymotic or pustular lesions are occasional. Large maculopapular lesions may have a bluish or gray central discoloration, but most papules and nodules are erythematous.

• DIAGNOSIS AND DIFFERENTIAL DIAGNOSIS •

Illness is usually present for several weeks before positive blood cultures establish the diagnosis. Many blood cultures obtained over several days may be necessary before the organism is isolated. Once positive, however, blood cultures tend to remain positive until treatment is started. Skin biopsies show perivascular infiltration predominantly of chronic inflammatory cells with only a few neutrophils. Cultures and stains for organisms in skin lesions are almost always negative.

The cutaneous findings of chronic meningococcemia are not distinctive; the clinical setting of relapsing fever, arthralgias, and a rash should suggest the possibility of the diagnosis. Still's disease can also cause joint complaints and an evanescent truncal eruption, but the fever is usually not relapsing. Other types of bacteremia, endocarditis, and vasculitis must also be considered in the differential.

• TREATMENT AND CLINICAL COURSE •

Chronic meningococcemia responds promptly to penicillin therapy. In penicillin-allergic patients, chloramphenicol is an alternative agent. With delayed diagnosis and therapy, meningitis or endocarditis may develop, but fatalities are rare.

Disseminated Gonococcal Infection

• PATHOGENESIS •

Disseminated gonococcal infection occurs in sexually active individuals in whom *Neisseria gonorrhoeae* enters the bloodstream, usually from the genital tract, urethra, rectum, or pharynx. In women, in whom it is more common, the disease typically occurs during menstruation or in the second and third trimesters of pregnancy, when changes in the endometrium presumably allow gonococci ready access to the systemic circulation. Some of the manifestations of the disorder, including skin lesions, result from bacteremia, but others may arise from the effects of circulating immune complexes.

• CLINICAL FEATURES •

Often the patient has no symptoms at the infected mucosal site from which the gonococci originated. Systemic manifestations of fever, malaise, or anorexia are present in some but not all patients. Joint pain is the most common symptom; it may involve a single joint, but most patients have polyarthralgia, which is often migratory and usually in the wrists, hands, and knees. In some, a frank septic arthritis develops, most often involving the knee, ankle, or wrist. Frequently, the rheumatic complaint is tenosynovitis of the ankle, wrist, or dorsum of the hand. This condition consists of pain, swelling, and erythema along the tendon sheaths, with discomfort and tenderness on resistant motion.

Skin lesions, present in 50% to 70% of patients with disseminated gonococcal infection, are usually sparse, painful, and confined to the distal extremities (Figs. 4.12, 4.13). They evolve from small red macules or petechiae into vesicles and pustules (Fig. 4. 14), typically with an erythematous or hemorrhagic base and, occasionally, a necrotic center. Sometimes, hemorrhagic bullae may occur.

• DIAGNOSIS AND DIFFERENTIAL DIAGNOSIS •

Blood or synovial fluid cultures (when arthritis is present) are positive in about 50% of cases. In the remaining patients, the diagnosis is clinical, buttressed in most circumstances by the isolation of gonococci from a mucosal surface (urethra, cervix, rectum, pharynx). Often, however, all cultures are negative, but the disease clears with appropriate antibiotic therapy.

Skin biopsies show substantial neutrophilic vasculitis and perivascular inflammation of both deep and superficial vessels, hemorrhage, and microthrombi. Stains and cultures reveal the organism in less than 5% of cases, although direct immunofluorescent antibody techniques show gonococcal antigen in most.

In hand-foot-and-mouth disease, most commonly due to coxsackie A 16 virus, vesicles and pustules resembling those of dis-seminated gonococcal infection appear on the distal extremities. This infection usually occurs in young children rather than young adults; arthralgia and arthritis are absent; and ulcerative lesions, not found in gonococcal disease, appear on the oral mucosa. Other septic disorders or vasculitic syndromes must also be considered in the differential diagnosis.

• TREATMENT AND CLINICAL COURSE •

Ceftriaxone is currently the drug of choice, although certain other antibiotics are also effective. Response to therapy is prompt; serious complications such as meningitis or endocarditis are rare. Septic arthritis usually resolves with antibiotic therapy and repeated arthrocenteses as necessary. Surgery is rarely warranted. Skin lesions, which often resolve within several days, even without therapy, disappear rapidly with therapy and usually leave no residual cutaneous abnormality.

Enteric Fever (Salmonellosis)

• PATHOGENESIS •

Enteric fever is usually caused by *Salmonella typhi* or *S. paratyphi*, organisms confined to humans and spread via food or water contaminated by feces. Other salmonella types, widespread among animals, less commonly cause enteric fever. After ingestion, organisms proliferate in the gut, entering the lymphatic system of the small intestine and then the bloodstream, causing a continuous, low-grade bacteremia. Later, the organisms, excreted in the bile, reenter the alimentary canal, and stool cultures become positive.

• CLINICAL FEATURES •

Headache, continuous fever, generalized aching, cough, and anorexia are the initial symptoms, which follow an incubation period of 1 to 2 weeks. Diffuse abdominal pain, constipation, splenomegaly, delirium or mental torpor, and relative bradycardia may develop during the second week of illness. Skin lesions known as rose spots occur in 10% to 60% of patients at this time (Fig. 4.15). They are 2- to 3-mm blanching pink papules that usually become brown and fade in 3 to 4 days. They usually appear on the central portion of the anterior part of the trunk, are uncommon on the extremities or back, and are more frequently noticed in light-skinned than dark-skinned patients.

• DIAGNOSIS AND DIFFERENTIAL DIAGNOSIS •

Blood cultures are positive in about 80% of untreated patients. Stool cultures, usually negative in the first week of illness, grow salmonellae in about 80% of patients during the second week. Bone marrow cultures are positive in about 90% of patients early in the course of disease, even in most patients who have received antibiotics.

Skin biopsies show capillary dilation, surrounding edema, and pericapillary infiltration with macrophages. Cultures of skin tissue specimens from rose spots are positive in more than 60% of cases, a yield that makes routine culture worthwhile.

Lesions resembling rose spots are occasionally seen in psittacosis, but the presence of pneumonia and a history of bird exposure should help distinguish the two diseases. *Pseudomonas aeruginosa* bacteremia may cause similar eruptions, but these patients are more acutely and severely ill than most of those with typhoid fever.

• TREATMENT AND CLINICAL COURSE •

The antimicrobial susceptibility of salmonellae varies, but potentially useful agents are chloramphenicol, ampicillin, sulfamethoxazole-trimethoprim, ceftriaxone, or a fluoroquinolone such as ciprofloxacin. The mortality for enteric fever is less than 5%. Relapses occur in about 15%.

Bacteremia From *Pseudomonas aeruginosa* and Other Enteric Gram-Negative Bacilli

• PATHOGENESIS •

Pseudomonas aeruginosa, a Gram-negative bacillus widely distributed in air, dust, soil, and water can colonize the moist regions of the skin folds and the external auditory canals. It is found in small numbers in the stools of 10% to 25% of normal persons. *Pseudomonas* bacteremia tends to occur in seriously ill patients with neutropenia, prolonged hospitalization, severe burns, or previous extensive antimicrobial therapy. The sites of entry are commonly the urinary tract, skin, lungs, and alimentary canal, especially in neutropenic patients.

• CLINICAL FEATURES •

The patient is usually seriously ill, febrile, and hypotensive. If pneumonia is present, respiratory insufficiency is common. Skin lesions, present in only a small minority of patients, can have several appearances. Ecthyma gangrenosum from *P. aeruginosa* usually begins as an area of erythematous swelling, often in the anogenital region or the axilla that evolves into a hemorrhagic blister, which later breaks down. The result is an erythematous swelling with a central area of bluish-black necrosis (Fig. 4.16). These lesions typically evolve during 12 to 24 hours (For further discussion, see Chapter 5). Another type of skin lesion in patients with *Pseudomonas* bacteremia consists of painful vesicles or bullae on erythematous bases that contain opalescent fluid, tend to occur in crops, and may become bloody. A third type is a rapidly advancing cellulitis accompanied by cutaneous hemorrhage and necrosis. Lesions resembling the rose spots seen in salmonellosis can also occasionally occur in *Pseudomonas* bacteremia, as can painful subcutaneous nodules or abscesses. Bacteremia from other Gram-negative bacilli, such as *Escherichia coli, Serratia marcescens* (Fig. 4.17), *Pseudomonas cepacia, Yersinia pestis* and *enterocolitica*, and *Aeromonas hydrophila* rarely cause skin lesions similar to those in *Pseudomonas* bacteremia. These organisms may also provoke disseminated intravascular coagulation and the accompanying cutaneous changes described in the next section, "Sepsis-Induced Hemostatic Disorders."

For a further description of cutaneous lesions caused by *Pseudomonas aeruginosa*, see Chapter 5.

• DIAGNOSIS AND DIFFERENTIAL DIAGNOSIS •

Blood cultures are usually positive. Gram's stains of skin aspirates commonly show many Gram-negative bacilli but few neutrophils, and cultures typically grow the organism.

Skin biopsies show vascular necrosis with bacteria invading the walls of small arteries and veins. The endothelial surfaces of the vessels are rarely damaged, and vascular thrombi are uncommon. Inflammation is usually slight, with few neutrophils visible. Extravasation occurs around the vessels, leading to extensive edema and bland necrosis in the perivascular and adventitial regions. Bullae, when present, are subepidermal.

Necrotic arachnidism caused by bites of spiders like the brown recluse can resemble ecthyma gangrenosum, but the lesions do not evolve as quickly, and the clinical setting is markedly different. Cutaneous vasculitis may also create similar lesions, but Gram's stain and culture of an aspirate will be negative; a biopsy will show more vascular inflammation; organisms will be absent; and cultures will be negative. As mentioned under the section on clinical features, bacteremia from other organisms may also simulate *Pseudomonas* sepsis.

• TREATMENT AND CLINICAL COURSE •

The therapy of choice is a combination of an aminoglycoside (gentamicin, tobramycin, amikacin) and an antipseudomonal penicillin (e.g., mezlocillin, ticarcillin, piperacillin). Alternatives, depending upon the organism's antimicrobial susceptibility, include ceftazidine, imipenem, or a fluoroquinolone, alone or in various combinations. The mortality resulting from Pseudomonas bacteremia is about 60% to 70%.

Sepsis-Induced Hemostatic Disorders

• PATHOGENESIS •

Bacteria may cause isolated thrombocytopenia

1. By inducing platelet aggregation;

2. By injuring the endothelium of vessels, which allows platelets to adhere to the exposed subendothelium;

3. By immunologically destroying platelets.

The mechanisms of immune-mediated platelet destruction include: (*a*) nonspecific binding of IgG to platelets damaged by bacteria, (*b*) specific IgG binding to bacterial fragments that adhere to platelets, or (*c*) specific IgG binding to bacterial fragments, producing immune complexes that attach to platelet Fc receptors.

Gram-positive organisms, such as pneumococci, can cause disseminated intravascular coagulation (the formation of fibrin thrombi within vessels), but Gram-negative bacteremia from meningococci or other Gram-negative bacilli produce this disorder much more commonly. The process can lead to hemorrhage because of depletion of platelets, fibrinogen, and various clotting factors.

• CLINICAL FEATURES •

With isolated thrombocytopenia from systemic bacterial infections, the platelet count is usually not sufficiently low to result in cutaneous or mucosal bleeding. Petechiae, purpura, or confluent ecchymoses may occur, however, with severe thrombocytopenia.

Petechiae and large ecchymoses, usually confined to the extremities and sometimes evolving into hemorrhagic bullae, are the most common lesions in disseminated intravascular coagulation (Fig. 4.18). Progressive painful subcutaneous hematomas may occur, and a few patients develop a non-blanching, symmetrical grayish discoloration of the hands, feet, ears, or nose that may transform into gangrene.

Purpura fulminans is a variously used term referring to a febrile illness with widespread, rapidly developing purpura that may evolve into hemorrhagic bullae and cutaneous gangrene. Common sites of involvement include the lower extremities, buttocks, arms, and abdomen. Young children are usually the victims, with the disease commonly appearing 1 to 4 weeks after a streptococcal, other bacterial, or viral infection. Purpura fulminans appears to be a type of disseminated intravascular coagulation with prominent skin findings.

• DIAGNOSIS AND DIFFERENTIAL DIAGNOSIS •

The usual definition of thrombocytopenia is a platelet count of less than 100,000 microliters (µ/L). Petechiae ordinarily do not form, however, until the count falls below 20,000 µ/L.

The laboratory diagnosis of disseminated intravascular coagulation depends on the presence of thrombocytopenia and evidence of generalized activation of thrombin and plasmin, indicated by elevated levels of fibrin degradation products, fibrinopeptide A, and D-dimer, diminished amounts of fibrinogen, and depletion of clotting factors such as factors V and VIII (most commonly shown by prolonged prothrombin and partial thromboplastin times) and antithrombin III. Positive protamine sulfate or ethanol gelation tests are also useful in confirming the diagnosis.

Biopsies of fresh petechiae and purpura demonstrate fibrin thrombi in the capillaries with extravasation of red blood cells. Little inflammation occurs. Older lesions show epidermal necrosis, formation of subepidermal bullae, and patchy necrosis of the eccrine glands and pilosebaceous apparatus. Extensive necrosis of the epidermis, dermis, and cutaneous appendages occurs in patients with gangrene.

• THERAPY AND CLINICAL COURSE •

The focus of therapy is treatment of the underlying infection. The effect of heparin remains unsettled, and some experts recommend only the replacement of depleted hemostatic factors when serious bleeding occurs. For surviving patients, amputation of gangrenous portions of the extremities may be necessary.

ANNOTATED BIBLIOGRAPHY

Benoit FL. Chronic meningococcemia: Case report and review of the literature. Am J Med 1963;35:103.

Despite its age, this paper remains the best review of chronic meningococcemia.

Bick RL. Disseminated intravascular coagulation. Hematol Oncol Clin North Am 1992;6:1259.

A comprehensive review, including a discussion of diagnostic tests and therapy.

Bodey GP, et al. Infections caused by *Pseudomonas aeruginosa*. Rev Infect Dis 1983;5:279.

An extensive review of the topic.

Cardullo AC, Silvers DN, and Grossman ME. Janeway lesions and Osler's nodes: A review of histopathologic findings. J Am Acad Dermatol 1990;22:1088.

Biopsies of purpuric pustules and hemorrhagic macules in a patient with *Staphylococcus aureus* endocarditis show neutrophilic vasculitis, abscess formation, and vascular thrombosis. The authors conclude that these lesions represent septic emboli.

Dallabetta G, Hook EW, III. Gonococcal infections. Infect Dis Clinics North Am 1987;1:25.

A thorough review of all aspects of gonococcal disease.

DeVoe W. The meningococcus and mechanisms of pathogenicity. Microbiol Rev 1982; 46:162.

A complete discussion of this organism.

Farrior JB, II, Silverman MD. A consideration of the difference between a Janeway lesion and an Osler's node in infectious endocarditis. Chest 1976;70:239.

Historical perspective on these lesions and their clinical differentiation.

Gilman RH, et al. Relative efficacy of blood, urine, rectal swab, bone marrow, and rose-spot cultures for recovery of *Salmonella typhi* in typhoid fever. Lancet 1975;1:1211.

A very helpful study demonstrating the yield of various cultures in patients with typhoid fever, many of whom had already received antimicrobial therapy.

Kingston ME, Mackey D. Skin clues in the diagnosis of life-threatening infections. Rev Infect Dis 1986;8:1.

Discussion of the pathological manifestations of a variety of infections that cause dermatologic disease.

Litwack KD, Hoke AW, Borchardt KA. Rose spots in typhoid fever. Arch Dermatol 1972;105:252.

A case report of a patient with typhoid fever and rose spots that includes photographs of the clinical and pathologic findings.

Musher DM, McKenzie SO. Infections due to *Staphylococcus aureus*. Medicine 1977;56:383.

A thorough review of staphylococcal infections.

O'Brien JP, Goldenberg DL, Rice PA. Disseminated gonococcal infection: A prospective analysis of 49 patients and a review of pathophysiology and immune mechanisms. Medicine 1983;62:395.

A prospective study that delineates the clinical findings.

Robboy SJ, et al. The skin in disseminated intravascular coagulation. Prospective analysis of 36 cases. Br J Dermatol 1973;88:221.

A prospective study of disseminated intravascular coagulation in which skin lesions are detected in 75% of cases. Excellent clinical description of the lesions and their frequency.

Spicer TE, Rau JM. Purpura fulminans. 1976;Am J Med 61:566.

A case report followed by a complete and discerning literature review.

Wilson JJ, Neame PB, Kelton JG. Infection-induced thrombocytopenia. Semin Thromb Hemost 1982;8:217.

A thorough discussion of the causes and mechanisms of thrombocytopenia caused by infections.

Yee J, McAllister CK. The utility of Osler's nodes in the diagnosis of infective endocarditis. 1987;Chest 92:751.

A description of a patient with endocarditis whose skin biopsy of an Osler's node grows *Streptococcus sanguis*. The authors conclude that these skin lesions represent septic emboli.

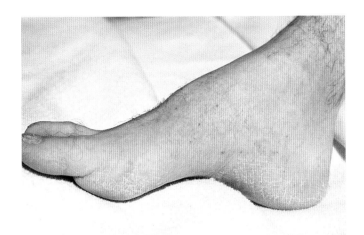

Figure 4.1.   Endocarditis. Endocarditis due to *Streptococcus viridans* petechial lesions of the medial aspect of the foot. (Courtesy of Dr. Charles V. Sanders)

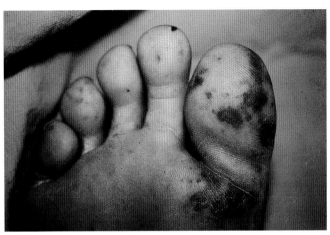

Figure 4.2.   Endocarditis. Endocarditis due to *Staphylococcus aureus.* Hemorrhagic and purpuric lesions of the toes.

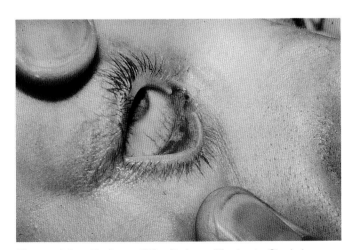

Figure 4.3.   Endocarditis. Endocarditis due to *Staphylococcus aureus.* Subconjunctival petechiae.

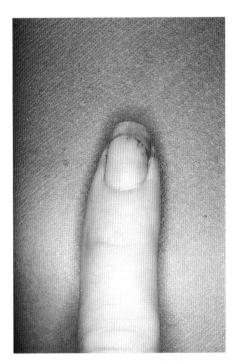

Figure 4.4.   Endocarditis. Endocarditis due to group B *Streptococcus.* Splinter hemorrhage in the nail bed and Osler's nodes on the side of the finger. (Courtesy of Dr. Gene Beyt)

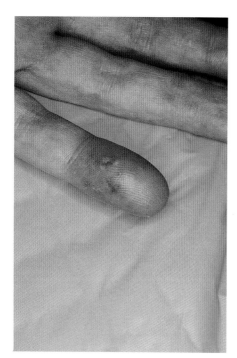

Figure 4.5.   Endocarditis. Endocarditis due to *Staphylococcus aureus*. Osler's nodes: tender, papulopustules on the pulp of the finger. (Courtesy of Dr. Charles V. Sanders)

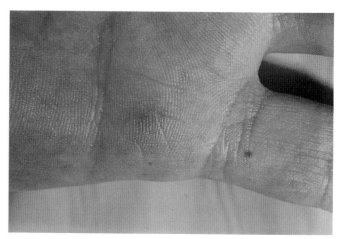

Figure 4.6.   Endocarditis. Endocarditis due to *Streptococcus bovis*. Janeway lesion on the palm.

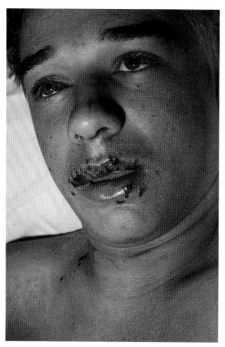

Figure 4.7.   Acute meningococcemia. Hemorrhagic lesions of the lips and conjunctivae. (Courtesy of Dr. Lee T. Nesbitt, Jr.)

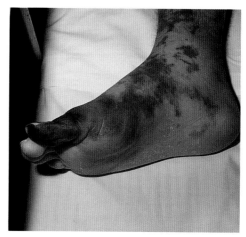

Figure 4.8.   Acute meningococcemia. Extensive purpura involving the foot and a gangrenous great toe. (Courtesy of Dr. Lee T. Nesbitt, Jr.)

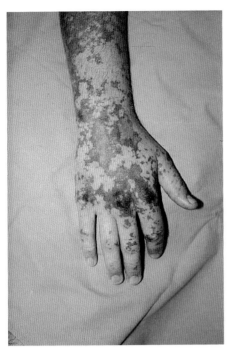

Figure 4.9.   Acute meningococcemia. Purpuric lesions on the hand and arm. (Courtesy of Dr. Charles V. Sanders)

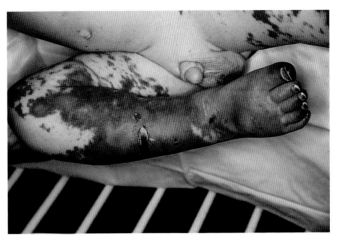

Figure 4.10.   Acute meningococcemia. Purpuric lesions due to disseminated intravascular coagulation. (Courtesy of Dr. Gene Beyt)

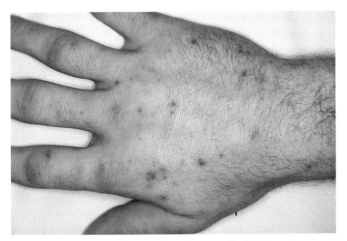

Figure 4.11.   Chronic meningococcemia. Erythematous maculopapules of the dorsal hand.

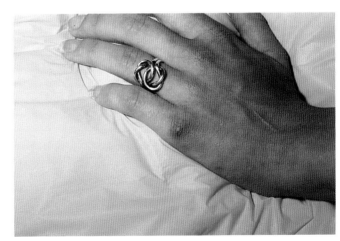

Figure 4.12.   Disseminated gonococcal infection. Pustule with surrounding erythema on the dorsum of the hand, a typical location. (Courtesy of Dr. Lee T. Nesbitt, Jr.)

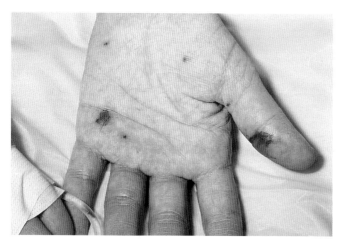

Figure 4.13. Disseminated gonococcal infection. Multiple purpuric areas on the palm. (Courtesy of Dr. Lee T. Nesbitt, Jr.)

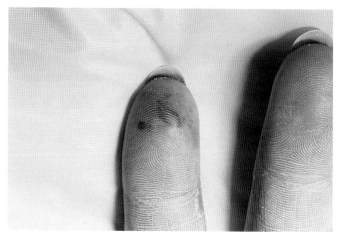

Figure 4.14. Disseminated gonococcal infection. Petechial lesions on the pulp of the fifth finger. The center of the larger lesion may be developing into a vesicopustule. (Courtesy of Dr. Lee T. Nesbitt, Jr.)

Figure 4.15. Rose spots. Pink, blanching macules on the abdomen of a patient whose blood cultures grew *Salmonella typhi*.

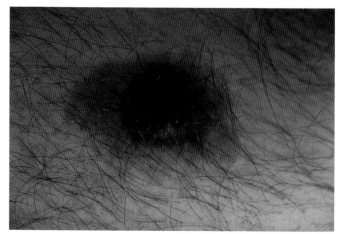

Figure 4.16. Ecthyma gangrenosum. Ecthyma gangrenosum due to bacteremia from *Pseudomonas aeruginosa*. Central necrotic eschar with surrounding erythema. (Courtesy of Dr. Gene Beyt)

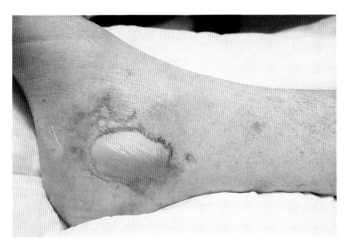

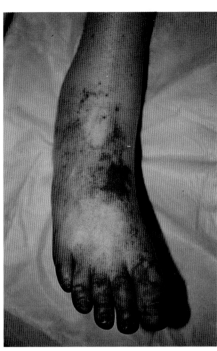

Figure 4.17.   *Serratia marcescens.* Bullae surrounded by ecchymotic borders in a patient with alcoholic cirrhosis and hypotension.

Figure 4.18.   *Staphylococcus aureus.* *Staphylococcus aureus* sepsis showing disseminated intravascular coagulopathy. (Courtesy of Dr. Charles V. Sanders)

CHAPTER **5**

Other Bacterial Infections

EDWARD J. SEPTIMUS and DANIEL M. MUSHER

This chapter covers miscellaneous bacterial infections, including various cutaneous manifestations of infection produced by Gram-negative enteric bacilli. The focus is on *Vibrio* and *Pseudomonas* species, encompassing a discussion of sepsis from these organisms.

Miscellaneous Gram-Negative Enteric Bacilli

Sepsis caused by Gram-negative enteric bacilli occasionally leads to secondary involvement of the skin and subcutaneous tissues. Four general patterns are seen:

1. Cellulitis or thrombophlebitis characterized by intense inflammatory changes, with bacteria not readily detectable microscopically;
2. Necrosis without clinical or histologic findings of inflammation but with profuse numbers of bacteria present in the lesions;
3. Disseminated intravascular coagulation and symmetric peripheral gangrene, in which few bacteria are seen and the inflammatory response is slight;
4. Peripheral lesions of endocarditis.

The interplay between host and bacterial factors is thought to determine the nature of the cutaneous involvement, but these factors generally are not well understood (1, 2). This chapter will discuss some of these patterns of cutaneous involvement, but bacterial endocarditis and disseminated intravascular coagulation are covered in Chapter 4.

VIBRIO SPECIES

• PATHOGENESIS •

Vibrio species other than *Vibrio cholerae* cause serious infections of the skin and soft tissues; organisms once called noncholera and/or halophilic vibrios but now properly speciated, are responsible. Of these, *V. vulnificus* is most commonly implicated in serious infection, although identical syndromes may be produced by a number of other species, including, for example, *V. damsela*, *V. parahaemolyticus*, or *V. alginolyticus*.

Vibrio vulnificus is commonly found in high concentrations in brackish water along the coasts of the Gulf of Mexico and, to a lesser extent, the southeast Atlantic. Infection of skin and soft tissues occurs either via a hematogenous route or by direct inoculation. When skin and soft tissue infection occur in the absence of any recognized local trauma, hematogenous spread from the gastrointestinal tract is usually responsible. Patients often have ingested shellfish in the preceding 12 to 48 hours and generally have developed diarrheal disease. The great majority of such patients have an underlying medical condition predisposing to this infection: alcoholism (especially if associated with cirrhosis of the liver) is by far the most common, followed by other hepatic dysfunctions, various forms of immunosuppression, and diabetes mellitus.

Localized infection due to inoculation of *Vibrio* species nearly always results from a break in the skin that occurs during fishing or water-related activities in an endemic area, or from a break in the skin in a person who prepares uncooked seafood that presumably has come from such an area. Seemingly normal hosts can be infected, although susceptibility greatly increases with underlying diseases.

The pathogenetic factors in *V. vulnificus* have not been fully characterized. *V. vulnificus* produces a number of tissue-destructive enzymes, but they are insufficient to explain the severity of disease caused by this species. Environmental isolates are susceptible to killing by relatively low concentrations of human serum and are readily opsonized for phagocytosis by leukocytes. In contrast, *V. vulnificus* isolated from the bloodstream of infected patients is not killed by human serum, and is phagocytosed only poorly. *Vibrio damsela* has been shown recently to cause necrosis that progresses even more rapidly than that caused by *V. vulnificus*. This organism produces a highly destructive toxin that is associated with beta hemolysis of sheep blood, and brief exposure of a blood-agar plate to involved tissue causes hemolysis even if no viable bacteria are present.

• CLINICAL AND HISTOLOGICAL FEATURES •

In most cases, intense inflammation predominates. Areas of erythema, erysipelas, or frank cellulitis with hemorrhagic bullous lesions appear, and rapid progression to fasciitis with necrosis of skin and subcutaneous tissues is characteristic (Figs. 5.1–5.3). Infection commonly involves the distal lower extremities, in which case the presenting symptoms and signs may be indistinguishable from deep-vein thrombophlebitis, with one or both calves involved. In cases of cellulitis or thrombophlebitis resulting from bacillary sepsis, the histologic appearance is that of an intense inflammatory exudate caused by polymorphonuclear leukocytes (PMNs). Whether cellulitis or thrombophlebitis predominates, clinical and histologic evidence of inflammatory changes may be found in the major vessels, often with thrombosis. Bacteria usually are not seen microscopically, although cultures of involved tissues may be positive. The fact that cultures remain positive despite antibiotic therapy probably reflects the intensity of the local inflammatory response and the compromise to blood supply.

In addition to this illness caused by the *Vibrio* species, a similar syndrome may be produced by *Campylobacter fetus* (in which a picture of deep-vein thrombophlebitis of the calf is especially likely), *Aeromonas hydrophila*, *Bacteroides* species, *Yersinia enterocolitica*, or *Serratia marcescens.*

In some cases, the inflammatory response is minimal and necrosis predominates. Discrete, round lesions appear singly or multiply anywhere on the body, although the extremities seem to be the areas most commonly involved. Lesions may begin as blisters filled with clear or bloody fluid followed by necrosis and sloughing of superficial tissues. Sometimes, lesions begin as dark red or purplish macules but progress rapidly to become papular and/or necrotic. (These lesions are called ecthyma gangrenosum—literally, gangrenous pustule—and are discussed in the following section on *Pseudomonas aeruginosa* and in Chapter 4.) On occasion, the appearance may suggest erythema multiforme. Histologic examination of these uninflamed lesions reveals profuse numbers of bacteria in and around vessels with a minimal or absent inflammatory response. If disseminated intravascular coagulation is present, peripheral symmetrical gangrene of toes, fingers, nose, and ears may also be observed. (Also see Chapter 4.)

In localized infection, intense inflammation extends from the area of insult proximally more than distally and with striking rapidity. Thus, a lesion of the hand can progress to involvement of the entire arm within 24 to 36 hours. Histologic examination reveals intense perivascular inflammation of connective tissues and skin with few bacteria being observed. Necrosis rapidly follows, resulting from compromise of the blood supply to superficial tissues. If any feature of cellulitis is characteristic of the *Vibrio* species, it is the extraordinary rapidity of progression.

In some patients, it is difficult to determine whether systemic or local invasion of tissues is responsible. The typical case is that of a fisherman who has been wading in coastal waters all day, using shrimp for bait, eating without washing his hands, and consuming alcohol, who is hospitalized because of rapidly progressive inflammation in the calf of one leg, with a Gram-negative organism such as *V. vulnificus* or *Aeromonas hydrophila* (Fig. 5.4) isolated from the bloodstream.

• DIAGNOSIS AND DIFFERENTIAL DIAGNOSIS •

Vibrio should be suspected in any immunocompromised patient, especially those with cirrhosis, who develop septic illness associated with rapidly spreading cellulitis days after ingesting oysters or patients developing cellulitis on extremities exposed to sea water. *Vibrio* grows well on media that contains sodium chloride as well as on selective TCBS (triosulfate, citrate, bile salts, sucrose) media. The differential diagnosis would include other forms of sepsis that produce necrosis of the skin.

• TREATMENT AND CLINICAL COURSE •

Treatment of severe cutaneous *Vibrio* infection requires both appropriate antibiotics (a tetracycline is regarded as first choice, with ampicillin, gentamicin, chloramphenicol, and cephalosporins also active) and surgical debridement. When the inflammatory component predominates, debridement and fasciotomy are nearly always required, even when the early findings have not been impressive. Small necrotic lesions are generally not debrided because they tend to slough. Treatment of disseminated intravascular coagulation is discussed in Chapter 4. In spite of treatment, the mortality rate for *V. vulnificus* sepsis is 50% to 60%, three times that of local wound infections from the organism.

PSEUDOMONAS AERUGINOSA

• PATHOGENESIS •

Pseudomonas aeruginosa infects skin and soft tissues via a hematogenous route or by direct inoculation. Cutaneous lesions develop as a result of hematogenous infection in the severely immunocompromised, usually granulocytopenic host, and, rarely, in patients who appear to be immunologically normal, as for example, those with *Pseudomonas* endocarditis. In addition, many local infections of nails, toe webs, the external ear, or other skin sites that are secondarily colonized may occur and will be discussed in this chapter.

• CLINICAL FEATURES •

The characteristic lesions in *Pseudomonas* sepsis are initially superficial and nodular, ranging in size from 0.5 cm to 3.0 cm and in color from red to purplish. Some lesions remain nodular, whereas others tend to progress rapidly to necrosis and ulceration and in some cases extend to cause large areas of tissue breakdown (Figs. 5.5, 5.6). The term "ecthyma gangrenosum" is classically used to describe the early lesions of *P. aeruginosa* sepsis, although it can be used to describe the entire syndrome. Lesions may be single or multiple, and can occur anywhere on the body.

Histological examination of these lesions shows profuse bacteria within the walls of, and surrounding, arterioles and venules. The inflammatory reaction is minimal or absent, in many instances reflecting the nature of the immune compromise that usually predisposes to this disease. Extravascular hemorrhage and intravascular thrombosis are part of the pathologic picture. These findings are sometimes designated

"*Pseudomonas* vasculitis," although this term is a misnomer because of the absence of inflammatory cells in blood vessel walls. Interestingly, similar clinical and pathologic abnormalities occur in *P. aeruginosa* colonization in burn patients.

Lesions with the above-described appearance are often assumed to be due to *P. aeruginosa*—i.e., the clinical diagnosis of ecthyma gangrenosum is often thought to imply a specific bacteriologic etiology. In fact, identical syndromes can be caused by other Gram-negative bacilli (Figs. 5.7, 5.8), such as *Vibrio, Xanthomonas, Serratia, Acinetobacter,* or *Aeromonas* species; Gram-positive bacteria, such as *Staphylococcus aureus, Corynebacterium* group JK (3); and fungi such as *Mucor, Aspergillus, Candida* (4), and *Fusarium* (5).

Pseudomonas aeruginosa is said to be the most common cause of osteomyelitis following puncture wounds of the feet; a selective effect of prophylactic drugs effective against *Staphylococcus aureus* but not against *Pseudomonas* may be partly responsible.

Diffuse folliculitis caused by *Pseudomonas aeruginosa* is now a well recognized entity. Exposure to a large inoculum of *Pseudomonas*, especially under pressure, as in a whirlpool bath, is responsible; in one outbreak, swimming in a *Pseudomonas*-contaminated pool led to *Pseudomonas* folliculitis only in persons who also used a whirlpool. Lesions appear within 48 hours of exposure (range of 8 hours to 5 days) as 2- to 5-mm inflamed papules at hair follicles (Fig. 5.9), although they may enlarge and, occasionally, result in frank pustules. The lesions occur primarily in areas of skin where hair is present and have special predilection for moist and/or traumatized areas, such as axillae, buttocks, waistband, and lateral aspects of the trunk; the swimsuit area also is generally involved. Interestingly, mastitis has been noted in 6% to 19% of affected persons, reflecting involvement of mammary glands or areolar apocrine glands of Montgomery (6).

Other characteristic localized lesions caused by *Pseudomonas* organisms include paronychial infections with green discoloration of the nail (Fig. 5.10), macerated areas between the toes with possible slight green discoloration, and macerated painful external otitis, often referred to as swimmer's ear. Predisposition to these infections occurs by chronic immersion in water or chronic wetness. Also, *P. aeruginosa* may colonize burns and leg ulcers, or may produce a severe chondritis following ear surgery. On occasion, the exudate in these infections may have what has been described as a "fruity" odor.

• DIAGNOSIS AND DIFFERENTIAL DIAGNOSIS •

For diagnosis and differential diagnostic considerations of *P. aeruginosa* sepsis, please see the discussion in Chapter 4. The diagnosis of *Pseudomonas* folliculitis can be made by history and physical examination. If the complete history is not elicited, lesions can be confused with those due to staphylococcal folliculitis, insect bites, scabies, contact dermatitis, or varicella. Other Gram-negative bacilli, including *Salmonella* and *Proteus,* have been noted to cause bacterial folliculitis, usually superimposed on preexisting acne vulgaris, and can be distinguished from *Pseudomonas* folliculitis by patient history and sites of involvement. Nail, toe web, and ear canal infections may also be confused with those caused by other bacteria, such as *Proteus*, and fungal organisms, including *Candida, Aspergillus*, and various dermatophytes.

• TREATMENT AND CLINICAL COURSE •

Pseudomonas folliculitis in immunocompetent patients is a self-limiting disease; therefore, no treatment is necessary. Spontaneous resolution usually occurs over a period of 7 to 14 days, although pustules may recur for a few months, and larger lesions may persist for weeks before resolving. Other localized skin and nail infections characterized by wetness should be treated with drying of the affected area and appropriate topical antimicrobial agents such as gentamicin. Serious concern should be given to the immunocompromised host with any infection due to *Pseudomonas*, no matter how superficial (6).

KLEBSIELLA RHINOSCLEROMATIS

• PATHOGENESIS •

Rhinoscleroma is a slowly progressive, mildly contagious disease caused by *Klebsiella rhinoscleromatis*, a Gram-negative rod with a gelatinous capsule. It is endemic in certain parts of Europe, Russia, Asia, Africa, and both Central and South America. The disease is acquired by direct or indirect contact with the nasal secretions of infected persons.

• CLINICAL FEATURES •

The disease begins insidiously with nasal secretions, followed by nodules and diffuse enlargement of the nose, upper lip, and palate. Sclerotic changes, ulceration, and hardened skin are followed later by marked disfigurement and mutilation. Nasal obstruction may be complete, and death due to obstructive sequelae may occur.

• DIAGNOSIS AND DIFFERENTIAL DIAGNOSIS •

Biopsy of affected tissue shows characteristic histological findings consisting of plasma cells, degenerating plasma cells (Russell bodies), and foamy macrophages containing the bacilli (Mikulicz cells) that can be visualized with the Warthin-Starry silver stain. Diffuse fibrosis is present in surrounding tissues. Clinically, the disease must be differentiated from leprosy, sarcoidosis, syphilitic gumma, leishmaniasis, tuberculosis, rhinosporidiosis, and keloid formation.

• TREATMENT AND CLINICAL COURSE •

The disease is only moderately responsive to antibiotic treatment; sensitivity studies are advisable. The tetracyclines are the usual drugs of choice, with cephalosporins, streptomycin, and trimethoprim-sulfamethoxasole being other choices. Systemic steroids may be added in some cases. Surgical procedures may be necessary to correct structural and functional abnormalities of the affected nasopharynx and nose.

Haemophilus influenzae

• PATHOGENESIS •

Haemophilus influenzae causes cellulitis of the face and neck in susceptible toddlers, children, and adults. Encapsulated organisms are always responsible, and nearly all documented cases have been due to infection with *H. influenzae* type B. Susceptibility is said to be determined by absence of antibody to the capsular polyribosome phosphate; lack of antibody to lipopolysaccharide and/or membrane proteins may also be partially responsible. Infection presumably results from direct spread of infective organisms via loose connective tissues from the pharynx to superficial tissues of the cheek, the face, or the lateral aspect of the neck; this hypothesis regarding pathogenesis is supported by the frequent simultaneous occurrence of epiglottitis.

• CLINICAL FEATURES •

Facial cellulitis is usually seen in young children. The patient usually presents with a warm, rapidly spreading, tender, reddish, macular lesion on the cheek or the periorbital region.

Recently, *Haemophilus influenzae* cellulitis has also been described in adults. These patients tend to be over age 50 and have a cellulitis of the neck and upper chest associated with bacteremia and epiglottitis (7). Bacteremia is documented in over 75% of these cases.

• DIAGNOSIS AND DIFFERENTIAL DIAGNOSIS •

Some authorities claim that facial cellulitis caused by *Haemophilus* demonstrates a distinctive purplish hue of involved tissues. Others have not observed this characteristic, stating that cellulitis caused by *Haemophilus* cannot be distinguished from that due to *Streptococcus pyogenes* and suggesting that cellulitis caused by other organisms may, on occasion, produce the same purplish discoloration. Therefore, the diagnosis depends on the isolation of *Haemophilus influenzae* from blood or the local skin lesion.

• TREATMENT AND CLINICAL COURSE •

Since 1980, the emergence of resistance mediated by ß-lactamases has greatly increased, probably now exceeding 40% in most areas of the country. In some regions, isolated resistance to chloramphenicol has also been reported. Therefore, routine susceptibility testing is essential. Current trends favor third-generation cephalosporins as initial therapy in serious *H. influenzae* infections. In patients with epiglottitis, maintenance of an adequate airway should be an urgent goal along with appropriate antibiotics. The incidence of serious infection caused by this organism has fallen drastically, thanks to widespread use of protein-conjugated *Haemophilus* vaccine.

Actinomycetes

ACTINOMYCOSIS

• PATHOGENESIS •

Actinomyces, often in association with other anaerobic or microaerophilic bacteria, causes localized abscesses in areas where mouth or intestinal flora are likely to find a break in mucocutaneous defenses, such as in the jaw, thorax, abdomen, or pelvis. In these cases, cutaneous manifestations of actinomycosis simply reflect extension of a deeper infection toward the surface. Rarely, disseminated infection causes an abscess, osteomyelitis, or septic arthritis in one or more peripheral sites, with cutaneous manifestations reflecting extension or metastatic infection to the skin or soft tissues. Given the capacities of *Actinomyces* to produce burrowing infections and to spread hematogenously, infection can appear almost anywhere in the body. Human actinomycosis is caused mainly by *A. israelii*.

• CLINICAL FEATURES •

Cervicofacial actinomycosis, so-called "lumpy jaw," is usually associated with odontogenic disease. The infection spreads slowly, eventually developing draining cutaneous fistulas. Thoracic actinomycosis from pulmonary infection is much less common. Infection follows either aspiration, esophageal perforation, or direct extension into the mediastinum from the neck. The disease is usually suspected when the patient develops a draining chest wall fistula. Rarely, abdominal actinomycosis can occur from perforation of the gastrointestinal tract or endometritis associated with intrauterine devices. Figure 5.11 shows an actinomycotic abscess of the chest wall, and Figures 5.12 and 5.13 show a cutaneous fistula reflecting underlying osteomyelitis of the jaw.

• DIAGNOSIS AND DIFFERENTIAL DIAGNOSIS •

Routine aerobic cultures do not grow the organism. *Actinomyces* species are microaerophilic and grow slowly. In disease states, they are usually recovered with other anaerobes. When actinomycosis is suspected, exudate or tissue must be cultured promptly under anaerobic conditions. Gram's stain of pus or exudate will show filamentous and beaded, branching Gram-positive rods that must be differentiated from *Nocardia*. This can usually be done, since *Nocardia* is aerobic and weakly acid-fast positive, whereas *Actinomyces* is not. The diagnosis of actinomycosis should also be considered if so-called "sulfur" granules (yellow grains that actually represent clumps of organisms) are observed in draining exudates. Figure 5.14 demonstrates "sulfur" granules in tissue.

Chronic osteomyelitis tumors and osteoradionecrosis can mimic chronic actinomycosis.

• TREATMENT AND CLINICAL COURSE •

Penicillin is the preferred drug for treatment of patients with actinomycosis, although tetracyclines are also effective. Since

Actinomyces species grow well in avascular tissues, debridement is often necessary. High doses of parenteral penicillin or a tetracycline are often given initially, after which oral penicillin or tetracycline is continued for a total of 3 to 6 months.

ACTINOMYCETOMA

• PATHOGENESIS •

Several species of aerobic actinomycetes, *Actinomadura*, *Nocardia*, and *Streptomyces*, are agents of actinomycetoma. The disease presents after trauma to exposed skin sites. Infection starts in the skin and soft tissue but spreads to involve deeper structures, destroying connective tissue and bone.

• CLINICAL FEATURES •

These species of actinomycetes usually produce a chronic suppurative infection that commonly involves the feet. The term "madura foot" is often used to describe the salient clinical features of an indolent, swollen, indurated limb with multiple draining sinuses (Figs. 5.15, 5.16). Osteomyelitis is reported in over half of the cases. The disease occurs mainly in tropical climates; in the United States, the majority of cases have appeared in Texas, Louisiana, and Florida. *Nocardia brasiliensis* is the most common cause of actinomycetoma in the Western Hemisphere; 86% of all cases reported from Mexico are *N. brasiliensis*.

• DIAGNOSIS AND DIFFERENTIAL DIAGNOSIS •

In endemic areas, an indurated swelling of the foot with sinus tract formation should be regarded as a mycetoma until proven otherwise. Once bone has been invaded, chronic bacterial osteomyelitis and botryomycosis can mimic madura foot. Tumors, cold abscesses, and Charcot's foot can all look similar if sinus tract formation is not evident.

The species of actinomycetes causing this process grow aerobically on either routine bacterial or fungal media and appear microscopically as clumped, beaded, Gram-positive filaments. Tissue Gram's stains will also detect the beading, branching filaments. In addition, *Nocardia* species are acid-fast-positive; species of *Actinomadura* and *Streptomyces* are not. Biopsy specimens are preferred since exudates from sinus tracts are often contaminated by surface bacteria. Hematoxylin and eosin-stained specimens of involved tissues reveal neutrophils mixed with epithelioid cells and multinucleated giant cells with areas of fibrosis.

True fungi can produce a similar type of mycetoma infection, called eumycetoma, which is discussed extensively in Chapter 15.

• TREATMENT AND CLINICAL COURSE •

Treatment of *Nocardia* species is reviewed under nocardiosis later in this chapter. Sulfonamides, trimethoprim-sulfamethoxazole, and tetracyclines are active against most strains of *Actinomadura*. Long-term therapy of 12 to 24 months is usually needed. Surgical debridement is frequently required as well.

Amputation is occasionally needed to control or cure this disease, especially if the infection is caused by true fungi or by *Actinomadura*.

NOCARDIOSIS

• PATHOGENESIS •

Nocardia asteroides and *N. brasiliensis* are both implicated as causes of infection of the skin and soft tissues. *Nocardia asteroides* may produce local infection by direct inoculation or by hematogenous dissemination, although the majority of cases result from local inoculation. Systemic infection due to *N. brasiliensis* is rare, and superficial infection nearly always results from local invasion. In the United States, the preponderance of cutaneous *Nocardia* lesions are caused by *N. brasiliensis*; a small proportion are caused by *N. asteroides*, and rare infections with *N. otitidiscaviarum* infection are seen.

The majority of cases of local infection caused by either *N. asteroides* or *N. brasiliensis* appear in the southern and southwestern United States and occur in apparently normal persons. These localized infections occur when a break in the skin is associated with soil contamination, as in abrasions resulting from motor vehicle accidents or penetrating injury caused by a thorn. No specific predisposing event is detectable in half of such patients, although patients often state that gardening is a hobby. Systemic *Nocardia* infection occurs almost exclusively in immunocompromised hosts and is nearly always due to *N. asteroides*; occasionally, involvement of skin and soft tissues results. Since PMNs and activated macrophages both contribute to host defense against infection by *Nocardia*, a wide range of factors that compromise immunity have been found to predispose to systemic infection, including corticosteroids, cancer chemotherapy, immunosuppressive regimens used in transplant patients, renal dialysis, and chronic granulomatous disease.

• CLINICAL FEATURES •

Patients with primary cutaneous nocardiosis may be afebrile or have persistent low-grade fever with minimal or absent systemic symptoms. Lesions can appear as a localized pyoderma or abscess similar to infections caused by *Staphylococcus aureus*. They are typically on the extremities, except in children where they frequently appear around the face or neck. Patients can also present with lymphangitic spread, having multiple subcutaneous nodules that can mimic sporotrichosis (Fig. 5.17). Dissemination from primary cutaneous disease is rare. Hematogenous dissemination is generally assumed to occur from a pulmonary focus, although, on occasion, no pulmonary focus is documented. The skin is the most common extrapulmonary site in disseminated disease.

• DIAGNOSIS AND DIFFERENTIAL DIAGNOSIS •

Nocardia grows well on media such as routine blood agar, Sabouraud's dextrose agar, and Löwenstein-Jensen (rarely used today). The organisms appear as beaded, branching filaments on Gram's stain and are weakly acid-fast. The differential diagnosis should include tuberculosis and other acid-fast infections as well as deep fungal infections.

• TREATMENT AND CLINICAL COURSE •

Sulfonamides have long been known to be effective in treating nocardiosis, and the addition of trimethoprim may increase activity against *Nocardia*. The combination of sulfamethoxazole 800 mg and trimethoprim 160 mg has been effective when given to adults 3 or 4 times daily in disseminated disease (although a half life of 10 to 12 hours should cause the drug to be equally effective with less frequent dosing) and twice daily in localized infections. In vitro susceptibility has been shown for minocycline, amikacin, cefuroxime, and cefotaxime, and one or more of these drugs have been added with modest success in cases of disseminated infection that fail to respond to sulfamethoxazole and trimethoprim. Several studies from Mexico have shown amikacin to be excellent for actinomycetomas caused by *Nocardia*. The treatment period has usually been 3 months for primary cutaneous disease and 6 months for disseminated disease, although shorter courses should be effective and need to be studied in a controlled fashion (8).

Corynebacteria

CORYNEBACTERIUM DIPHTHERIAE

• PATHOGENESIS •

Although uncommon in the United States due to widespread immunization, *Corynebacterium diphtheriae*, the causative agent of human diphtheria, can produce three kinds of involvement of skin and soft tissues:

1. Colonization or infection of preexisting skin lesions;

2. Primary skin ulcer;

3. Cellulitis of the neck in association with diphtheritic pharyngitis.

This organism can colonize the skin if its integrity has been damaged in any way—for example, by wounds, abrasions, preexisting dermatologic disease, or bacterial (e.g., staphylococcal or streptococcal) infections. Colonization may serve as a reservoir for endemic or even epidemic diphtheria in a susceptible population (9). Two of the three subtypes of *C. diphtheriae*—var. *mitis* and *intermedius*—have generally been implicated in skin infections in the United States, while the third subtype—*gravis*—has not. In cases of cellulitis associated with diphtheritic pharyngitis, bacterial production of hyaluronidase as well as diphtheria toxin in a susceptible host is thought to be partly responsible.

• CLINICAL FEATURES •

Infection of the skin by *C. diphtheriae* causes a spectrum of involvement that is indistinguishable from other bacterial infections, including infected abrasions and wounds, impetigo, ecthyma, pyoderma of the scalp, and infected insect bites. Of importance for public health reasons is the observation that most strains isolated in this circumstance are toxigenic, i.e., capable of producing diphtheritic pharyngitis. In tropical climates, *C. diphtheriae* may cause ulcers that have clearly demarcated margins and clean or fibrin-covered bases; this clinical picture has been observed occasionally in the southern United States. The presentation of an indolent ulcer in which *C. diphtheriae* is isolated is rarely associated with systemic symptoms.

In a small proportion of cases of diphtheritic pharyngitis, the area of involvement may extend from the tonsils and pharynx to the lymph nodes and soft tissues under the mandible and into the anterior aspect of the neck, producing what has traditionally been called a "bull-neck" appearance. The tissues are red, hot, tender, and markedly swollen. In a 1970 outbreak in Texas, one-third of patients developed a slightly different picture in which edema of the lower part of the neck obliterated the borders of the sternocleidomastoid muscle, the clavicle, and to a lesser extent, the mandible (10).

• DIAGNOSIS AND DIFFERENTIAL DIAGNOSIS •

Primary diagnosis of pharyngeal diphtheria must be based on clinical findings because therapy cannot wait for laboratory confirmation. Cultures should be obtained from the throat or from skin lesions. Swabs should be cultured on Loeffler's or tellurite-containing media. All isolates of *C. diphtheriae* should be tested for toxin using in vitro guinea pig lethality or in vitro ELEK immunodiffusion test.

Cutaneous lesions may simulate impetigo or ecthyma caused by staphylococci or streptococci.

• TREATMENT AND CLINICAL COURSE •

Isolates of *C. diphtheriae* are frequently toxigenic and can serve as a source of infection to others. The risk of treating cutaneous diphtheria with diphtheria antitoxin must be balanced against the low risk of toxin-mediated complications. Both erythromycin and penicillin are effective antimicrobials. For pharyngeal diphtheria, diphtheria antitoxin remains the backbone of therapy. Antitoxin is effective only if administered before circulating toxin binds to tissues. Although antibiotics do not alter the course of pharyngeal diphtheria, they should be administered to terminate toxin production and prevent spread of the organism.

CORYNEBACTERIUM MINUTISSIMUM

• PATHOGENESIS •

Erythrasma is a superficial bacterial infection due to *Corynebacterium minutissimum*. This organism is widespread and is commonly found on both normal and abnormal human skin. Infection begins with a proliferation of bacteria on the surface of the skin and invasion of the stratum corneum.

• CLINICAL FEATURES •

Skin lesions tend to be reddish-brown with scaly macular patches usually present in the axillary and genital areas (Figs.

5.18, 5.19). The infection can range from an asymptomatic form to a generalized form with intense pruritus and periodic exacerbations. The disease is more common in obese diabetic patients, and tends to be seen more commonly in the tropics.

• DIAGNOSIS AND DIFFERENTIAL DIAGNOSIS •

Gram's stain of the skin usually shows large numbers of Gram-positive bacilli. A characteristic coral red fluorescence under Wood's lamp confirms the diagnosis (Fig. 5.20). Tinea versicolor on the trunk and tinea cruris should be considered in the differential diagnosis.

• TREATMENT AND CLINICAL COURSE •

Treatment with oral erythromycin for approximately 1 week is usually adequate, with resolution within several weeks. Topical treatment with erythromycin or clindamycin has occasionally been successful as well.

REFERENCES

1. Musher DM. Cutaneous and soft-tissue manifestations of sepsis due to Gram-negative enteric bacilli. Rev Infect Dis 1980;2:854.
2. Kingston ME, Mackey D. Skin clues in the diagnosis of life- threatening infections. Rev Infect Dis 1986;8:1.
3. Dan M, Somer I, Knobel B, Gutman R. Cutaneous manifestations of infection with *Corynebacterium* group JK. Rev Infect Dis 1988;10:1204.
4. Silverman RA, Rhodes AR, Dennehy PH. Disseminated intravascular coagulation and purpura fulminans in a patient with *Candida* sepsis: Biopsy of purpura fulminans as an aid to diagnosis of systemic *Candida* infection. Am J Med 1986;80:679.
5. Richardson SE, et al. Disseminated fusarial infection in the immunocompromised host. Rev Infect Dis 1988;10:1171.
6. Gustafson TL, Band JD, Hutcheson RH, Jr, Schaffner W. *Pseudomonas* folliculitis: an outbreak and review. Rev Infect Dis 1983;5:1.
7. Drapkin MS, Wilson ME, Shrager SM, Rubion RH. Bacteremic *Haemophilus influenzae* type B cellulitis in the adult. Am J Med 1977;63:449.
8. Wallace RJ, Jr, et al. Use of trimethoprim-sulfamethoxazole for treatment of infections due to *Nocardia*. Rev Infect Dis 1982;4:315.
9. Harnisch JP, et al. Diphtheria among alcoholic urban adults. Ann Intern Med 1989;111:71.
10. McCloskey RV, et al. 1970 epidemic of diphtheria in San Antonio, Texas. Ann Intern Med 1991;75:495.

ANNOTATED BIBLIOGRAPHY

Dan M, Somer I, Knobel B, Gutman R. Cutaneous manifestations of infection with *Corynebacterium* group JK. Rev Infect Dis 1988;10:1204.
    A useful review of infections caused by group JK corynebacteria.
Drapkin MS, Wilson ME, Shrager SM, Rubion RH. Bacteremic *Haemophilus influenzae* type B cellulitis in the adult. Am J Med 1977;63:449.
    Description of adult soft tissue infection due to *H. influenzae* type B.
Gustafson TL, Band JD, Hutcheson RH, Jr, Schaffner W. *Pseudomonas* folliculitis: An outbreak and review. Rev Infect Dis 1983;5:1.
    One of a number of good reviews of this subject.
Harnisch JP, et al. Diphtheria among alcoholic urban adults. Ann Intern Med 1989;111:71.
    Review of a diphtheria outbreak in urban alcoholic persons associated with poor hygiene, crowding, and underlying skin disease. Cutaneous infection was an important epidemiologic feature.
Kingston ME, Mackey D. Skin clues in the diagnosis of life-threatening infections. Rev Infect Dis 1986;8:1.
    Discussion of the pathogenesis and manifestations of a variety of infections that cause dermatologic disease.
Musher DM. Cutaneous and soft-tissue manifestations of sepsis due to Gram-negative enteric bacilli. Rev Infect Dis 1980;2:854.
    Discussion of the pathogenesis and manifestations of a variety of infections that cause dermatologic disease.
Richardson SE, et al. Disseminated fusarial infection in the immunocompromised host. Rev Infect Dis 1988;10:1171.
    Description of the cutaneous manifestations of serious fungal infection.
Silverman RA, Rhodes AR, Dennehy PH. Disseminated intravascular coagulation and purpura fulminans in a patient with *Candida* sepsis: Biopsy of purpura fulminans as an aid to diagnosis of systemic *Candida* infection. Am J Med 1986;80:679.
    Description of the cutaneous manifestations of serious fungal infection.
Tight RR, Bartlett MS. Actinomycetoma in the United States. Rev Infect Dis 1981;3:1139.
    Good review on the medical and surgical management of actinomycetomas.
Wallace RJ Jr, et al. Use of trimethoprim-sulfamethoxazole for treatment of infections due to *Nocardia*. Rev Infect Dis 1982;4:315.
    An extensive review of *Nocardia* infections and their treatment.

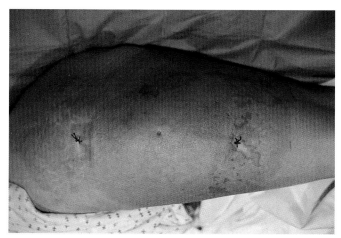

Figure 5.1. *Vibrio vulnificus.* Irregular areas of necrosis in the left thigh plaque. (Courtesy of Dr. Charles V. Sanders)

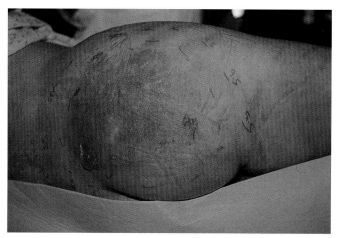

Figure 5.2. *Vibrio vulnificus.* Rapid advancement of cellulitic process in the right buttock. (Courtesy of Dr. Charles V. Sanders)

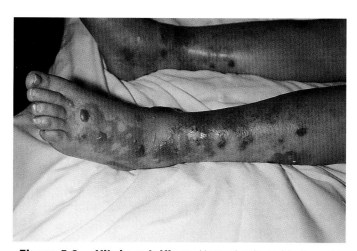

Figure 5.3. *Vibrio vulnificus.* Hemorrhagic and bullous skin lesions of the feet and lower legs, also showing hemorrhagic necrosis of the dorsum of the left foot. (Courtesy of Dr. Charles V. Sanders)

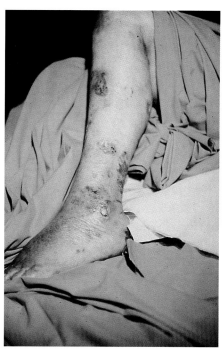

Figure 5.4. *Aeromonas hydrophila* **sepsis.** Multiple purpuric and ulcerative lesions of the leg and foot. (Courtesy of Dr. Charles V. Sanders)

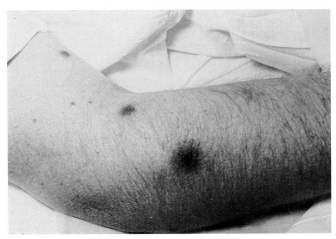

Figure 5.5.   *Pseudomonas.* Pseudomonas sepsis, causing small necrotic lesions (ecthyma gangrenosum). (Courtesy of Dr. Gerald Bodey)

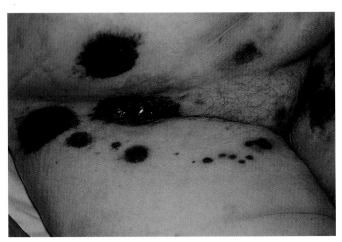

Figure 5.6.   *Pseudomonas.* Pseudomonas sepsis, causing large areas of necrosis. (Courtesy of Dr. Gerald Bodey)

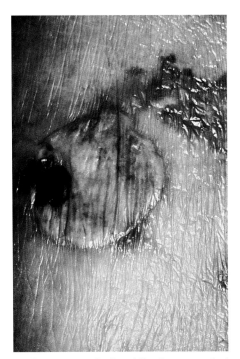

Figure 5.7.   *Aeromonas hydrophila.* Aeromonas hydrophila sepsis, causing necrosis of the tissues of the lower leg with minimal or absent inflammatory changes.

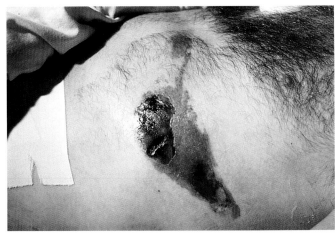

Figure 5.8.   *Acinetobacter.* Purpuric and necrotic lesion in left upper quadrant with ulceration and sloughing of superficial skin. (Courtesy of Dr. Charles V. Sanders)

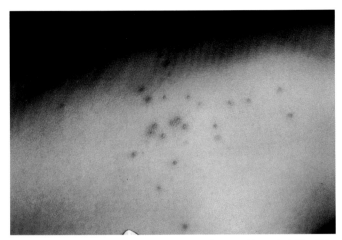

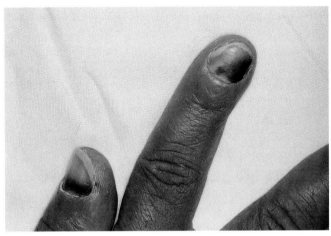

Figure 5.9. *Pseudomonas aeruginosa.* Hot tub folliculitis, caused by *Pseudomonas aeruginosa.* (Courtesy of Dr. Charles V. Sanders)

Figure 5.10. *Pseudomonas aeruginosa.* Green nail syndrome caused by localized *Pseudomonas aeruginosa* infection. (Courtesy of Dr. Lee T. Nesbitt, Jr.)

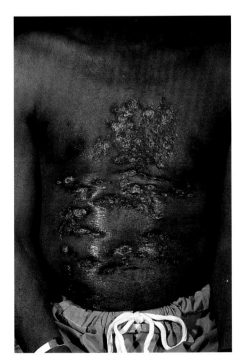

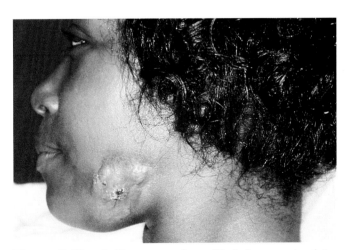

Figure 5.11. *Actinomyces israelii.* Thoracic actinomycosis due to *Actinomyces israelii* with multiple draining sinuses of the thoracic wall. (Courtesy of Dr. Charles V. Sanders)

Figure 5.12. *Actinomyces israelii.* Actinomycosis of the mandible due to *Actinomyces israelii.*

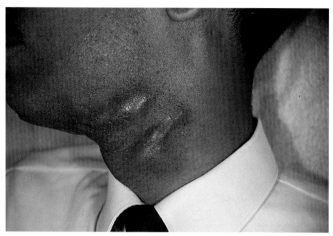

Figure 5.13. *Actinomyces israelii.* Cervicofacial actinomycosis due to *Actinomyces israelii*, producing "lumpy jaw." (Courtesy of Dr. Lee T. Nesbitt, Jr.)

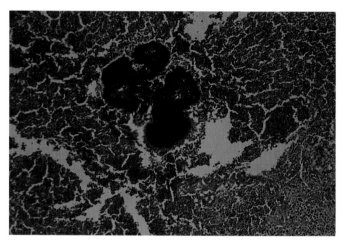

Figure 5.14. **Actinomycosis.** Sulfur granules in tissue. (Courtesy of Dr. Lee T. Nesbitt, Jr.)

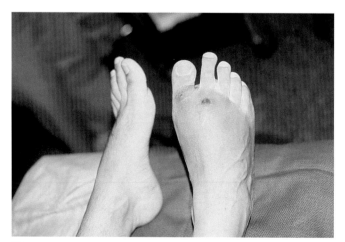

Figure 5.15.   Madura foot. Due to *Actinomadura madurae.* (Courtesy of Dr. Terry Satterwhite)

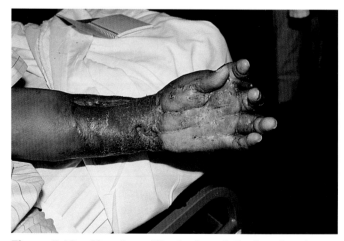

Figure 5.16.   Mycetoma-like lesion of the hand and arm. Due to *Nocardia asteroides.* (Courtesy of Dr. Lee T. Nesbitt, Jr.)

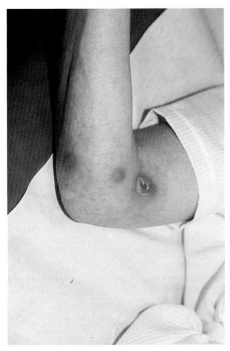

Figure 5.17. Nocardiosis. Lymphocutaneous form due to *Nocardia brasiliensis.*

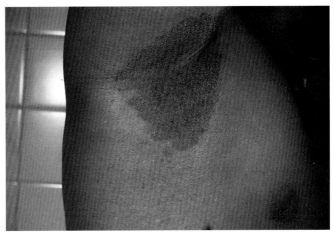

Figure 5.18. Erythrasma of the axillae. Noninflammatory hyperpigmented patch, produced by *Corynebacterium minutissimum.* (Courtesy of Dr. Lee T. Nesbitt, Jr.)

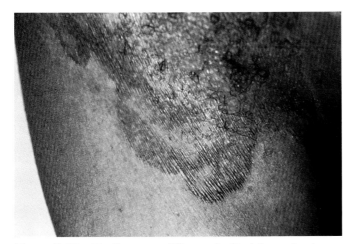

Figure 5.19. Erythrasma of the groin. Noninflammatory hyperpigmented patch, produced by *Corynebacterium minutissimum.* (Courtesy of Dr. Lee T. Nesbitt, Jr.)

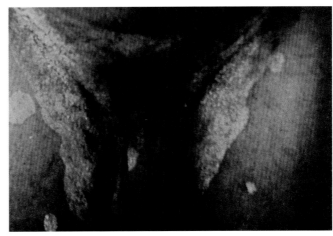

Figure 5.20. Erythrasma of the groin. Produced by *Corynebacterium minutissimum,* showing positive coral red fluorescence under Wood's light. (Courtesy of Dr. Lee T. Nesbitt, Jr.)

CHAPTER 6

Necrotizing and Gangrenous Soft Tissue Infections

MICHAEL K. HILL and CHARLES V. SANDERS

Overview of Necrotizing Infections and Their Management

Necrotizing soft tissue infections are a group of potentially life-threatening illnesses produced by a variety of organisms that may cause massive local tissue damage, progressive gangrene, profound systemic toxemia, and death. These infections are more frequently seen in compromised hosts, and they may occur following minor puncture wounds, lacerations, surgery, blunt trauma, abrasions, or hypodermic injections. They may appear on any part of the body, but they more frequently involve the extremities, abdomen, groin, and perineum.

The wide variety of clinical presentations makes it difficult to distinguish between the many types of necrotizing soft tissue infections. Most classifications have been based on anatomic structure, infecting organisms, and clinical presentation. However, some infections involve several components of soft tissue, and different bacterial species can produce infections with similar clinical appearances. Currently, the trend is toward regrouping the syndromes according to the depth of soft tissue destruction. This classification has been proposed by Sapico (1) and will be used here with some modification (Table 6.1). This simplified classification is based on the anatomic location of the disease process, the microbial etiology of the disease, and the presence or absence of vascular disease and/or diabetes mellitus. It includes only those disease processes accompanied by significant tissue necrosis or tissue death.

The key to successful management of necrotizing infection is early diagnosis and, in most cases, prompt radical surgical intervention. Morbidity and mortality can be reduced with aggressive debridement of all necrotic tissue combined with proper antimicrobial therapy, nutritional support, control of underlying diseases, such as diabetes mellitus, and close monitoring of organ functions.

Surgical intervention is usually diagnostic as well as therapeutic, since early clinical differentiation between necrotizing cellulitis, necrotizing fasciitis, and myonecrosis is difficult. All necrotic debris should be removed and the wound irrigated and

Table 6.1. Classification of Necrotizing Soft Tissue Infections

I. Superficial infections (not involving deep compartments)

    A. Infections involving epifascial soft tissue
        1. Anaerobic cellulitis
            a. clostridial
            b. nonclostridial
        2. Bacterial synergistic gangrene (mixed infection)
        3. Chronic undermining ulcer (of Meleney)

    B. Infections involving the superficial fascia—necrotizing fasciitis

        1. Monomicrobial
            a. *Clostridium* species
            b. *Streptococcus pyogenes*
            c. *Staphylococcus aureus*
            d. Group B *Streptococcus*
            e. *Vibrio* species
            f. Other organisms

        2. Polymicrobial (aerobes and anaerobes)

        3. Fournier's gangrene

II. Infections involving deep muscle compartments

    A. Monomicrobial
        1. *Clostridium species* (clostridial myonecrosis or classic gas gangrene)
        2. *Peptostreptococcus* species (anaerobic streptococcal myonecrosis)
        3. *Streptococcus pyogenes*
        4. *Staphylococcus aureus*
        5. Ecthyma gangrenosum (*Pseudomonas aeruginosa*)
        6. Other microorganisms (including *Vibrio vulnificus*, fungi causing cutaneous mucormycosis)

    B. Polymicrobial, also known as synergistic nonclostridial anaerobic myonecrosis (synergistic necrotizing cellulitis); mixed aerobic and anaerobic.

III. Other Infections

    A. Infected vascular gangrene
    B. Peripheral diabetic gangrene (no demonstrable large-vessel disease)
    C. Pyoderma gangrenosum

Modified from Sapico FL. Infect Dis Clin Practice 1993;2:330.

packed. In most cases, especially when there is massive tissue destruction, serial debridement is required. The wound should not be closed until healthy granulation tissue has been established. A necrotizing infection of anorectal origin often requires a diverting colostomy to prevent recurrent fecal soiling if the perineum or perianal tissues are involved.

Antibiotic selection is made difficult by the changing antibiotic susceptibility pattern of aerobes along with the proliferation of antibiotics. Moreover, anaerobic susceptibility testing has not been standardized and is not available in most hospitals. Before antimicrobial therapy is initiated, adequate aerobic and anaerobic tissue cultures and Gram's stain of clinical material should be obtained. Culture and Gram's stain of fluid aspirated from bullous lesions, areas of fluctuation, or wound exudate may be helpful. However, cultures from superficial swabs of ulcerative lesions or necrotic tissues are useless and provide misleading culture data, since many necrotic lesions become colonized with numerous bacteria.

In most necrotizing infections, therapy must be directed at a polymicrobial flora, which consists of anaerobes, aerobic streptococci, and, frequently, aerobic Gram-negative bacilli. Traditionally, combination therapy has consisted of ampicillin, gentamicin, and clindamycin (or metronidazole). The newer ß-lactam/ß-lactamase inhibitor combinations such as ampicillin/sulbactam, ticarcillin/clavulanate, and piperacillin/tazobactam provide excellent anaerobic and aerobic coverage. Piperacillin/tazobactam has the broadest aerobic Gram-negative bacilli activity, including the best *Pseudomonas aeruginosa* coverage, followed closely by ticarcillin/clavulanate. Ampicillin/sulbactam has no anti-*Pseudomonas* activity. In addition, these combination antibiotics also have good activity against methicillin-sensitive, ß-lactamase-producing staphylococci and streptococci. Ampicillin/sulbactam and piperacillin/tazobactam have much better enterococcal coverage than ticarcillin/clavulanate. Imipenem/cilastatin has the broadest coverage of currently available parenteral antibiotics. It provides coverage very similar to that of piper-acillin/tazobactam, but has better stability to type I chromosomal ß-lactamases found in many nosocomial Gram-negative bacilli, particularly *Enterobacter* species, *Citrobacter* species, *Acinetobacter* species, *Proteus vulgaris, Pseudomonas aeruginosa,* and *Serratia marcescens.* In many cases, the ß-lactam/ß-lactamase inhibitors and imipenem/cilastatin can be used as monotherapy to treat necrotizing skin and soft tissue infections, avoiding the potential nephrotoxicity of aminoglycoside therapy. The current available fluoroquinolones have good aerobic Gram-negative coverage and activity but are poor against anaerobic and aerobic streptococci, thus precluding their use as single-agent therapy in polymicrobial necrotizing infections. In penicillin-allergic patients, who are at high risk of developing aminoglycoside-associated nephrotoxicity, combination therapy with an antipseudomonal third-generation cephalosporin such as ceftazidime and metronidazole or clindamycin may be effective.

Since severe illness and stasis predisposes to venous thrombosis, prophylactic low-dose subcutaneous heparin should be given after surgical debridement. The benefits of nutritional therapy are well known, but have only been documented in uncontrolled studies. Hyperbaric oxygen (HBO) treatment has been advocated for treatment of necrotizing soft tissue infections. Although it has been suggested that early HBO treatment together with antibiotic administration and surgical debridement reduce the extent of infection, carefully controlled studies investigating the impact of variations in clinical presentations and therapy in humans have not been performed. Experimental evidence regarding the efficacy of HBO in animal models is often conflicting and inconclusive. Recently, a murine model of clostridial myonecrosis that mimicked the salient features of gas gangrene in humans was utilized to evaluate HBO therapy (2). HBO significantly improved the survival rate when combined with metronidazole or penicillin, but did not enhance the survival rate with clindamycin alone. The results of this study suggest that HBO therapy may be useful when treatment is delayed or the inoculum is large.

Superficial Infections Not Involving Deep Compartments

INFECTIONS INVOLVING EPIFASCIAL SOFT TISSUE

Anaerobic Cellulitis

Necrotizing soft tissue infections usually only include those disease processes that involve significant tissue necrosis or tissue death. Infections that involve epifascial tissue, such as anaerobic cellulitis, are included in this classification because they involve devitalized tissue and have the ability to spread rapidly.

• PATHOGENESIS •

Clostridial anaerobic cellulitis is usually due to infection of devitalized subcutaneous tissues, without associated fasciitis or myositis. Clostridial species, particularly *C. perfringens*, are introduced into subcutaneous tissue through trauma, surgical contamination, or a preexisting localized infection. Gas formation is common and usually extensive. The incubation period is usually several days as opposed to the shorter incubation period of only 1 or 2 days for clostridial myonecrosis. Although the onset is gradual, once established in the tissue, the infection spreads rapidly.

Nonclostridial anaerobic cellulitis is the result of infection with a variety of nonspore-forming anaerobic bacteria such as *Bacteroides* species, peptostreptococci, and peptococci, either alone or as part of a polymicrobial infection. The anaerobic bacteria may be present along with facultative species, such as aerobic Gram-negative bacilli, various streptococci, and staphylococci in a mixed infection. Predisposing factors for infection are similar to those for clostridial anaerobic cellulitis.

• CLINICAL FEATURES •

The clinical features of these two entities are similar (Figs. 6.1–6.3). Common sites of involvement are: epifascial soft tissues of the extremities, perineum, abdominal wall, retroperitoneum, buttocks, hips, thorax, or neck. The deep fascia is usually not significantly involved. The lesions usually appear clean or have superficial exudate. There is usually no evidence of tissue necrosis or systemic toxicity. Although pain may be the first symptom, it is usually mild. Gas may be readily detected by palpation or radiographic studies (Fig. 6.4).

• DIAGNOSIS AND DIFFERENTIAL DIAGNOSIS •

It is often difficult to distinguish clinically between anaerobic cellulitis and clostridial gas gangrene. Frequently, there is a characteristic thin, foul-smelling drainage emanating from the wound that is characterized as gas gangrene. Frank crepitus may extend widely from the involved area. Gram-stained smears of area drainage show numerous blunt-end, thick, Gram-positive bacilli and a variable number of polymorphonuclear neutrophils. Although *Clostridium perfringens* is the usual cause of the infection, *Clostridium septicum* and other clostridial species have been isolated occasionally along with other facultative organisms. Many incisions and wounds, when cultured, may yield clostridial species that are often mixed with other saprophytic bacteria.

The ultimate differentiation between anaerobic cellulitis and clostridial gas gangrene takes place at surgery when the viability and appearance of the muscles are observed. The muscle is unaffected in anaerobic cellulitis, but grossly discolored and necrotic in clostridial myonecrosis.

• TREATMENT AND CLINICAL COURSE •

These wounds require close observation for signs of tissue necrosis or infection. Aggressive surgical debridement and institution of broad-spectrum parenteral antibiotics are the mainstays of treatment. In some cases, serial debridement of necrotic tissue may be necessary.

Bacterial Synergistic Gangrene (Mixed Infections)

• PATHOGENESIS •

Bacterial synergistic gangrene is characterized by a chronic gangrenous infection of the skin and subcutaneous tissue, usually in conjunction with an ileostomy or colostomy at the exit of a fistulous tract or in proximity to a chronic ulceration. Although synergistic gangrene is primarily the result of group A streptococci infection, it can also be caused by a variety of non-spore-forming anaerobic bacteria (various *Bacteroides* species and *Peptostreptococcus* species) along with facultative species (aerobic Gram-negative bacilli, streptococci, or staphylococci) in a mixed infection.

• CLINICAL FEATURES •

Progressive bacterial synergistic gangrene usually begins as an indurated erythematous lesion that subsequently ulcerates. The painful, shaggy ulcer gradually enlarges and is characteristically encircled by a margin of gangrenous skin. Peripherally, a violaceous zone fades into an outer pink edematous border. If untreated, the ulcer progressively expands (Fig. 6.5). The major symptoms are extreme pain and tenderness. Usually, there is little systemic reaction and the patient is generally well.

• DIAGNOSIS AND DIFFERENTIAL DIAGNOSIS •

The diagnosis is generally made at the time of surgical debridement. The involvement of skin and soft tissue as well as the indolent nature of the infection distinguishes this clinical entity from anaerobic cellulitis.

• TREATMENT AND CLINICAL COURSE •

Although surgical debridement is usually necessary, cures have occasionally been accomplished with antimicrobial therapy alone. Broad-spectrum antibiotics are usually instituted until tissue cultures are available. When group A streptococci are causative, penicillin G should suffice.

Chronic Undermining Ulcer (of Meleney)

Chronic undermining ulcer (of Meleney) is a particular type of synergistic gangrene, now rarely seen. It is characterized by a slowly progressive infection of the subcutaneous tissue associated with ulceration of the overlying skin.

• PATHOGENESIS •

Although it may be associated with any wound or incision, Meleney's ulcer has occurred most frequently following lymph node surgery in the neck, axilla, or groin and, occasionally, after colon or female genital tract surgery. The causative organism is classically microaerophilic streptococci and infrequently anaerobic bacilli and streptococci.

• CLINICAL FEATURES •

The initial lesion is usually erythematous and tender, but systemic reaction is minimal. If untreated the lesion spreads gradually. Multiple ulcers and sinuses may develop at a distance from the original ulcer with undermining of the intervening skin and destruction of subcutaneous supporting tissues. There is little tendency for the lesions to heal spontaneously.

• DIAGNOSIS AND DIFFERENTIAL DIAGNOSIS •

Chronic undermining ulcer should be considered when one sees slowly progressive infection of the subcutaneous tissue associated with ulceration involving the overlying skin. The differential diagnosis would include other causes of gangrene.

• TREATMENT AND CLINICAL COURSE •

Debridement and drainage are important. Although in most cases penicillin G is effective, broad-spectrum agents should be employed until tissue cultures are available in order to cover ß-lactamase-producing anaerobic bacteria.

Infections Involving the Superficial Fascia—Necrotizing Fasciitis

Necrotizing fasciitis is an uncommon, severe infection that is characterized by widespread necrosis of fascia and deep subcutaneous tissue that usually spares the skin and muscle. This process spreads along the superficial fascial plane, unlike non-clostridial anaerobic myonecrosis, which involves the muscle underneath the deep enveloping fascia. The overall mortality rate is reportedly as high as 47%, but diagnosis made within 4 days of the onset of symptoms reduces the risk to 12%. Despite improved surgical techniques and antimicrobial therapy, the morbidity and mortality rates have not improved significantly since the condition was described in 1924.

• PATHOGENESIS •

Necrotizing fasciitis may be caused by several different monomicrobial infections, including *Clostridium* species, *Streptococcus pyogenes, Staphylococcus aureus*, group B streptococcus, and *Vibrio vulnificus*. It may also be caused by polymicrobial infections that include anaerobic bacteria, such as *Bacteroides* species and *Peptostreptococcus* species, in association with one or more facultative streptococci and a number of *Enterobacteriaceae*, such as *Escherichia coli, Enterobacter* species, *Klebsiella* species, *Proteus* species, *Clostridium* species, *Streptococcus* species, and *Vibrio vulnificus*. These infections are characterized by a rapidly spreading subcutaneous infection with thrombosis of nutrient vessels and resultant slough of the overlying skin. It usually occurs on the extremities, although the perineum, face, and other parts of the body may be involved. The infection typically occurs in the setting of some minor operation or injury.

Necrotizing fasciitis from intestinal sources may extend along the psoas muscle to the lower extremity, groin, or abdominal wall (via a colocutaneous fistula) and is usually polymicrobial. Anecdotal reports have linked the fulminant form to the use of nonsteroidal antiinflammatory drugs (3). Underlying clinical conditions may include diabetes mellitus, alcoholism, and parenteral drug abuse. Necrotizing fasciitis of the vulva has occurred following episiotomy.

Acute necrotizing fasciitis is rare in childhood but has been reported after surgery or trauma. In newborns, necrotizing fasciitis can be a serious complication of omphalitis, with periumbilical necrosis extending over the anterior abdominal wall and surrounding area. Acute necrotizing fasciitis of the scalp has been reported in premature infants, secondary to infiltration of intravenous fluid into the subcutaneous region of the scalp.

• CLINICAL FEATURES •

The initial signs are pain and marked swelling at the site of the wound, chills, fever, toxemia, and a rapidly spreading, painful cellulitis that undergoes bullous formation and eventual patchy skin necrosis. Bacteremia is common in this setting (4). Necrotizing fasciitis spreads rapidly along the superficial fascia. Initially, the skin may appear normal, but as the blood sup-ply to the skin becomes compromised, the skin becomes erythematous and edematous. Skin anesthesia develops as the subcutaneous gangrene progresses. Within a day or so, skin color changes from red-purple to patches of blue-gray. Skin breakdown with bullae (containing thick pink or purple fluid) occurs within 3 to 5 days of onset. Frank cutaneous gangrene resembling a thermal burn eventually develops (Figs. 6.6–6.9).

• DIAGNOSIS AND DIFFERENTIAL DIAGNOSIS •

Histologically, polymorphonuclear (PMN) leukocyte infiltration is pronounced in the deep dermis and fascial planes, and obliterating vascular thrombosis is usually extensive where microorganisms and microabscesses are plentiful. The characteristic pathologic changes seen in necrotizing fasciitis include severe and extensive necrosis of the superficial fascia and subcutaneous tissue with widespread destruction and liquification of fat. Early on, the process typically spares the overlying skin and underlying muscle, but in the latter stages, occlusion of the nutrient vessels causes progressive necrosis and gangrene of the skin.

In many cases, the clinical distinction between anaerobic cellulitis and necrotizing fasciitis can be made only after surgical inspection of the involved area. On probing the lesion with a hemostat through a limited incision, one can easily pass the instrument along a plane just superficial to the deep fascia. This would not be possible with ordinary cellulitis. Frozen section examination of biopsy specimens of the subcutaneous tissue and fascia have also been helpful in establishing the diagnosis (5).

Leukocytosis is common. Gram's stain smear of the exudate usually reveals polymicrobial infection or, in the case of streptococcal gangrene, chains of Gram-positive cocci. Drainage may not be foul-smelling. Blood cultures may be positive. Hypocalcemia may occur when there is extensive fat necrosis, causing production of calcium soaps. Soft tissue roentgenograms and computed tomography (CT) scans may show extensive soft tissue gas (6).

• TREATMENT AND CLINICAL COURSE •

Once the diagnosis is established, prompt surgical intervention should proceed. Treatment should focus on early and extensive surgical debridement of all nonviable fascia and tissue. This is best accomplished with extensive incisions through the skin and subcutaneous tissue, going beyond the area of involvement until normal tissue is found. This is noted when the hemostat can no longer separate skin and subcutaneous fascia from the deep fascia. Amputation of the limb is rarely necessary since the necrosis usually remains superficial to the deep fascia.

Local wound care consists of diligent cleansing and application of loose packs of gauze soaked with a topical agent such as Dakin's solution, an antibiotic solution, or normal saline. A sterile, gloved finger should check all areas of the wound to determine whether dissection has occurred, requiring additional drainage.

Antibiotics should be administered immediately after cultures are obtained. Broad-spectrum antibiotics are warranted until culture results are available, after which coverage can be modified.

Fournier's Gangrene

Fournier's gangrene is a form of necrotizing fasciitis that initially affects male perineum and genitalia, sometimes extending to the scrotum and abdominal wall.

• PATHOGENESIS •

Predisposing factors associated with this syndrome include diabetes mellitus, alcohol abuse, local trauma, paraphimosis, periurethral extravasion of urine, perirectal or perianal infection, and surgery, including circumcision and hernioplasty.

• CLINICAL FEATURES •

The infection commonly starts as cellulitis adjacent to the portal of entry. The involved area becomes progressively indurated, tender, and painful. As scrotal gangrene develops, swelling and crepitance of the scrotum quickly increases, and dark purple areas develop and coalesce. Granulocytopenic patients may not have local signs of inflammation. Mixed bacterial flora is usually present, including aerobic Gram-negative bacilli, streptococci, and anaerobic bacteria, such as *Bacteroides fragilis* and *Clostridium* species (Fig. 6.10).

• DIAGNOSIS AND DIFFERENTIAL DIAGNOSIS •

The diagnosis is usually made clinically and confirmed by histopathology. Histopathologic findings are similar to those mentioned for necrotizing fasciitis. Tissue cultures usually yield polymicrobial flora, including Enterobacteriaceae, enterococci, anaerobic microaerophilic streptococci, and anaerobic bacteria, particularly *Bacteroides, Fusobacterium*, and *Clostridium*. Group A streptococcal gangrene may rarely involve the male genitalia area.

• TREATMENT AND CLINICAL COURSE •

After blood, urine, and local cultures are obtained for both aerobic and anaerobic organisms, broad-spectrum antibiotic therapy should be initiated. Aggressive surgical debridement is also a necessity. Wide incision and drainage of all involved areas and removal of all devitalized tissue should be initiated as soon as possible. A transverse loop colostomy and suprapubic cystostomy may be needed for fecal and urinary diversion. The need for orchiectomy is rare, since the testes have their own blood supply independent of the compromised fascia and cutaneous circulation of the scrotum.

Infections Involving Deep Muscle Compartments

MONOMICROBIAL

Clostridium Species

• PATHOGENESIS •

Clostridial myonecrosis, also known as gas gangrene, is a rare, rapidly advancing, sometimes lethal infection characterized by muscle necrosis and severe toxin-related systemic toxicity. It is usually preceded by trauma or surgery, including soft tissue trauma, penetrating injuries, septic abortion or delivery, and soft tissue lesions associated with vascular insufficiency. Intestinal gas gangrene and spontaneous gas gangrene may also occur.

Some 80% to 90% of cases of clostridial myonecrosis are caused by *Clostridium perfringens*, with the occasional involvement of other clostridial species, including *Clostridium novyi, Clostridium septicum, Clostridium histolyticum, Clostridium fallax*, and *Clostridium bifermentans*. In some cases, more than one species of clostridia can be isolated from the infected site.

Many of the clinical manifestations of this disease are probably toxin-mediated. Enterotoxins produced by clostridia are often lethal when injected into mice. The most important toxin is thought to be an alpha toxin, which when injected intravenously into experimental animals produces massive hemolysis, platelet destruction, and widespread capillary damage. Their systemic absorption presumably accounts for the dramatic sequence of events in gas gangrene.

• CLINICAL FEATURES •

The usual incubation period from time of injury to the onset of symptoms is 1 to 4 days. The onset is heralded by intense, progressive muscular pain. The skin initially appears pale and then progresses to a bronze discoloration, often followed by the appearance of hemorrhagic bullae (Figs. 6.11–6.13). A thin, dirty-brown, serosanguineous discharge with a characteristic offensive odor is distinctly different from the usual anaerobic putrid discharge. Microscopic examination of the watery wound discharge usually reveals numerous red blood cells with only a few white blood cells along with many Gram-positive boxcar-shaped bacilli. Gas may be present but is frequently unrecognized, particularly in the early course of the disease.

Systemic findings include diaphoresis, low-grade fever, tachycardia, and in many cases, toxic delirium. The patient becomes incoherent and disoriented, and may develop hypotension, profound weakness, and pallor as the disease progresses. Late complications include hemolytic anemia, hypotension, and renal failure. Jaundice is rarely seen except when there is bacteremia and intravascular hemolysis. The patient eventually becomes moribund, and the entire body may develop the typical bronze or magenta color.

• DIAGNOSIS AND DIFFERENTIAL DIAGNOSIS •

Spontaneous clostridial myonecrosis is usually accounted for by hematogenous seeding of muscle groups. This condition may be misdiagnosed because of lack of a penetrating injury or obvious underlying process predisposing to gas gangrene. *Clostridium septicum* and *Clostridium perfringens* are equally responsible, and anaerobic blood cultures are frequently positive. Gastrointestinal malignancy is often present, although any process that disrupts bowel mucosa may be responsible. The clinical picture is similar to that of myonecrosis associated with wounds.

Since gas gangrene cannot be detected by laboratory tests, diagnosis hinges on clinical clues: severe toxicity and, with the exception of "spontaneous" gas gangrene, the occurrence of this infection after injury or trauma. The typical soft tissue and skin changes with the characteristic exudate are usually seen only after irreversible changes have occurred. Computed tomography or magnetic resonance imaging may show muscle compartment involvement. When gas gangrene is suspected, immediate surgical exploration is indicated. Necrotic muscle is typically dark and cold; it does not bleed when incised or contract when stimulated by electric current.

• TREATMENT AND CLINICAL COURSE •

The successful management of clostridial myonecrosis includes aggressive surgical debridement, which frequently requires multiple incisions and fasciotomy or amputation. Traditional therapy has been intravenous penicillin G, 12 to 24 million units daily, given in divided doses every 4 hours; however, some strains are beginning to show diminished susceptibility in vitro to penicillin (7). Although used for decades, intravenously administered polyvalent gas gangrene antitoxin has not been clinically validated and is no longer available. Intravascular hemolysis warrants exchange transfusion. While the usefulness of HBO is still unclear, it can be tried in cases involving the trunk or those in which extensive excision of involved muscle would be mutilating.

Peptostreptococcus Myositis

• PATHOGENESIS •

Myonecrosis may also be caused by anaerobic and microaerophilic streptococci, which are almost always found in association with other organisms, including *Streptococcus pyogenes* and *Streptococcus aureus*. Although *Bacteroides* is occasionally the major pathogen, there is usually a mixture of anaerobic bacteria and facultative bacteria (*Klebsiella* species, *Enterobacter* species, *Escherichia coli*, and *Proteus* species).

• CLINICAL FEATURES •

Its clinical presentation is similar to clostridial myonecrosis, although more subacute. The incubation period is usually 3 to 4 days. Pain typically occurs later in the disease, but may be very severe. Edema and a seropurulent exudate are common. Gas may be present but is less prominent than in clostridial myonecrosis. Although the muscle may be edematous and discolored, in the early course of the disease it is still viable and reactive to stimuli. There is usually marked systemic toxicity and elevations of serum creatinine phosphokinase and muscle compartment pressure. Mortality in reported cases is high.

• DIAGNOSIS AND TREATMENT •

Diagnosis is made at the time of surgery. Treatment is incision, aggressive debridement, and broad-spectrum antimicrobials.

Ecthyma Gangrenosum

• PATHOGENESIS •

This condition is classically described as a skin lesion caused by bacteremia from *Pseudomonas aeruginosa* with emboli to the skin. Although most commonly associated with *P. aeruginosa*, ecthyma gangrenosum has also been reported in sepsis due to other pseudomonal species, *Aeromonas hydrophila*, *Candida* species, *Serratia marcescens*, *Staphylococcus aureus*, *Aspergillus* species, and *Mucor* species. The lesion has also originated from vasculitis or malignant skin infiltration. The typical patient is immunocompromised, often neutropenic, or critically ill after chemotherapy. Ecthyma gangrenosum rarely occurs in the absence of sepsis.

• CLINICAL FEATURES •

The lesion may be discrete or multiple and appear anywhere on the body. It begins as a painless, round erythematous macule with or without an adherent vesicle that soon becomes indurated and develops into a hemorrhagic bluish bulla. Later, the lesion sloughs to form a gangrenous ulcer with a gray-black eschar and surrounding erythema. The skin lesions evolve over a period of 12 to 24 hours.

• DIAGNOSIS AND DIFFERENTIAL DIAGNOSIS •

Histologically, ecthyma gangrenosum is characterized by bacterial invasion of the media and adventitia of vein walls deep in the dermis, sparing the intima and lumen. Bacterial invasion results in marked fibrin exudation and frank hemorrhage, followed by ballooning of the upper dermis with resulting bullous formation. Finally, necrosis of the dermis occurs. Bacteria are readily visible in biopsy samples and can be demonstrated in Gram-stained material scraped from the base of the lesion.

In the early stages, before there is skin necrosis, the lesions may appear maculopapular and may be difficult to distinguish from skin lesions associated with *Candida* septicemia or staphylococcal bacteremia, which also occur in neutropenic patients. However, as the lesion progresses and the typical skin necrosis occurs, the diagnosis of ecthyma gangrenosum can usually be made.

• TREATMENT AND CLINICAL COURSE •

Therapy usually includes the combination of an antipseudomonal ß-lactam antibiotic such as piperacillin, ceftazidime, or imipenem/cilastatin and an aminoglycoside antibiotic. Despite the prolonged antibiotic therapy, these lesions may contain viable bacteria weeks after the blood has been cleared from infection. The absence of fluctuance may be due to either the lack of pus in neutropenic patients and/or the deep location of the abscess. Therapy usually also requires incision and debridement of skin lesions. Four weeks or more of antimicrobial therapy is the rule. Significant improvement usually does not occur until the neutropenia is resolved.

Streptococcus pyogenes and *Staphylococcus aureus*

Infections caused by *Streptococcus pyogenes* and *Staphylococcus aureus* are discussed in Chapter 3.

Other Organisms

Vibrio Vulnificus Infections. *Vibrio vulnificus* is an uncommon cause of life-threatening necrotizing skin lesions.

• PATHOGENESIS •

Vibrio vulnificus may cause necrotic skin lesions either by direct inoculation into the skin and soft tissue or by hematologic spread after a primary bacteremia that follows ingestion of contaminated shellfish. Wound infections are almost always associated with direct contact with seawater or shellfish, often the result of a deep puncture wound sustained while cleaning crabs, peeling shrimp, shucking oysters, or exposing a preexisting wound to seawater.

• CLINICAL FEATURES •

The initial wound appears to be trivial, but skin lesions quickly develop into an intense subcutaneous cellulitis, extending into the dermis and muscle, with overlying hemorrhagic bullae. Within hours, these areas may infarct, causing large areas of devitalized tissue. Patients who are immunocompromised, especially those with liver disease (cirrhosis or renal failure) are more likely to develop progressive cellulitis, myositis, or fasciitis.

• DIAGNOSIS AND DIFFERENTIAL DIAGNOSIS •

The diagnosis of *Vibrio vulnificus* should be considered when the physician encounters a case of rapidly progressive cellulitis with bullae formation following a seawater or shellfish-related injury or when a patient presents with multiple bullous skin lesions after eating raw or poorly cooked shellfish.

A Gram's stain aspirate of bullae and wounds may reveal curved Gram-negative bacilli suggestive of *Vibrio* infection, and culture of these areas should confirm the diagnosis. In primary septicemia, blood cultures are positive in 70% to 100%, compared to a third of wound infections.

Differential diagnosis includes group A streptococcal ecthyma gangrenosum, erysipelas, necrotizing fasciitis, other *Vibrio* infections, and brown recluse spider bite.

• TREATMENT AND CLINICAL COURSE •

It is important to distinguish infection due to *Vibrio vulnificus* from other causes of necrotizing soft tissue infection. Evidence of injury related to handling seafood or ingestion of raw oysters, particularly in an immunocompromised host, should arouse clinical suspicion of *Vibrio vulnificus*. As with other types of necrotizing soft tissue infections, aggressive debridement and medical support are crucial, and amputation of an involved limb may be life-saving. Intravenous tetracycline has been the traditional antibiotic of choice. A recent clinical study suggests that ceftazidime may be efficacious as well (8).

More information on *Vibrio* infections is found in Chapter 5.

Cutaneous Mucormycosis. Cutaneous mucormycosis may represent a primary or metastatic skin lesion. It is seen most commonly in immunosuppressed persons.

• PATHOGENESIS •

Mucormycosis is the common name given to several different diseases caused by the fungi of the order Mucorales. The taxonomy of this group is complicated. Although the label mucormycosis is not taxonomically correct, it is ingrained in the medical literature as the term describing a particular group of clinical presentations. These fungi are well known to cause invasive and often lethal rhinocerebral, pulmonary, gastrointestinal, or disseminated necrotizing skin lesions. Cutaneous mucormycosis has been described in burn victims, particularly after the use of intense topical antibacterial chemotherapy. Infection may also develop when there is inoculation of the organism from major or minor trauma. Diabetes is a predisposing factor in these patients. A nationwide epidemic of cutaneous mucormycosis occurred as a result of the use of elastic bandages in the 1970s. Cellulitis occurred under the bandage when fungi was directly inoculated into the skin that was occluded by the adhesive. The use of sterilized bandages and dressings has eliminated this problem.

• CLINICAL FEATURES •

Cutaneous mucormycosis usually involves the epidermis and dermis. Necrosis develops secondary to vascular invasion and tissue necrosis. The clinical course may be subacute with slowly progressive, gangrenous cellulitis with extensive tissue necrosis within a week of onset. The lesion is characterized as a black necrotic area with a margin of red-to-purple edematous cellulitis (Fig. 6.14).

• DIAGNOSIS AND DIFFERENTIAL DIAGNOSIS •

Diagnosis depends on histologic examination of the infected tissues. These fungi are ubiquitous, occasionally cultured from normal skin, and are frequent laboratory contaminants. However, even in proven cases, isolation of the organism can be difficult. It is important, therefore, to obtain an adequate biopsy specimen from the margin of the lesion. Scrapings or swabs are inadequate for isolation or identification.

The key to diagnosis is a high index of suspicion and early deep tissue biopsy and culture. Since the organisms invade deeply into tissue, swab wound cultures may only reveal colonizing bacterial contamination. Tissue sections usually demonstrate nonseptate hyphae invading blood vessels and viable tissue. Because the hematoxylin and eosin stain does not reliably identify fungi in tissue sections, period-acid-Schiff (PAS) and methenamine-silver stain are employed.

Aspergillus may produce a similar lesion and may be confused histologically with cutaneous mucormycosis. The hyphae of *Aspergillus* may be differentiated on the basis of their medium width, numerous septae, and characteristic acute, dichotomous branching. On rare occasions, patients with acute leukemia have developed skin lesions identical to ecthyma gangrenosum, which is more commonly due to *Pseudomonas aeruginosa.*

• TREATMENT AND CLINICAL COURSE •

When bacteriologic examination of tissue confirms cutaneous mucormycosis, treatment must begin immediately. The cornerstone of therapy is wide surgical debridement with the margins of resection extending into healthy tissue. Amputation of the involved extremity may be required when the infection involves muscles or extends across fascial planes. Amphotericin B is the drug of choice if the initial surgical debridement fails to control the disease. Anecdotal reports suggest that HBO therapy may be useful in severe cases; however, there is little experimental evidence to suggest that HBO, at a dose tolerable to humans, is effective against these pathogens.

POLYMICROBIAL INFECTIONS

Polymicrobial infections involving deep muscle compartments are also known as synergistic nonclostridial anaerobic myonecrosis (synergistic necrotizing cellulitis), mixed aerobic and anaerobic.

• PATHOGENESIS •

This is a variant of myonecrosis due to monomicrobial infection; however, there is usually extensive involvement of the skin, subcutaneous tissue, and fascia, as well as muscle. Predisposing factors include diabetes mellitus, obesity, cardiopulmonary disease, renal insufficiency, and advanced age.

• CLINICAL FEATURES •

The most common sites of occurrence are the lower extremities and perineum (Figs. 6.15–6.19). The lesion typically begins as small skin ulcers draining foul-smelling, reddish-brown or dishwater-colored pus. Circumscribed areas of blue-gray gangrene surround these draining sites; however, the intervening skin appears deceptively normal despite extensive necrosis involving underlying subcutaneous tissue, fascia, and muscle. There is usually exquisite pain and tenderness at the site of involvement and the patient appears toxic. Tissue gas is present in about a quarter of the patients and bacteremia in half.

Deep tissue cultures usually show a mixture of anaerobic bacteria, such as anaerobic streptococci and *Bacteroides*, along with facultative bacteria, such as *Klebsiella, Enterobacter, Escherichia coli,* and *Proteus.*

• DIAGNOSIS AND DIFFERENTIAL DIAGNOSIS •

Diagnosis is suspected based on the clinical syndrome and is usually confirmed at the time of surgery. Differential diagnosis includes necrotizing fasciitis as well as bacterial synergistic gangrene and chronic undermining ulcer of Meleney.

• TREATMENT AND CLINICAL COURSE •

Radical surgical debridement is frequently required because of extensive involvement of the deep fascia and muscle, and amputation may be required. Therapy involves the use of broad-spectrum antibiotics that have activity against aerobic Gram-negative and anaerobic bacilli.

Other Infections

INFECTED VASCULAR GANGRENE

• PATHOGENESIS •

Infected vascular gangrene is the result of secondary infection of muscle and soft tissue devitalized primarily from circulatory insufficiency associated with diabetes mellitus. This infection is usually caused by a mixture of anaerobes, facultative anaerobes, and Gram-negative rods. Common pathogens isolated include *Proteus* species, *Bacteroides* species, and anaerobic streptococci. *Bacillus cereus* infection has been associated with myonecrosis after thrombosis of arterial grafts.

• CLINICAL FEATURES •

Gas production may be considerable. The infection may involve part or all of an extremity, mostly the legs, and usually does not spread beyond devitalized tissue. Tissue necrosis usually begins at the distal part of the affected extremity (usually the toes) and progresses proximally (Fig. 6.20). Acute toxemia is rare.

• DIAGNOSIS AND DIFFERENTIAL DIAGNOSIS •

Clinical diagnosis is usually not difficult once extensive tissue destruction has occurred.

• TREATMENT AND CLINICAL COURSE •

In the very early stages of tissue necrosis, surgical debridement and restoration of tissue perfusion to affected tissue may reverse tissue necrosis. Broad-spectrum antibiotics play a very limited role, but should be used early in the treatment course. Once extensive tissue necrosis and gangrene occur, the necrotic extremity must be amputated.

REFERENCES

1. Sapico FL. Commentary: Necrotizing soft tissue infections. Infect Dis Clin Practice 1993;2:330.
2. Stevens DL, et al. Evaluation of therapy with hyperbaric oxygen for experimental infection with *Clostridium perfringens.* Clinic Infect Dis 1993;17:23.
3. Rimailho A, Riou B, Richard C, Auzepy P. Fulminant necrotizing fasciitis and non-steroidal anti-inflammatory drugs. J. Infect Dis 1987;155:143.
4. Majewski JA, and Alexander JN. Early diagnosis, nutritional support, and immediate extensive debridement improve survival in necrotizing fasciitis. Am J Surg 1983; 145:784.
5. Barker FG, Leppard BJ, Seal DV. Streptococcal necrotizing fasciitis: Comparison between histologic and clinical features. J Clin Pathol 1987;40:335.

6. Kaldican LC, Andriole VT. Necrotizing fasciitis: use of computerized tomography for non-invasive diagnosis. Infect Dis Clin Practice 1993;2:325.
7. Marrie TJ, et al. Susceptibility of anaerobic bacteria to nine antimicrobial agents. A demonstration of decreased susceptibility testing to *Clostridium perfringens* to penicillin. Antimicrob Agents Chemother 1981;19:51.
8. Chuang YC, et al. *Vibrio vulnificus* infection in Taiwan: Report of 28 cases and review of clinical manifestations and treatment. Clin Infect Dis 1992;15:271.

ANNOTATED BIBLIOGRAPHY

Bessman AN, Wagner W. Nonclostridial gas gangrene: Report of 48 cases and review of the literature. 1975;JAMA 233:958.

In a group of diabetic patients, nonclostridial gas gangrene occurred more commonly than clostridial gas gangrene. The most common bacteria isolated were aerobic and anaerobic Gram-negative bacilli, enterococcus, and streptococci.

Clayton MD, Fowler JE, Sharifi R, Pearl RK. Causes, presentation and survival of fifty-seven patients with necrotizing fasciitis of the male genitalia. Surg Gyncol Obstet 1990;170:49.

Survival of necrotizing fasciitis of the male genitalia was associated with young age, BUN less than 50 mg/dl, absence of sepsis, and decreased complications after debridement.

Feingold DS. The diagnosis and treatment of gangrenous and crepitant cellulitis. In: Remington JS, Swartz MN, eds. Current clinical topics in infectious diseases. New York: McGraw Hill, 1981:259.

Discusses the clinical features that distinguish the different types of necrotizing skin and soft tissue infections. Diabetes is present in a significant number of patients.

Fisher JR, Conway MJ, Takeshita RT, Sandoval R. Necrotizing fasciitis. Importance of roentgenographic studies for soft-tissue gas. 1979;JAMA 241:803.

Crepitance was found in only 5 of 26 patients with necrotizing fasciitis while roentgenograms of the involved site disclosed gas in every patient subsequently found to have gas at surgery. This underscores the significance of the roentgenographic studies to enhance earlier diagnosis and treatment.

George WL. Other infections of skin, soft tissue, and muscle. In: Feingold SM, George WL, eds. Anaerobic Infections in Humans. New York: Academic Press, 1989:485.

A good overview and clinical classification of skin, soft tissue, and muscle infections.

Golde S, Ledger W. Necrotizing fasciitis in postpartum patients: A report of four cases. 1977;Obstet Gynecol 50:670.

The first report of necrotizing fasciitis in an obstetric patient.

Hill MK, Sanders CV. Localized and systemic infections due to *Vibrio* species. Infect Dis Clin North Am 1987;3:687.

The major clinical syndrome of *Vibrio vulnificus* infections in this study included primary septicemia, wound infection, and gastrointestinal illness without septicemia or wound infection. Epidemiologic features are discussed.

MacLennen JD. The histotoxic clostridial infections of man. Bact Rev 1962;26:177.

Discusses the toxins and their role in clostridial infections.

Majeski JA, Alexander JN. Early diagnosis, nutritional support, and immediate extensive debridement improve survival in necrotizing fasciitis. Am J Surg 1983;145:784.

Rapid diagnosis followed by immediate surgical intervention and nutritional support improves survival of necrotizing fasciitis.

Parfey NA. Improved diagnosis and prognosis of mucormycosis. Medicine 1986;65:113.

A study of 33 cases of mucormycosis over 5 decades suggests the incidence is increasing. Improvement of outcome is directly related to early diagnosis and treatment.

Patino JF, Castro D. Necrotizing lesions of soft tissues: A review. World J Surg 1991;15:235.

Proposes a simple classification of necrotizing soft tissue infections. Discusses pathology, diagnosis, and treatment of necrotizing skin and soft tissue infections.

Riseman JA, et al. Hyperbaric oxygen therapy for necrotizing fasciitis reduces mortality and the need for debridement. Surgery 1990;108:847.

The addition of HBO therapy to the surgical and antimicrobial treatment of necrotizing fasciitis reduced mortality and wound morbidity, especially in nonclostridial infections.

Rogers JM, Gibson JV, Farrar E, Schabel SI. Usefulness of computerized tomography in evaluating necrotizing fasciitis. South Med J 1984;77:782.

CT scanning provides a much more accurate and earlier picture of the extent of tissue involvement than traditional roentgenogram.

Sanders CV, Aldridge KE. Current antimicrobial therapy of anaerobic infections. Eur J Clin Microbiol Infect Dis 1992;11(11):999.

A comprehensive review of antimicrobial therapy for anaerobic infections. Underscores the need to take into account the site of infection and thus the bacteria most likely to be found when choosing antimicrobial therapy.

Smith RJ, Berk SC. Necrotizing fasciitis and non-steroidal anti-inflammatory drugs. South Med J 1991;84:785.

A review of four reports and other case studies of necrotizing fasciitis in association with nonsteroidal anti-inflammatory drugs.

Stamenkovic I, Lew D. Early recognition of potentially fatal necrotizing fasciitis: The use of frozen-section biopsy. N Engl J Med 1984;310:1689.

Frozen section biopsy may facilitate the diagnosis of necrotizing fasciitis and subsequent treatment.

Stevens DL, et al. Spontaneous, non-traumatic gangrene due to *Clostridium septicum*. Rev Infect Dis 1990;12:286.

Clostridium septicum appears to be more capable of initiating infection in the absence of obvious tissue damage. Gastrointestinal carcinoma, diabetes, and leukopenia are predisposing factors.

Sudarsky LA, Laschinger JC, Coppa GF, Spencer FC. Improved results from a standardized approach in treatment of patients with necrotizing fasciitis. Ann Surg 1987;206:661.

Standardized treatment—including aggressive resuscitation, surgical debridement with mandatory reexploration at 24 hours, intravenous antibiotics, nutritional support, and early soft tissue coverage—resulted in favorable clinical conditions in the majority of cases.

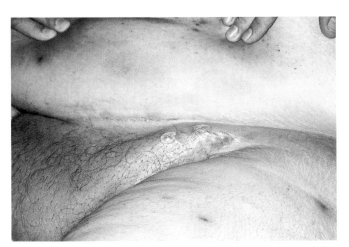

Figure 6.1   Cellulitis. In the left groin of an obese patient, cellulitis due to mixed aerobic/anaerobic infection. Note "orange peeling" and bullous lesions. (Courtesy of Dr. Charles V. Sanders)

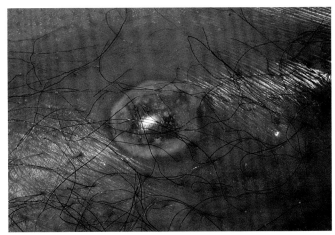

6.2.   Cellulitis. In the left groin of an obese patient, cellulitis due to mixed aerobic/anaerobic infection. Note "orange peeling" and bullous lesions. (Courtesy of Dr. Charles V. Sanders)

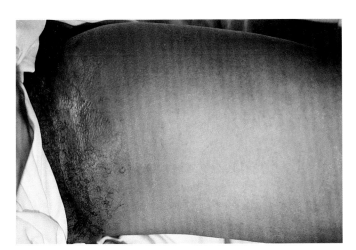

Figure 6.3.   Cellulitis. Mixed aerobic/anaerobic infection in the medial aspect of the left upper thigh. Note the swelling and erythema. (Courtesy of Dr. Charles V. Sanders)

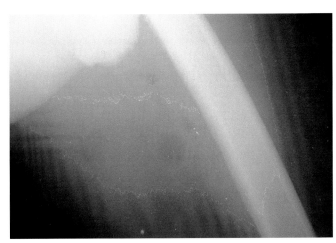

Figure 6.4.   Cellulitis. Radiograph shows gas in the tissue of the patient with cellulitis. (Courtesy of Dr. Charles V. Sanders)

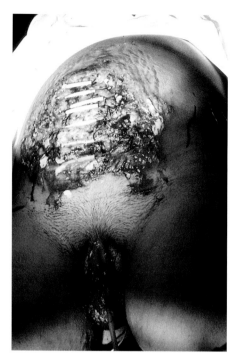

Figure 6.5. **Postoperative synergistic bacterial gangrene.**
Gangrene following a cesarean section. Note the triple zone of necrosis.
(Courtesy of Dr. Charles V. Sanders)

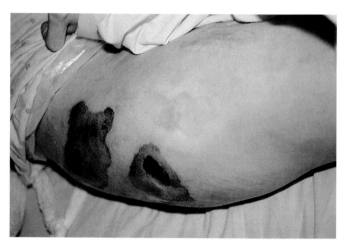

Figure 6.6. **Necrotizing fasciitis and myonecrosis.** A mixed
aerobic/anaerobic infection. (Courtesy of Dr. Charles V. Sanders)

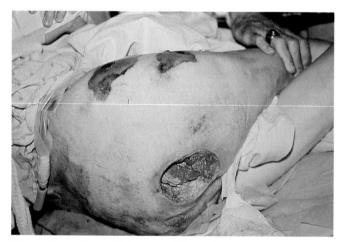

Figure 6.7. **Necrotizing fasciitis and myonecrosis.** A mixed
aerobic/anaerobic infection. (Courtesy of Dr. Charles V. Sanders)

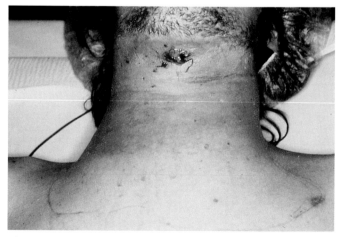

Figure 6.8. **Necrotizing fasciitis.** Secondary to periodontal
infection. Note the marked erythema and swelling of the neck. (Courtesy
of Dr. Michael Zide and Dr. Eric Dierks)

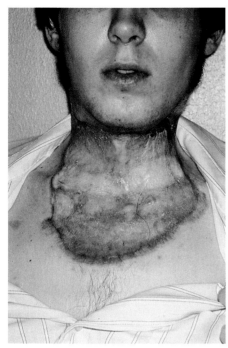

Figure 6.9.   Necrotizing fasciitis. Postoperative view of patient in Figure 6.8. Note marked loss of skin over anterior neck secondary to severe necrotizing fasciitis. (Courtesy of Dr. Michael Zide and Dr. Eric Dierks)

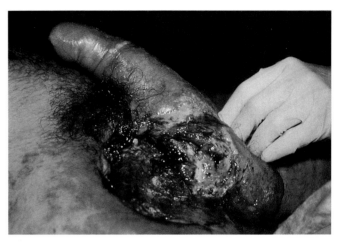

Figure 6.10.   Fournier's gangrene. A mixed aerobic/anaerobic infection. (Courtesy of Dr. Gene Beyt)

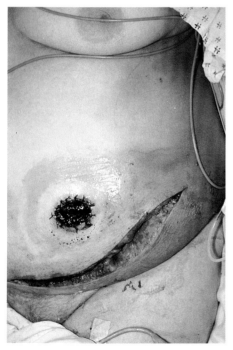

Figure 6.11.   Clostridial myonecrosis. Clostridial myonecrosis that developed after resection of a leiomyosarcoma of the rectum. (Courtesy of Dr. Charles V. Sanders)

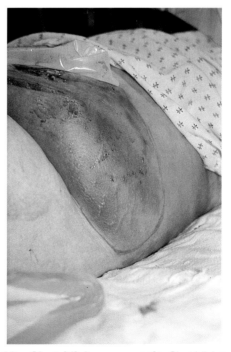

Figure 6.12.   Clostridial myonecrosis. Clostridial myonecrosis that developed after resection of a leiomyosarcoma of the rectum. (Courtesy of Dr. Charles V. Sanders)

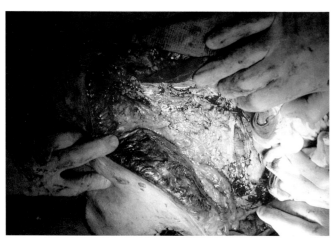

Figure 6.13.   Clostridial myonecrosis. Clostridial myonecrosis that developed after resection of a leiomyosarcoma of the rectum. (Courtesy of Dr. Charles V. Sanders)

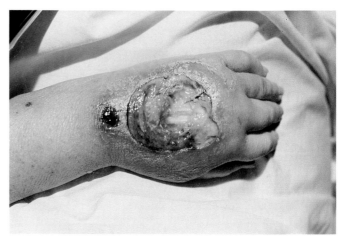

Figure 6.14.   Gangrenous lesion. Large gangrenous lesion with exposed tendon sheaths on the dorsum of the right hand of a diabetic. The infection, caused by *Mucor* species, developed at a venipuncture site. (Courtesy of Dr. Charles V. Sanders)

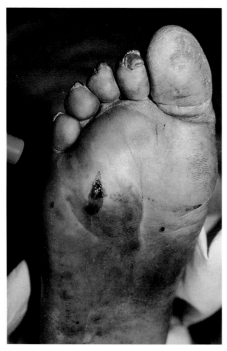

Figure 6.15.   Mixed gangrenous infection. Infection following a puncture wound to the foot of a patient with diabetes. (Courtesy of Dr. Charles V. Sanders)

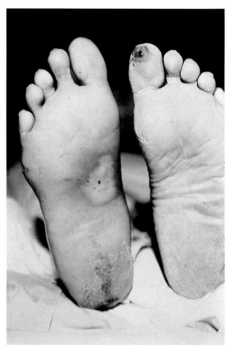

Figure 6.16.   Synergistic necrotizing cellulitis. The lesion led to amputation. Note abscess with surrounding erythema and callous lesion of the left toe. (Courtesy of Dr. Charles V. Sanders)

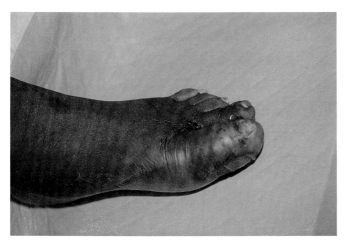

Figure 6.17. Gas-forming cellulitis. Same patient as Figure 6.16, some years later. Gas-forming cellulitis, which began as a callous lesion, led to transmetatarsal amputation. (Courtesy of Dr. Charles V. Sanders)

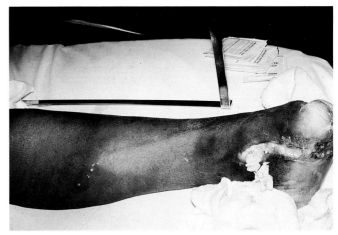

Figure 6.18. Abscess. Note prominence of the superficial vein due to a mixed aerobic/anaerobic infection. *Bacteroides fragiles* was cultured from the blood. (Courtesy of Dr. Charles V. Sanders)

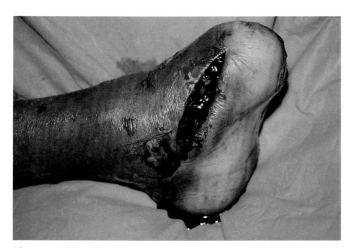

Figure 6.19. Synergistic necrotizing cellulitis. In a patient after transmetatarsal amputation. (Courtesy of Dr. Charles V. Sanders)

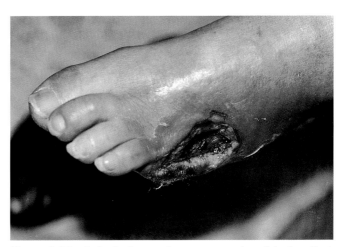

Figure 6.20. Infected vascular gangrene. In a diabetic patient. (Courtesy of Dr. Keith Van Meter)

CHAPTER 7

Skin Signs of Infectious Zoonoses

JOY D. JESTER

The infectious zoonoses are generally defined as bacterial or spirochetal infections acquired through contact with animals or animal products. The source of infection may be obvious, as in an animal bite, or indirect, such as introduction of rat feces-contaminated water into an open abrasion. Better hygiene and more careful handling of food and other organic materials have reduced the incidence of many of these diseases, but have not eradicated them.

Anthrax

Most cases of anthrax today are reported from endemic areas in Western Asia (especially Iran, Afghanistan, and Turkey) and West Africa. Currently, in the United States the infection is rare, despite the fact that the bacillus is endemic in the soil of some areas of Louisiana, Oklahoma, and Colorado. Industrial cases comprise 80% of all reports in the United States, involving such sources as goat hair, wool, cashmere, and bones. Agricultural cases in endemic areas result from direct contact with dying livestock or ingestion of infected meat. Rare arthropod-borne cases are described, and one case of mother-to-infant transmission has been reported (1).

• PATHOGENESIS •

The causative bacteria is *Bacillus anthracis*, a Gram-positive encapsulated rod that sporulates. The bacteria produces two exotoxins, lethal factor and edema factor, both of which are dependent on a third protein, protective factor, for biologic activity. The protective factor, additionally, is effective alone as an anthrax vaccine.

Anthrax spores are generally introduced through minor abrasions of the skin. The organisms grow and reproduce rapidly, releasing toxins that create marked tissue edema and necrosis. In the more unusual cases of intestinal, inhalation, or oropharyngeal anthrax, the spores are phagocytized by macrophages and carried to local lymph nodes. Bacteremia may follow with intravascular multiplication of organisms.

• CLINICAL FEATURES •

More than 95% of cases are cutaneous, with incubation periods of 1 to 3 days following inoculation. In the common and relatively innocuous "dry" form, an elevated hemorrhagic area quickly turns into a necrotic eschar (Figs. 7.1, 7.2). The edematous "malignant" form initially presents as a painless papule that rapidly enlarges and vesiculates, developing a wide surrounding zone of brawny, gelatinous, nonpitting edema (Fig. 7.3). Malaise and low-grade fever accompany the lesion. Bacteremia with high fever and hypotension may follow. Lesions of anthrax are most commonly seen on the face, hands, and arms. Multiple lesions may occur, and many heal without scarring. Initially, the lesions may be pruritic.

Noncutaneous forms of anthrax tend to have marked systemic symptoms and are commonly fatal. These include intestinal anthrax secondary to ingestion of infected meat, inhalational anthrax, and oropharyngeal anthrax.

• DIAGNOSIS AND DIFFERENTIAL DIAGNOSIS •

The differential diagnosis of cutaneous anthrax includes orf, staphylococcal pyoderma, tularemia, and plague. The bacteria is reliably cultured from blister fluid of edematous lesions. Gram's stains of edematous lesions usually show many large Gram-positive rods, but the characteristic "box car" appearance is seen only in culture. It may be difficult to identify the organisms in crusted, necrotic lesions. Biopsies of lesions show marked subcutaneous edema with a diffuse neutrophilic cellulitis. Single organisms may be seen in tissue. Direct immunofluorescence and EIA (enzyme immunoassay) may also be used to diagnose the infection.

• TREATMENT AND CLINICAL COURSE •

Cutaneous lesions of anthrax should not be incised or debrided, as bacteremia can result. The treatment of choice is parenteral penicillin; tetracycline is an alternative in the penicillin-allergic patient. Rare cases of penicillin-resistant anthrax are reported (2). About 20% of untreated cutaneous cases are fatal, but fatalities are rare after antibiotic treatment.

Immunization against anthrax is useful in occupations at risk. Animals may also be vaccinated. Proper care of animal carcasses and steam sterilization of wool helps prevent infection.

Tularemia

The bacteria, *Francisella tularensis*, is prevalent throughout the Northern hemisphere, except in the United Kingdom. It has been identified in about 100 species of wild animals, several domestic animals, birds, amphibians, and fish. The organism has also been found in ticks, deer flies, mosquitoes, and mud from streams and wells. In the United States, the reservoir is predominantly rabbits, hares, ticks, and muskrats.

Fewer than 200 cases a year are reported in the United States, mostly in Arkansas, Missouri, Oklahoma, Texas, Utah, and Tennessee. Adult males have generally accounted for about 75% of cases, but more children are being seen with the rise in tick-bite-associated disease.

• PATHOGENESIS •

Francisella tularensis is a small Gram-negative coccobacillus that is extremely virulent. As few as 10 organisms can initiate an infection. The bacteria most likely enters through breaks in the skin or the mucosa, although it reportedly can also penetrate intact skin. It is highly resistant to desiccation and can also be transmitted by fomites. Contact with tissues or body fluid of an infected animal or an arthropod bite are the usual modes of contracting the disease. Less often, bites of animals such as cats, squirrels, or coyotes are responsible, or the bacteria is ingested. Bacteremia is common, and the bacilli become entrapped in the reticuloendothelial system where they survive within cells indefinitely.

• CLINICAL FEATURES •

The onset of disease is abrupt in most patients, with sudden development of fever, chills, malaise, and fatigue. Ulceroglandular disease accounts for 75% to 85% of all cases, displaying ulcerated skin lesions and lymphadenopathy (Figs. 7.4–7.7). Rarely, lymphangitis or a sporotrichosis pattern may occur. The fingers and hands are the site of skin lesions in more than 90% of cases. Lesions of tick-borne disease are seen more commonly on lower extremities, the perineum, or on the heads of children.

The glandular type accounts for 5% to 10% of cases, consisting of fever and tender lymphadenopathy with no ulcer. Typhoidal disease comprises 5% to 10% of cases, involving fever, prostration, and weight loss. Oculoglandular disease occurs in 1% to 2%, marked by unilateral, painful, purulent conjunctivitis with preauricular and cervical lymphadenopathy (Fig. 7.8). Sometimes periorbital edema or small nodules or ulcerations of the conjunctivae may be seen. Pneumonia is seen in 30% to 50% of typhoidal and 10% to 15% of ulceroglandular cases.

Aside from the ulceroglandular lesions, other cutaneous manifestations appear from 3 days to several weeks after the onset of disease. Rashes are described as macular, maculopapular, papulovesicular, or pustular. The papulovesicular rash is pruritic, occurs on arms and legs, and tends to resolve by the end of the second week. Erythema nodosum occurs later and is often associated with pulmonary disease. The lesions appear on arms and legs, may be few or numerous, and usually resolve in 2 weeks. Lesions of erythema multiforme tend to be large (3 to 4 cm) and favor the upper back, shoulders, and proximal extremities. Several cases of concomitant erythema nodosum and erythema multiforme have been reported (3). Acne-like eruptions, urticarial eruptions, and leukocytoclastic vasculitis have also been seen.

• DIAGNOSIS AND DIFFERENTIAL DIAGNOSIS •

The ulcerative skin lesions of tularemia are not distinctive. Included in the differential are staphylococcal and streptococcal infections, plague, cat-scratch disease, anthrax, lymphogranuloma venereum, *Pasteurella* infection, and sporotrichosis.

Biopsies of early lesions show necrosis surrounded by neutrophils and macrophages. Collections of epithelioid cells with lymphocytes appear, but with late lesions possibly exhibiting caseating granulomas.

Gram's stains of skin and sputum are rarely positive, and cultures of routine media are usually negative, as the bacteria grows poorly. On a cysteine-containing media, the organism forms smooth colonies with pleomorphic Gram-negative coccobacilli. Most cases are diagnosed serologically with either a 4-fold rise in agglutination titer, or a single convalescent titer of at least 1:160. Serology is negative in the first week of infection with 50% to 70% converting after 2 weeks and maximum titers at 4 to 8 weeks. Titers may remain elevated for many years.

• TREATMENT AND CLINICAL COURSE •

Intramuscular streptomycin is the drug of choice, but intramuscular or intravenous gentamicin is also used. Treatment with tetracycline or chloramphenicol commonly results in relapses, especially when given for less than 14 days. With treatment, mortality is less than 1%. Immunity is usually lifelong. A vaccine is available.

Rat-Bite Fever

Rat-bite fever is a febrile illness that is usually acquired by direct contact with infected rodents. The disease is seen worldwide, and the typical organism and clinical features may differ by locale. Most cases in the United States are caused by *Streptobacillus moniliformis*, whereas infections with *Spirillum minor* are primarily seen in Asia. "Haverhill fever" is an epidemic form of disease secondary to ingestion of products, such as raw milk, that are contaminated with *Streptobacillus moniliformis*.

Streptobacillus moniliformis can be found in the oropharynx of at least 50% of healthy wild and laboratory rats. It can also be found in mice, turkeys, and guinea pigs. *Spirillum minor* is found in about 25% of rats. Certain foods, such as raw milk and ice cream, presumably contain *Streptobacillus moniliformis* secondary to rodent contamination. *Streptobacillus* disease incidence is highest in urban areas with poor sanitation and in laboratories with rats and mice.

• PATHOGENESIS •

Streptobacillus moniliformis is a nonmotile, pleomorphic, Gram-negative aerobe (Fig. 7.9). L-forms have been isolated in human and rat blood; these cell-wall-deficient variants are resistant to penicillin. *Spirillum minor* is a spirochete that is Gram-negative and tightly curled with polar flagella.

Infection is usually initiated from a bite or scratch of a rodent, but some cases involve only close contact with cats, dogs, pigs, squirrels, or dead rats. Cases with no clear history of exposure may represent ingestion of contaminated food.

• CLINICAL FEATURES •

The onset of disease with *Streptobacillus moniliformis* is abrupt and usually occurs within 10 days (commonly 2 to 3 days) of rodent exposure. High fever and chills are followed by headache, vomiting, myalgia, and marked muscle tenderness. The white blood cell count may range from normal to as high as 30,000/mm^3, and a coagulopathy with thrombocytopenia may develop. About 25% of patients have a false-positive VDRL. Within 2 to 4 days after the onset of symptoms, 90% of patients develop a rash and 50% of patients develop joint symptoms. By then, the wound is usually healed without lymphangitis. The eruption is usually generalized, often involving the palms and soles (Figs. 7.10, 7.11). It may be morbilliform, pustular, or petechial. Desquamation occurs in 20% of cases during resolution. Arthralgias are common, often with full-blown arthritis and effusions. All symptoms tend to resolve within 2 weeks, but, in the absence of treatment, a relapsing course may be seen at irregular intervals over a period of weeks to months. Other systemic disease complications, such as endocarditis, pneumonia, pericarditis, and abscess formation are described. Weight loss and diarrhea are common in children and chorioamnionitis may be seen in pregnant women.

"Haverhill fever" has similar features, commonly presenting with fever, rash, joint complaints, chills, and vomiting. A rash is seen in over 90% of cases, usually within 3 days of disease onset. The eruption may present as flat red papules, pustules, blotchy macules, or vesicles. It is commonly seen on anterior and lateral extremities, occasionally on palms and soles, and it may generalize. The rash may appear as other symptoms abate and may desquamate on resolution.

Infection with *Spirillum minor* also begins abruptly, but the incubation is longer at 1 to 4 weeks. Myalgias are less frequent and arthritis is rare. The bite may initially heal but later ulcerate into a chancre-like lesion with prominent lymphangitis and lym-

phadenopathy. Chills, fever, and photophobia are commonly seen. A rash, either generalized or localized to extremities, is present in about half the cases, consisting of large, reddish-brown macules. Roseolar or urticaria-like eruptions are also described. The eruption may spread centrifugally from the area of the bite. The white blood cell count is variably elevated and half of the patients have a false-positive VDRL. Fever disappears in a few days but may recur in a relapsing fashion for 1 or 2 months, and, occasionally, for years.

• DIAGNOSIS AND DIFFERENTIAL DIAGNOSIS •

If there is no history of rat exposure, the diagnosis is often made by culture or Gram's stain of blood, joint fluid, or abscess material. In cases involving *Streptobacillus moniliformis*, the bacteria grows on standard media, but enrichment with horse serum is optimum. Inhibition of growth is reported with media containing sodium polyanethol sulfonate (4).

Spirillum minor cannot be cultured and is identified via dark-field examination of clinical material or animal inoculation. Agglutination antibodies to *Streptobacillus moniliformis* develop within 10 days of initial disease. A titer of ≥1:80 is diagnostic.

• TREATMENT AND CLINICAL COURSE •

Untreated cases of *S. moniliformis* have a 10% mortality rate, usually secondary to endocarditis or pneumonia; 6.5% of untreated *Spirillum minor* infections are fatal. Both organisms are sensitive to penicillin with the exception of L-forms, which respond to tetracycline. Patients appear well within a week of treatment, but antibiotics should be continued for at least 10 to 14 days.

Plague

The plague bacillus, *Yersinia pestis*, entered the United States around the turn of the century. Historically, cases were concentrated in port cities and associated with rats. Now, about 20 cases a year are reported with greater than half in New Mexico and others in Arizona, Colorado, Utah, or California. Cases commonly involve exposure to sciuroid rodents, such as chipmunks, ground and rock squirrels, and prairie dogs carrying infected fleas. North American Indians in the endemic area account for 30% of cases. Today, plague is most common in the Far East, India, Africa, and South and Central America.

• PATHOGENESIS •

During feeding, an infected flea vector regurgitates a large number of organisms into the host. Bacilli are readily phagocytized by leukocytes but not destroyed. The inflammatory response to bacterial antigens may produce the lymph node changes of bubonic plague, the "bubo" (Fig. 7.12). Septicemic plague is a nonlocalized form of disease that occurs when the inflammatory response within lymph nodes is minimal. Transient bacteremia is common in bubonic plague, however, and may also lead to hypotension and disseminated intravascular coagulation. Inhalation of encapsulated bacteria from infected humans causes primary pneumonic plague, a rapidly progressive form that caused epidemics in the past but is rare today.

• CLINICAL FEATURES •

The incubation period is 2 to 7 days in the bubonic or septicemic forms of plague and 2 to 3 days in primary pneumonic plague. About 90% of cases are of the bubonic form with fever and painful lymphadenopathy, with or without overlying erythema and edema. Malaise, nausea, vomiting, and diarrhea may be seen. About 10% to 15% of cases are septicemic and present as an acute febrile illness without adenopathy; within a few days, signs of sepsis may develop. In primary pneumonic plague, pneumonia develops within 27 hours of onset, often accompanied by meningitis and disseminated intravascular coagulation (DIC). The disease is often fatal by day 2 or 3.

Bacteremic patients may also present with a variety of skin lesions: erythematous macules, petechial or purpuric lesions, vesicles, pustules, ecthyma gangrenosum-like lesions, and even massive cutaneous edema. "Plague carbuncles" are described as similar in appearance to anthrax (Fig. 7.13). Gangrenous skin lesions of the digits are especially common in septicemic disease and are the source of the term "The Black Death."

• DIAGNOSIS AND DIFFERENTIAL DIAGNOSIS •

The diagnosis is often made with Gram's stains of aspirations of buboes; two-thirds of cases show Gram-negative rods. Skin pustules may also have positive Gram's stains. Giemsa-stained peripheral blood smears show bipolar staining rods in 10% to 40% of septicemic cases. A fluorescent antibody can also be used on clinical tissue. Cultures grow somewhat slowly and should be held a minimum of 72 hours. About 80% of patients with bubonic disease have positive blood cultures.

• TREATMENT AND CLINICAL COURSE •

Chemoprophylaxis is mandatory for all people exposed to patients with plague pneumonia and for all household contacts of flea-borne cases. Contacts are usually treated with tetracycline or sulfonamides. Patients with bubonic disease respond to a variety of antibiotics, including streptomycin and other aminoglycosides, tetracycline, chloramphenicol, and sulfonamides. Strict isolation should be enforced for 48 hours. Overall mortality in untreated cases is 50% to 60%, but, in the United States, early treatment has lowered the mortality rate to about 10%.

Melioidosis

Human melioidosis is caused by the motile Gram-negative bacillus *Pseudomonas pseudomallei*, which is endemic in Southeast Asia but also occurs sporadically elsewhere. Most United States cases have been Vietnam veterans who acquired the infection overseas. About 1% of healthy, nonwounded veterans had significant hemagglutination titers on returning to the United States. Elevated titers were even more likely after injury, occurring, for example, in up to 32% of burn patients (5).

• PATHOGENESIS •

Most cases are thought to occur secondary to contaminations of skin abrasions, but contraction by inhalation also occurs and probably explains the increased incidence in veterans who worked with helicopter landings. No arthropod-mediated transmission has been reported.

• CLINICAL FEATURES •

Clinically, there are subacute, acute, and chronic forms. Many cases are probably subacute local skin infections that resolve spontaneously in 1 to several weeks. Acute localized suppurative infections present as a nodule or eschar-like lesion with acute local lymphangitis and fever. This form may progress rapidly to the acute septicemic form. Acute pulmonary infection is very common, occurring as a primary disease or secondary to bacteremia. It varies from mild bronchitis to severe, necrotizing pneumonia. Acute septicemic disease can occur in normal hosts, but narcotic addiction, diabetes mellitus, systemic steroids, and chemotherapy are predisposing factors. The onset is usually abrupt with pneumonitis, disorientation, headache, pharyngitis, diarrhea, and, commonly, pustular skin lesions scattered over the head, trunk, and extremities. Usually, the course is rapidly progressive. Rarely, chronic suppurative disease is limited to the skin and lymph nodes, with chronic abscess and sinus formation. More often, the lung is involved, and the striking cavitation of upper lungs mimics tuberculosis. Recrudescent melioidosis can be seen as a septicemic or pulmonary form years after the patient has resided in endemic areas. It is precipitated by burns, chemotherapy, or severe injuries.

• DIAGNOSIS AND DIFFERENTIAL DIAGNOSIS •

The diagnosis should be considered in any person who has been in an endemic area who presents with fulminant pulmonic disease, widespread pustular or necrotic skin lesions, or an X-ray-like tuberculosis with no recoverable tubercle bacilli. Wright's stain of exudate from lung, joint fluid, or skin abscess may reveal poorly staining Gram-negative bacilli with a bipolar staining pattern. The organism grows on most ordinary media within 24 to 48 hours. Hemagglutination, agglutination, and complement fixation may also be helpful.

• TREATMENT AND CLINICAL COURSE •

Patients with active infection will probably require prolonged therapy, especially those with extrapulmonary suppurative lesions. A variety of drugs (tetracycline, chloramphenicol, kanamycin, ceftazidime, sulfadiazine) have been successful, but combinations often are best. The organism is resistant to penicillin and streptomycin. Drainage of abscesses should supplement antibiotics.

Before the advent of antibiotics, mortality of apparent infection was said to be 95%. Even with antibiotics, the mortality rate in septicemic patients is at least 50%, but other forms have a much better prognosis.

Glanders

Glanders is an ancient disease of equine animals caused by *Pseudomonas mallei*, which, occasionally, is transmitted to man. The disease is rare worldwide but is endemic in horses of Asia and South America.

• PATHOGENESIS •

Human disease probably results from inoculation of skin abrasions or nasal mucosa with contaminated discharges. Inhalation is probably another mode of transmission and likely accounts for many cases in laboratory workers.

• CLINICAL FEATURES •

Clinical manifestations of the disease are quite variable and depend on the route of infection. Inoculation of skin results in a nodule, with lymphangitis within 5 days. The area of cellulitis may break down to form chronic, irregular ulcers with a purulent hemorrhagic discharge, lymphadenopathy, and sinus development. Infection of mucous membranes produces a mucopurulent discharge of eyes, nose, or lips that may develop into extensive ulcerating granulomas. Destruction of the septum or palate can occur. Localized disease may give rise to septicemia, which often is associated with a generalized papular, pustular, or bullous eruption. Infection by inhalation after an incubation period of 10 to 14 days results in chills, myalgia, headaches, photophobia, and pleuritic chest pain. Acute pulmonary disease resembles bronchopneumonia or multiple lung abscesses.

• DIAGNOSIS AND DIFFERENTIAL DIAGNOSIS •

The organism can be cultured on most meat infusion media. Blood cultures are usually negative except in terminal cases. Gram's stains of exudate may reveal scanty small Gram-negative bacteria. Agglutination titers rise rapidly and are ≥1:640 by the second week, but patients without apparent infection have had titers up to 1:320. Other diagnoses in the differential include pyoderma and, especially, sporotrichosis.

• TREATMENT AND CLINICAL COURSE •

Sulfadiazine is the treatment of choice and probably should be given for 3 weeks. Penicillin is ineffective. Isolation is recommended, as human-to-human transmission does occur. Surgical drainage is usually necessary. Septicemic forms are uniformly fatal within 7 to 10 days, but localized and chronic forms have a better prognosis.

Brucellosis

Brucellosis occurs worldwide secondary to occupational exposure or ingestion of contaminated dairy products. While 500,000 cases are reported each year, the World Health Organization estimates the real incidence to be much greater. In the United States, the number of cases has fallen from 6,000 to fewer than 200 annually. Brucellosis is seen in all 50 states, but most cases are reported from Texas, California, Iowa, and Virginia, mostly among meat processing workers, farmers, dairymen, veterinarians, and laboratory workers. Ingestion of goat cheese has also been implicated (6).

• PATHOGENESIS •

Different strains of *Brucella* produce varying patterns of human disease. *Brucella abortus* produces self-resolving granulomas, *B. suis* indolent abscesses, and *B. melitensis* some abscesses but also systemic toxic reactions. *Brucella* bacteria tend to persist in the cells of the reticuloendothelial system, giving rise to chronic and relapsing disease. The intracellular bacteria are protected from the lethal effects of serum and antibiotics. Cell-mediated immunity appears to play a large role in host resistance as evidenced by the increased prevalence of the disease in patients with lymphoma.

• CLINICAL FEATURES •

Human brucellosis can be categorized as subclinical, acute/subacute, relapsing, or chronic. Asymptomatic or subclinical disease is diagnosed by serology and may occur at up to 12 times the frequency of clinically apparent infection. Acute brucellosis has an incubation period of weeks to months. It may be a mild, transient illness or an explosive, toxic one, particularly if *B. melitensis* is the agent. Chills, fever, malaise, and weakness may appear suddenly or gradually, but few localizing physical signs occur. Relapsing brucellosis presents by symptoms similar to, although often more severe than, the acute disease. Some patients with chronic disease may present with localized disease such as epididymo-orchitis. But about 85% of patients are relatively asymptomatic and complaints tend to be nonspecific.

The skin is involved in about 10% of cases in a variety of ways. Cutaneous lesions occur predominantly with acute or relapsing disease and tend to resolve quickly with treatment. Disseminated violaceous-erythematous papulonodular eruptions of the trunk and extremities may coincide with positive blood cultures, especially *B. melitensis*. Biopsies show focal granuloma and sometimes necrosis. Erythema nodosum-like lesions are thought to represent an immune reaction, as the histopathologic changes (granulomas and necrosis) are similar to those seen with *Brucella* vaccine. Other eruptions are described as roseola-like, papular urticarial, scarlatiniform, malar lupus-like, psoriasiform, erysipelas-like, eczematous, pityriasis rosea-like, or edematous. Disseminated abscesses are seen, as well as vasculitis.

Contact dermatitis, "erythema brucellum," occurs in veterinarians after delivery of infected calves. A rapid onset of pruritus is followed by contact urticaria, then eczematous and vesicular eruptions of the forearms. Indolent ulcers can occur with bacteria inoculated at the time of injury; this is seen most commonly with accidental self-inoculation of vaccine.

Different strains of bacteria are associated with different patterns of disease. *Brucella abortus* tends to produce noncaseating granulomas but often is a mild, self-limited disease rarely associated with chronic suppurative or disabling complications. *Brucella suis* (endemic in the midwestern United States) produces destructive suppurative lesions. *Brucella melitensis* causes severe acute disease and tends to be more disabling; it is also the strain most commonly associated with nonspecific secondary skin findings. *Brucella canis* often results in insidious, mild disease and accounts for many pediatric cases.

• DIAGNOSIS AND DIFFERENTIAL DIAGNOSIS •

Because of special culture requirements (such as 10% CO_2) and the slow growth of the organism (greater than 7 days), the Gram-negative coccobacillus of *Brucella* is only cultured out in about 15% to 20% of cases. However, in acute disease, particularly with *B. melitensis*, up to 85% of blood cultures may be positive. Bone marrow cultures may be helpful as well. Usually, the diagnosis is made with standard tube agglutination of ≥1:160 or a 4-fold rise in titer. Titers may persist, and special tests for immunoglobulin G (IgG) alone are more specific for acute disease. Radioimmunoassay and enzyme-linked immunosorbent assays may be more sensitive.

• TREATMENT AND CLINICAL COURSE •

Tetracycline has been used for years but has significant relapse rates and is less successful in children. Prolonged therapy as well as drug combinations can reduce relapses. Streptomycin, gentamycin, trimethoprim-sulfamethoxazole, and rifampin may all be helpful. Vaccination is effective in animals.

Pasteurella Multocida Infection

The *Pasteurella* species are predominantly animal pathogens. Most human infections are secondary to bites, scratches, or exposure to animals. *Pasteurella multocida* ("killer of many [species]") is seen worldwide and can be identified in the nasopharynx or gastrointestinal tract of numerous domestic and wild mammals and birds. It is a rapidly lethal infection in some animals. *Pasteurella haemolytica* is primarily seen in cattle, sheep, goats, and fowl. *Pasteurella pneumotropica* is another less frequent isolate from dogs and cats.

• PATHOGENESIS •

Up to 17% of all persons reporting to hospitals for animal bites or scratches develop *P. multocida* infection. Virulence is closely related to encapsulation. Cytotoxins, endotoxins, and enzymes such as hyaluronidase may correlate with virulence and types of clinical lesions.

• CLINICAL FEATURES •

Within a few hours to several days the patient experiences acute erythema, pain, and swelling (Figs. 7.14–7.16). Serosanguineous drainage, regional lymphadenopathy, and low-grade fever may occur. Local complications of osteomyelitis, tenosynovitis, and arthritis occur predominantly on the hands. Rarely, small children with bites on the head have developed brain abscesses.

In patients with no history of bites, *Pasteurella* infection is expressed as airway disease (60%), intraabdominal disease (17%), and central nervous system infections or soft tissue infections of the extremities. Chronic lung disease and cirrhosis may be predisposing factors.

• DIAGNOSIS AND DIFFERENTIAL DIAGNOSIS •

Pasteurellae are nonsporeforming, bipolar-staining, Gram-negative coccobacilli that grow on ordinary media. Gram's stains of sputum, pus, or cerebrospinal fluid (CSF) may demonstrate the organism.

Pasteurella should be suspected in any patient who develops acute cellulitis less than 24 hours after a bite or scratch. When the incubation period is longer, the differential includes staphylococcal and streptococcal infections, tularemia, cat-scratch disease, and bubonic plague.

• TREATMENT AND CLINICAL COURSE •

Penicillin is considered the drug of choice. In the rare case of resistance, tetracycline, chloramphenicol, and fluoroquinolones are alternatives. Oral first- and second-generation cephalosporins are only effective intravenously. The prognosis is excellent except in patients with underlying illness, such as cirrhosis or malignancy.

Erysipeloid

Infection with *Erysipelothrix rhusiopathiae*, also known as "erysipeloid of Rosenbach," is an occupational risk for fish handlers, fishermen, meat and poultry workers, butchers, and veterinarians. The organism can be detected in numerous fish, birds, and domestic and wild mammals.

• PATHOGENESIS •

Most human infections are acquired through minor skin wounds during the handling of infected organic material, producing marked inflammation with epidermal edema, necrosis, and exocytosis. Rarely, the organism enters the blood stream to cause systemic infection.

• CLINICAL FEATURES •

Following an incubation period of 1 to 4 days, the inoculation site slowly becomes dusky-violaceous, edematous, hot, painful, or pruritic (Fig. 7.17). The eruption spreads peripherally, usually within 10 cm, with central clearing and, occasionally, with vesicles (Figs. 7.18, 7.19). Lymphadenitis, lymphangitis, and fever can sometimes be seen. The lesions tend not to suppurate or become umbilicated, and usually resolve spontaneously in about 2 weeks. Septicemia can occur in patients with predisposing illness and is often associated with endocarditis. The erysipeloid skin lesion may have healed before the endocarditis is apparent. Rarely, a diffuse cutaneous form occurs, which may resemble a gyrate erythema. It is self-limited and is not associated with bacteremia. The eruption progresses proximally from the inoculation site with central clearing and an advancing pink border.

• DIAGNOSIS AND DIFFERENTIAL DIAGNOSIS •

The differential diagnosis includes streptococcal and staphylococcal cellulitis, anthrax, and erythema multiforme. In a lesion that vesiculates, herpetic whitlow could be considered. The diagnosis is usually made with the clinical appearance and exposure history, or with a culture of the lesion.

• TREATMENT AND CLINICAL COURSE •

Penicillin is the drug of choice, but erythromycin, tetracycline, and cephalosporins are also effective. No vaccine is available.

Listeriosis

Listeria monocytogenes is a ubiquitous bacterium found in soil, water, sewage, almost all animals, and many asymptomatic humans. Some symptomatic human cases involve contact with animals, but contaminated food is the usual presumed source. The bacteria survives refrigeration, desiccation, and fairly high salinity. Epidemics of listeriosis are described in pregnant women and neonates. Other adult cases tend to occur in persons with gastrointestinal disease or immunosuppression, although it is uncommon in patients with AIDS.

• PATHOGENESIS •

The organism can invade the eye and skin after direct exposure, but most cases probably originate from gastrointestinal sources. Patients with decreased gastric acidity or intestinal disease seem especially vulnerable. Cellular-mediated immunity is important in resistance, but immune globulins and complement may also play a role. The bacteria survive and multiply in macrophages, enterocytes, and hepatocytes, which accounts for the common carrier status.

• CLINICAL FEATURES •

Clinical findings are variable. A transient, carrier state with little or no symptoms is the most common. Infections during pregnancy occur most often in the third trimester with flu-like symptoms of chills, fever, and back pain. Amnionitis, premature labor, and septic abortions may follow.

"Granulomatosis infantiseptica" is the grave illness of neonates who have been infected transplacentally. These infants present with pneumonia, septicemia, and disseminated abscesses and granulomas of the placenta, internal organs, and skin. Skin lesions typically appear on the trunk or extremities and are papular, pustular, or ulcerative. Meningitis also occurs late in the neonatal period; these infants tend not to have the skin findings. Fatality rates among neonates are high.

Focal skin infections are particularly common in veterinarians, ranchers, and laboratory workers; vesicular or ulcerative lesions at the inoculation site are the usual findings. Purulent conjunctivitis can also be seen as a localized form of disease.

In immunocompromised patients, sepsis is the usual presentation with or without meningoencephalitis.

• DIAGNOSIS AND DIFFERENTIAL DIAGNOSIS •

The diagnosis is made with culture of blood, CSF, skin lesions, meconium, or conjunctival drainage. Gram's stains may reveal Gram-positive rods. Other laboratory tests are not useful. Because the organism may resemble skin contaminant diphtheroids found in laboratory workers, correlation with clinical symptoms in such personnel should arouse suspicion of listeriosis. The differential diagnosis includes other septicemias presenting with scattered lesions.

• TREATMENT AND CLINICAL COURSE •

Ampicillin and penicillin are most effective and are sometimes used in combination with gentamycin. Tetracycline, erythromycin, and chloramphenicol are alternatives. Early treatment in pregnant women is imperative because their treatment greatly impacts neonatal mortality, which ranges from 33% to 100% in untreated neonates. In immunocompromised adults, the mortality rate is about 12% to 43%.

Leptospirosis

Infections with the spirochete, *Leptospira interrogans*, are seen primarily in wild and domestic animals. Humans are occasionally infected through contact with infected animals or urine-contaminated soil or water. The disease was once thought to be primarily an occupational risk in laborers such as sewer workers, but many recent patients have no obvious risk factors. Worldwide, rats are the usual source; in the United States, dogs and livestock also are common sources.

• PATHOGENESIS •

The spirochetes penetrate intact mucosal membranes or skin abrasions, enter the bloodstream, and are carried rapidly throughout the body, including the central nervous system and eye. These normally sheltered sites may be breached with the help of hyaluronidase or the burrowing motility of the spirochete. Leptospires may cause tubular damage in the kidney secondary to hypoxemia or a toxic effect, but most of the later symptoms of the disease are the result of circulating immune complexes and vasculitis.

• CLINICAL FEATURES •

Subclinical infection is common in meat processing workers and veterinarians. Among symptomatic patients, 90% have the milder, anicteric form of disease and 5% to 10% have the severe form with jaundice known as "Weil's disease" (Fig. 7.20). Often the disease follows a biphasic pattern. Following an incubation period of 7 to 12 days, the "septicemic" phase presents with nonspecific flu-like symptoms. At this time, leptospires can be detected from the blood and CSF. After about a week, there is defervescence, and the second "immune" stage begins, lasting a month or longer. At this stage, leptospires can be detected only in the urine, kidney, and aqueous humor, but there is circulating antibody and a variety of symptoms, including meningitis with severe headache, uveitis, photophobia, rash, and, in Weil's disease, hepatic and renal involvement.

The rash is highly variable. A blotchy to slightly raised rash of the pretibial area is said to be characteristic, but also described are truncal rashes that are macular, maculopapular, erythematous, patchy, urticarial, or hemorrhagic. The rash may persist for several days or only a few hours. Alopecia also may occur.

• DIAGNOSIS AND DIFFERENTIAL DIAGNOSIS •

The diagnosis of leptospirosis is usually made with serologic tests, such as slide agglutination tests or ELISA (enzyme-linked immunoadsorbent assay). Agglutinins appear on day 6 to 12 and peak at the 3rd to 4th week. False-negatives can occur if the causative leptospire is an unusual serotype not in the testing material. Leptospires can be seen with dark-field examination of tissue, but the number of organisms is small. Special culture media are required for culture.

Leptospirosis is often not recognized during the septicemic phase because the symptoms are flu-like and fever resolves within a week or less. The immune stage may be characterized only by aseptic meningitis, which may be misdiagnosed as viral meningitis. Ocular findings such as conjunctival infection and hemorrhage are common, however, and may help make the diagnosis. The severe form of leptospirosis, Weil's disease, may be confused with septicemia accompanied by disseminated intravascular coagulation; the presence of ocular findings and rash, or a history of animal exposure and biphasic illness, may suggest leptospirosis.

• TREATMENT AND CLINICAL COURSE •

Tetracyclines are probably the drug of choice; doxycycline in particular has been useful as a prophylactic and therapeutic agent. Penicillins may not eliminate the leptospires from the kidneys but have been used. Antibiotics work best when administered within the first 3 days of infection. Steroids are of no benefit in the immune phase.

Cat-Scratch Disease

Cat-scratch disease (CSD) is a self-limited bacterial disease typically presenting with chronic regional lymphadenopathy fol-
lowing contact with a kitten. The etiologic agent remained elusive for years. Earlier studies documented *Afipia felis* in a number of patients, but recent serologic studies and polymerase chain reaction analysis have confirmed that *Rochalimaea henselae* is usually responsible.

About 22,000 cases of CSD are reported annually in the United States and over 2,000 of these patients are hospitalized. Cases peak in the fall and winter; the seasonality corresponds with breeding patterns of cats, since CSD is usually transmitted by kittens who remain infectious for about 2 weeks. Rarely, dogs are reported to transmit the disease—as are some sharp objects, such as thorns and bones. *Rochalimaea henselae* has also been identified in fleas from the cats of some CSD patients. About 80% of cats have antibodies to the organism but no evidence of disease.

• CLINICAL FEATURES •

About 3 to 10 days following inoculation a papule or pustule develops at the site. Within 2 to 3 days it may crust or ulcerate and usually heals without scarring within days to weeks. Approximately 1 to 6 weeks after the primary lesion is seen, regional lymphadenopathy and the inoculation lesion may have resolved. The lymphadenopathy may be multiple but generally consists of a single enlarged node (1 to 5 cm), which is initially tender and suppurates uncommonly (Fig. 7.21). The adenopathy usually subsides within 2 to 4 months but may persist for up to a year. Because the hand or forearm are common inoculation sites, axillary nodes are usually involved, but cervical, submandibular, or preauricular lymphadenopathy can also occur, depending on the site of the primary lesion.

About one-third of patients experience concomitant low-grade fever and malaise. Less common findings include headache, anorexia, nausea, vomiting, and splenomegaly.

About 5% of cases exhibit a variety of rashes, including erythema nodosum, erythema multiforme, erythema annulare, urticaria, or maculopapular and petechial eruptions. These eruptions are thought to be an immunologic response to infection and may be associated with peripheral eosinophilia.

Parinaud's oculoglandular syndrome, which also has been used to describe oculoglandular tularemia, is seen in 2% to 17% of cases. It consists of granulomas of the conjunctivae or lid with preauricular lymphadenopathy. Another uncommon manifestation is encephalopathy that starts with headaches and progresses to altered mental status, delirium, seizures, and neurologic deficits. Diffuse neurologic deficits are most common and are reversible; focal deficits are rarer but are more likely to have long-term sequelae. Hepatitis, pneumonia, osteolytic lesions, and thrombocytopenia have also been described.

• DIAGNOSIS AND DIFFERENTIAL DIAGNOSIS •

Diagnosis is usually made with the combination of clinical lymphadenopathy and a history of inoculation. Biopsies of lymph nodes may be helpful. Early involved lymph nodes demonstrate reticulum cell hyperplasia and stellate necrotic granulomas, sometimes with giant cells. Multiple microabscesses may coalesce to form large suppurative foci. These findings are similar to those of tuberculosis and tularemia owing to delayed-type hypersensitivity. Bacteria may be seen within blood vessel walls, in macrophages, and in microabscesses. Rarely are organisms seen within extensive areas of necrosis, and the number of bacteria decline with time. Two forms of bacteria occur at different sites of the disease. The vegetative form is found only at the inoculum site. A cell-wall-deficient form is found in the lymph nodes; this form is extremely difficult to culture and is so small that only stains such as Warthin-Starry render it visible by light microscopy.

The skin test is fairly specific (79% to 100%) and very sensitive, with greater than 95% of affected patients demonstrating a positive reaction. False negatives can occur if the test is given in the first 1 to 2 weeks before an antibody response has occurred, if the antigen is not pooled, and if the patient is immunosuppressed. Asymptomatic family members of affected individuals and veterinarians commonly have positive tests. Recently, serology to *R. henselae* has been shown to be at least 85% sensitive and 94% specific.

The differential diagnosis includes bacterial adenitis, infectious mononucleosis and other viral disorders, tuberculosis, rat-bite fever, lymphogranuloma venereum, sarcoidosis, lymphoma, and histocytosis. In the oculoglandular syndrome of Parinaud, tularemia differs from CSD by its characteristic pain, tenderness, and purulence.

• TREATMENT AND CLINICAL COURSE •

Antibiotics have been relatively ineffective in treating routine CSD. However, in atypical cases with systemic disease, various antibiotics, especially gentamicin, have been helpful. In cases of suppurative nodes, aspiration is recommended rather than incision to avoid fistula formation. In general, the usual patient with CSD can be expected to recover spontaneously with minimal sequelae within about 2 months.

REFERENCES

1. Sekhar P, et al. Outbreak of human anthrax in Ramabhadrapuram village of Chittoor district in Andhra Pradesh. Indian J Med Res 1990;(A)91:448.
2. Bradaric N, Punda-Polic V. Cutaneous anthrax due to penicillin-resistant *Bacillus anthracis* transmitted by an insect bite. Lancet 1992;340:306.
3. Syrjalla H, Karronen J, Salminen A. Skin manifestations of tularemia: A study of 88 cases in northern Finland during 16 years, 1967–1983. Acta Derm Venereol 1984;64:513.
4. Holroyd KJ, Reiner AP, Dick JD. *Streptobacillus moniliformis* polyarthritis mimicking rheumatoid arthritis: An urban case of rat bite fever. Am J Med 1988;85:711.
5. Mandell GL, Douglas RG, Bennett JE. Principles and practice of infectious diseases. 2nd ed. New York: Churchill Livingston, 1985:125.
6. Taylor JP, Perdue JN. The changing epidemiology of human brucellosis in Texas, 1977–1986. Am J Epidemiol 1989;130(1):160.

ANNOTATED BIBLIOGRAPHY

The following texts and review articles offer good summaries of the zoonoses:

Anthrax

Dutz W, Kohout-Dutz E. Anthrax. Int J Dermatol 1981;20:203.

Brucellosis

Young EJ. Human Brucellosis. Rev Infect Dis 1983;5(5):821.

Cat-Scratch Disease

Shinall E. Cat-scratch disease: A review of the literature. Pediatr Dermatol 1990;7(1):11.

Erysipelothrix

Mandell GL, Douglas RG, Bennett JE. Principles and practice of infectious diseases. 3rd ed. New York: Churchill Livingstone, 1990.

Leptospirosis

Domm BM. Human leptospirosis. Medicine 1960;39:117.

Listeriosis

Kluge RM. Listeria–problems and therapeutic options. J Antimicrob Chemother 1990;25:887.

Melioidosis and Glanders

Howe C, Sampath A, Spotaitz M. The pseudomallei group. J Infect Dis 1971;124(6):598.

Pasteurella

Tindall JP, Harrison CM. *Pasteurella multocida* infections following animal injuries, especially cat bites. Arch Dermatol 1972;105:412.

Plague

Craven RB, Barnes AM. Plague and tularemia. Infect Dis Clin North Am 1991;5(1):165.

Rat-Bite Fever

McHugh TP, Bartlett RL, Raymond JI. Rat-bite fever: Report of a fatal case. Ann Emerg Med 1985;14(11):1116.

Tularemia

Evans ME, Gregory DW, Schaffner W, McGee ZA. Tularemia: A 30-year experience with 88 cases. Medicine 1985;64(4):251.

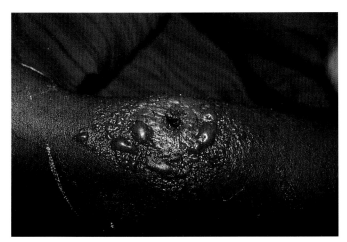

Figure 7.1. **Anthrax.** Edematous lesion of the arm with central eschar, surrounding edema, and vesicle formation.

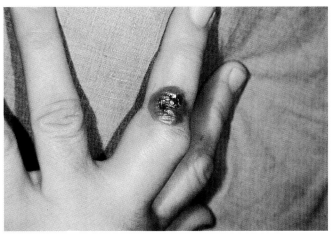

Figure 7.2. **Anthrax.** Lesion with central eschar on the finger of a wool worker.

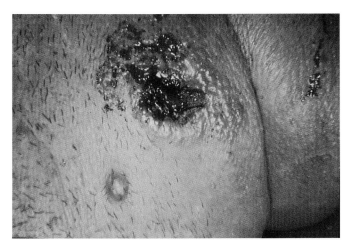

Figure 7.3. **Anthrax.** Malignant pustule with eschar.

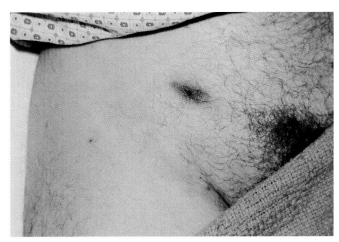

Figure 7.4. **Tularemia.** Primary inoculation site showing ulcerated erythematous nodule. (Courtesy of Dr. Charles Stratton)

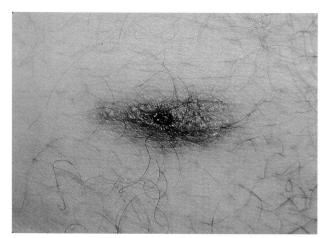

Figure 7.5.   Tularemia. Erythematous nodule with hemorrhagic necrotic center, close-up view. (Courtesy of Dr. Charles Stratton)

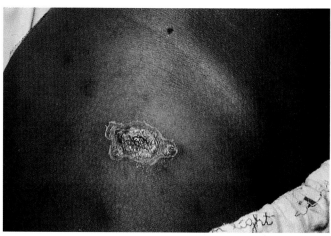

Figure 7.6.   Tularemia. Primary inoculation site, showing ulcerated nodule with associated lymphadenopathy. (Courtesy of Dr. Charles V. Sanders)

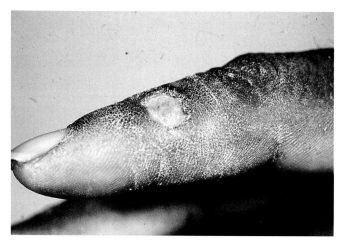

Figure 7.7.   Tularemia. Ulcerative lesion of the finger. Patient had associated lymphadenopathy. (Courtesy of Dr. Barbara Hanna)

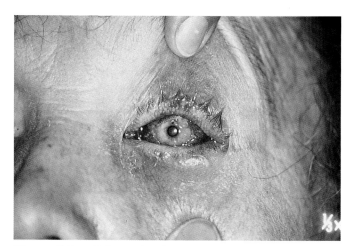

Figure 7.8.   Tularemia. Oculoglandular tick-borne form with severe conjunctival and periorbital edema. (From Guerrant RL. Arch Intern Med 1976;136:811.)

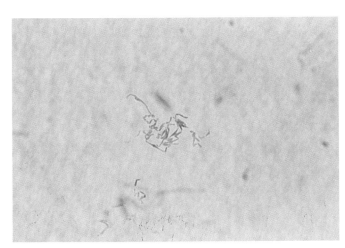

Figure 7.9. Rat-bite fever, streptobacillary form. *Streptobacillus moniliformis* in tissue.

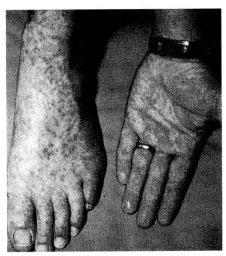

Figure 7.10. Rat-bite fever. Multiple petechial lesions on the palm and dorsum of the foot. (From Cole JS, Stoll RW, Bulger RJ. Ann Intern Med 1969;71:979.)

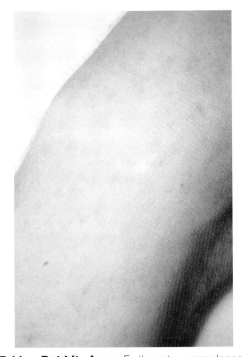

Figure 7.11. Rat-bite fever. Erythematous maculopapular eruption on the antecubital area.

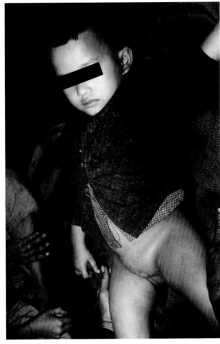

Figure 7.12. Plague. Bubo of inguinal area.

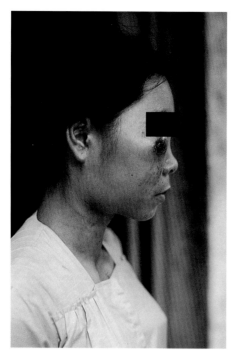

Figure 7.13.   Plague. Edematous nodular lesion below the eye with overlying eschar, typical of "plague carbuncle."

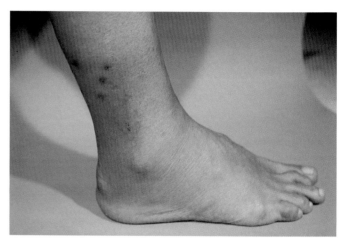

Figure 7.14.   *Pasteurella multocida* infection. Puncture wound with surrounding cellulitis of the lower leg following cat bites. (Courtesy of Dr. Charles V. Sanders)

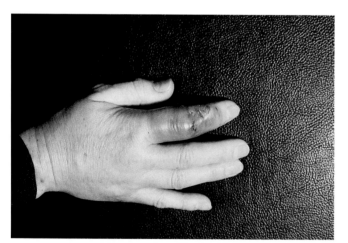

Figure 7.15.   *Pasteurella multocida* infection. Infection following a cat bite, showing erythematous induration of the index finger. (Courtesy of Dr. Charles V. Sanders)

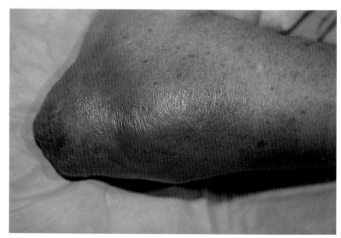

Figure 7.16.   *Pasteurella multocida* infection. Erythematous induration of the arm surrounding a lesion of gout on the elbow. (Courtesy of Dr. Charles V. Saunders)

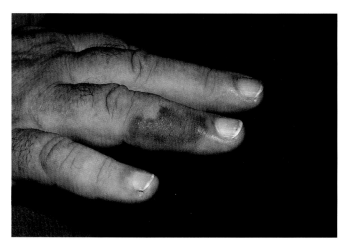

Figure 7.17. Erysipeloid. Violaceous maculopapular lesions of the fingers that developed after cleaning fish. (Courtesy of Dr. Lee T. Nesbitt, Jr.)

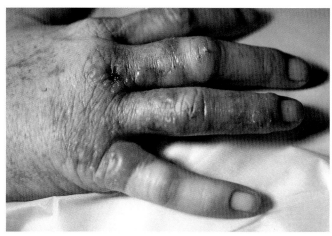

Figure 7.18. Erysipeloid. Erythematous induration and bulla formation on the dorsum of the hand and fingers. (From Park CH. South Med J 1976;69:1101.)

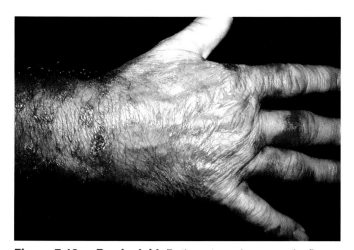

Figure 7.19. Erysipeloid. Erythematous plaques on the fingers and wrist. (From Barnett JH. J Am Acad Dermatol 1983;9:116).

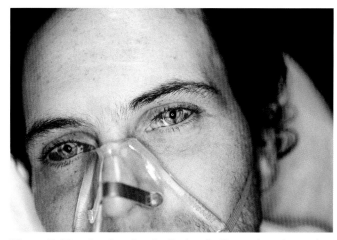

Figure 7.20. Leptospirosis. Conjunctival hemorrhage in a patient with Weil's disease, the most severe form. (Courtesy of Dr. Gene Beyt)

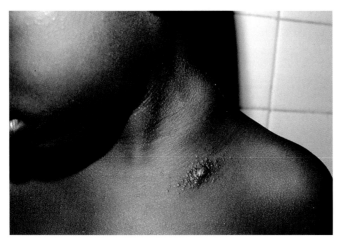

Figure 7.21.   Cat-scratch disease. Cervical lymphadenopathy
with primary inoculation lesion.

CHAPTER **8**

Sexually Transmitted Diseases

DAVID H. MARTIN and TOMASZ F. MROCZKOWSKI

Skin lesions can be produced by almost all traditional vene-real diseases, such as syphilis and gonorrhea, and by many "new" sexually transmitted diseases (STDs), including AIDS. In some STDs, skin lesions are the only signs of disease; in others, skin signs occur only as the result of disseminated infection or a local complication.

This chapter is organized into three sections: sexually transmitted diseases producing genital ulcerations, diseases primarily involving the genitourinary tract, and other sexually transmitted diseases.

Sexually Transmitted Diseases Producing Genital Ulcerations

SYPHILIS

• PATHOGENESIS •

Syphilis is a chronic disease caused by the spirochete *Treponema pallidum*. It is most commonly contracted through intimate skin-to-skin contact, usually sexual intercourse. However, accidental infections through contact with infected materials have also been reported. The disease can be transmitted transplacentally and also by blood transfusion (extremely rare in recent times). Biologically, the disease evolves through three distinct clinical stages—primary, secondary, and tertiary. These stages, however, frequently overlap each other and clinical manifestations can be extremely variable.

• CLINICAL FEATURES •

Primary Syphilis

Treponema pallidum is probably capable of penetrating an intact mucosa but may depend on a small cut or abrasion to invade the skin. The incubation period varies from 9 to 90 days, usually about 3 weeks. The primary lesion, the first physical manifestation of syphilis infection, appears at the site of inoculation as a small papule that quickly erodes and ulcerates. This ulcer, also called the "primary chancre," classically is described

as painless, rounded or oval, with a clean granular base (Table 8.1). The typical primary chancre is usually single and has well-defined raised and smooth borders often surrounded by a dull red areole (Fig. 8.1). On palpation, the base of the ulcer is button-like and hard, and, when squeezed, does not change its shape. Prolonged pressure on the lesion produces serous exudate that contains spirochetes. If not treated, the chancre of primary syphilis will heal within a few weeks, leaving no trace or a faint atrophic scar.

In men, the primary chancre occurs most commonly on the penis with the coronal sulcus, glans penis, and the inner surface of the prepuce most frequently affected. Homosexual men are more likely to have primary lesions around the anal margin, on the skin of the perineum, and in the oral cavity. In women, the most common sites are the labia minora but primary chancres may also appear on the labia majora, the fourchette, the clitoris, the cervix, the urethra, and less often on the perineum (Fig. 8.2). Primary syphilis in women is less conspicuous than in men, especially if the primary chancre is located in the cervix or on the vaginal wall. Women, therefore, are less likely to seek medical attention during the primary stage of the disease.

Exceptions to the typical clinical features of primary chancre are common. In fact, about half of primary chancres may present atypically. Primary syphilis in men can sometimes present as balanoposthitis (Follman's balanitis), phimosis or para-

---

Table 8.1. Characteristics of Primary Chancre[a]

- Usually single (multiple lesions less common)
- Most commonly on genitalia
- Indolent, persists for several weeks before healing
- Usually regular in shape: round or oval
- Painless, unless secondarily infected
- Slightly raised, well-defined, smooth borders
- Clean, hard, indurated, and finely granular base
- Shape unchanged when squeezed; serous discharge produced
- Heals without scar or a faint atrophic scar
- Associated with firm but painless and nontender regional lymphadenopathy

[a]Fewer than half of primary chancres are atypical.

phimosis with various degrees of swelling of the glans and the prepuce. In alcoholics or patients with impaired immune systems, primary chancre can be deep and large. Some patients may have multiple, very small chancres resembling the superficial erosions caused by genital herpes. Secondarily infected, the primary chancre can be painful and may have undermined or ragged edges and a necrotic base covered with pus or bloody discharge. About 5% of primary chancres are extragenital in site. They have been found in or on the oral cavity, tonsils, skin of the chin, eyelids, fingers, nipple, and umbilicus.

Regional lymphadenopathy follows the appearance of the primary chancre. Since over 90% of primary chancres appear on the genitalia or anogenital region, inguinal adenopathy, either unilateral or bilateral, is most common. On palpation, the nodes appear firm and rubbery, separated from one another, movable (not fixed to surrounding tissue), and nontender. They do not suppurate.

Secondary Syphilis

About 6 to 8 weeks after the primary stage begins, the first symptoms and signs of the secondary stage appear. In up to 30% of cases, the primary chancre is still present. While patients with primary syphilis rarely have systemic complaints, patients with secondary syphilis may complain of flu-like symptoms. Generalized lymphadenopathy frequently develops with lymph nodes that are characteristically discrete, nontender, firm and rubbery, and palpable for several weeks. An occasional patient also develops hepatosplenomegaly.

Although at this stage *T. pallidum* can be found in any organ of the body, the most prominent clinical feature of secondary syphilis is the skin rash. About 80% of patients have lesions of the skin or mucocutaneous junctions, and about 33% have lesions in the mouth or throat. The skin lesions of secondary syphilis resemble a wide array of common skin conditions, hence the label "the great imitator." Nonetheless, certain features of secondary syphilis are characteristic (Table 8.2).

The macular or roseolar rash (roseola syphilitica) is usually the first eruption to appear, occurring initially on the internal aspects of the trunk and later spreading over the chest, abdomen, and shoulders. The limbs, especially the flexor surfaces, are frequently affected. Whether the rash is localized to the trunk or generalized, the palms, soles, and face are usually spared except for perioral lesions. The lesions, which may be sparsely distributed, are often so delicate that they are invisible in artificial light. They last from a few hours to a few days,

occasionally developing into the papular rash. In dark-skinned persons the roseolar rash may leave a slight postinflammatory hyperpigmentation resembling pityriasis versicolor, which lasts only a few days. Rarely, after macular exanthema disappears, a patchy depigmented area can be observed.

Papular or maculopapular eruptions are the most common and most characteristic cutaneous expressions of secondary syphilis (Figs. 8.3, 8.4). In contrast to the early macular lesions, the papular lesions are generally fewer in number, larger, and often darker, dusky-red to brown. The lesions may be widely distributed over the trunk, arms, legs, palms, soles, perineum, and face. Papules that develop along the hairline may resemble a crown and are called "corona veneris." The lesions may be isolated or grouped, forming annular or arcuate lesions. Arcuate lesions are more common in black patients and have rolled, raised borders and centers that are darker than the edges. They occur most frequently on the face, anogenital areas, palms, and soles. Annular lesions frequently resemble coins, and are sometimes referred to as "nickel and dime" lesions. Papular rashes of secondary syphilis frequently resemble other skin diseases and have been described as psoriasiform, lichenoid, pityriasic, etc.

Papular or maculopapular lesions on the palms and soles are very characteristic of secondary syphilis (Figs. 8.5, 8.6). The papules remain flat or only slightly raised because of the tough, horny nature of the overlying epithelium. Since few other dermatologic conditions occur in this distribution, such lesions always suggest the diagnosis of secondary syphilis.

Pustular rash in secondary syphilis is seen in fewer than 2% of all cases (Fig. 8.7). Occasionally, a papular rash is accompanied by pustular lesions, most commonly on the face and scalp. A generalized pustular rash is usually associated with immunodeficiency (e.g., in HIV-positive patients) as is the occasional nodular rash.

Where skin surfaces are opposed, papules may become macerated. These moist papules may become eroded or fissured or may become elevated and condylomatous. Condylomata lata, or "broad condylomata," are hypertrophic, broad-based, exuberant papules with flat (in contrast to condylomata acuminata) moist tops, dull red to grayish in color. The surface slough is shed, leaving an eroded surface that oozes a thick mucoid secretion packed with spirochetes. Condylomata lata may remain as separate lesions or may form round, fleshy masses. Typically, these lesions appear on the labia in women (Fig. 8.8), around the anus and between the buttocks in men and women, and on the lateral surfaces of the scrotum in men. They also have been found on the inner thigh, in the groin, and around the mouth, but rarely in other parts of the body. They are considered the most infectious lesions of secondary syphilis.

Mucous membrane lesions occur in about one-third of cases of secondary syphilis. The most typical lesions are the so-called "mucous patches" that appear in conjunction with the papular skin rash. They can be found on the inner part of the lips, buccal surfaces, tongue, fauces, tonsils, and in the pharynx and larynx. The typical mucous patch is sharply marginated, flat or slightly raised, faintly inflammatory, and covered with a white or gray-

---

Table 8.2. General Characteristics of Skin Eruption in Secondary Syphilis

- Usually bilateral, symmetrical, and nonpruritic
- Macular, papular, papulosquamous, or rarely pustular
- More heavily distributed on flexural surfaces
- Predilection for palms and soles, near mucosal surfaces
- Different types of lesions may be seen at the same time (polymorphism)
- May persist for months untreated or be inconspicuous and transient
- Can be recurrent

ish membrane (Fig. 8.9). On the soft palate and fauces the lesions may be grouped into an elongated ulceration, the so-called "snail track ulcer." Lesions on the tongue lack papillae, and those in the nose and larynx occasionally give rise to a husky voice. Lesions may also appear on the mucous membranes of the genitals, most commonly the vulva, glans of the penis, and inner side of the prepuce. Mucous membrane lesions are usually painless unless secondarily infected. They are highly infectious and are more likely than skin lesions to recur during relapse.

Less common manifestations of secondary syphilis include syphilitic alopecia and syphilitic leukoderma. They occur later in the course, usually after 6 months. The hair loss in syphilis is usually patchy, producing a characteristic "moth-eaten" appearance, especially on the sides and back of the head (Fig. 8.10). Rarely, diffuse thinning of the scalp hair occurs. Syphilitic alopecia may also affect the eyebrows, eyelashes, beard, and occasionally, body hair. As the rash resolves, patchy areas of hypopigmentation may persist on the neck for a variable period of time. This condition, known as leukoderma colli, or "collar of Venus," is seen mainly in dark-complexioned female patients.

Untreated, the rash of secondary syphilis fades but may recur (relapsing secondary syphilis), sometimes several times within a year of initial infection. The lesions in this stage are usually asymmetrically distributed and fewer in number. "Corymbose syphilid," a common form of this rash, appears as one or a few groups of papules with a large central papule surrounded by many smaller papules resembling satellite lesions. It occurs most frequently on the back, shoulders, abdomen, and extensor surfaces of the arms.

Tertiary Syphilis

The first manifestations of tertiary (late) syphilis may appear as early as 3 years and as late as 15 years after the primary stage. Adequate treatment of the earlier stages of disease usually prevents development of late syphilis, which had become relatively rare until the advent of the AIDS epidemic.

Although lesions of tertiary syphilis may appear anywhere in the body, the most common forms are mucocutaneous, osseous, cardiovascular, neural, and visceral. These forms may occur separately or in combination.

The two major types of mucocutaneous lesions of tertiary syphilis, nodular or nodulo-ulcerative (Fig. 8.11) and gummas, may appear separately or may coexist. The nodular or nodulo-ulcerative lesions appear no earlier than 5 to 10 years after infection. The lesions are small, painless nodules that develop gradually and regress even more slowly. They are dull red in color, and, unlike skin lesions in secondary syphilis, they are localized and asymmetrical. They tend to be arranged in groups as rings, semicircles, or horseshoe shapes (Fig. 8.12) usually on the face, extremities, and scapular or interscapular areas. Most lesions are indurated, deeply rooted in the dermis, and involve the whole thickness of the skin. Over the course of several months some nodules heal while new ones appear, usually at the periphery of the original group, resulting in a circular or serpiginous appearance that is pathognomonic for this stage of the disease. Healing may result in residual hyperpigmentation and/or formation of a scar.

The gumma is a granulomatous lesion of tertiary syphilis that usually occurs as a single lesion. It may be restricted to the skin or originate in the subcutaneous tissue and secondarily involve the skin. The individual lesion begins as a painless nodule, often at a point of trauma. Gradually, the subcutaneous nodule grows, becomes attached to the overlying skin, and then breaks down to form a deep, punched-out ulcer that discharges gummy material. The ulcer may extend peripherally or may heal slowly and spontaneously. Gummas have a predilection for the skin over the sternum, the sternoclavicular joints, the legs below the knees, the face, and the scalp. Gummas of the mucous membranes most often involve the mouth, tongue, and soft and hard palates. Involvement of the posterior pharynx may result in deformity and/or destruction of the soft palate and uvula. The hard palate may perforate as a result of gummatous infiltration of the roof of the mouth or the floor of the nose. Destruction of the nasal septum leads to a characteristic deformity of the nose, and gummas in the larynx may cause a permanent voice change.

Congenital Syphilis

Congenital syphilis is transmitted from the infected mother to the fetus through the hematogenous route, resulting in clinical manifestations which, with the exception of bullous eruption, may resemble acquired secondary syphilis in adults. The clinical manifestations of congenital syphilis are categorized as early congenital syphilis, late congenital syphilis, and stigmata.

Early congenital syphilis becomes manifest before 2 years of age. Infants may be born with full-blown disease or may appear normal at birth, developing typical lesions in 2 to 3 weeks. The characteristic vesicular or bullous eruptions, sometimes referred to as "syphilitic pemphigus," consist of groups of vesicles or bullae distributed symmetrically on the palms, soles, and occasionally other body parts. The fluid in the bullae may be hemorrhagic or contain serous or seropurulent fluid swarming with spirochetes. Treatment may be futile for the seriously ill infants with these clinical signs.

Other skin manifestations resemble those of acquired syphilis, with a few characteristics typical for congenital syphilis. The rashes are usually widespread and symmetrical with predilection for the face, the napkin area, and the palms and soles. Hypertrophic papules may develop at mucocutaneous junctions (condylomata lata), dehydration and weight loss may produce facial wrinkling, and the skin may be yellowish-brown, or tinted "cafe au lait." Patchy hair loss may even involve the eyebrows and eyelashes. Nails may be loose or absent and new nail growth may be abnormal.

Mucous membranes most frequently involved are the nose, mouth, throat, and larynx. A purulent discharge (syphilitic rhinitis) blocking the nose may signify destructive changes in the nasal supporting tissue, leading to perforation of the nasal septum. Mucous patches in the larynx may cause aphonia or a thin or hoarse cry or cough. Anal and perioral lesions may become fissured and produce permanent radiating scars (rhagades). For information on late manifestations of congenital syphilis and stigmata, which usually involve organs other than skin or mucous membranes, the reader is referred to the bibliography.

• DIAGNOSIS AND DIFFERENTIAL DIAGNOSIS •

The diagnosis of syphilis depends on a combination of clinical observation, epidemiologic investigation, and laboratory testing. Dark-field microscopy is required to demonstrate *T. pallidum* in exudates from lesions and is the definitive diagnostic test. Unfortunately, few clinical laboratories have the skill necessary to perform this study satisfactorily. Therefore, the diagnosis is most often supported by positive syphilis serologic tests. These are divided into two groups: the relatively nonspecific cardiolipin or reagent tests (VDRL, RPR, etc.) or the specific treponemal tests (FTA-ABS, MHA-TP, etc). Extensive discussions of syphilis diagnosis have been published elsewhere (see Annotated Bibliography).

The differential diagnosis of primary syphilis depends on the site of the primary chancre. A primary chancre on the genitalia should be distinguished from genital herpes, chancroid, lymphogranuloma venereum, donovanosis, scabies, Behçet's syndrome, balanitis/balanoposthitis, squamous cell carcinoma, and traumatic lesions (Table 8.3). A primary chancre on the lips should be distinguished from herpes labialis, squamous cell carcinoma, aphthous ulcer, and angular cheilitis. A primary chancre on the finger may be mistaken for herpetic whitlow, paronychia, traumatic ulcer, and anthrax pustule. In the anorectal region, differential diagnosis includes anal fissure, anal wart, squamous cell carcinoma, hemorrhoids, and Bowen's disease.

The macular rash of secondary syphilis must be distinguished from measles, rubella, tinea versicolor, drug reaction, seborrheic dermatitis, mononucleosis, erythema multiforme, and typhoid fever. The papular secondary syphilis rash may be confused with pityriasis rosea, lichen planus, psoriasis, and parapsoriasis. Annular lesions may mimic erythema multiforme, ringworm, granuloma annulare, and annular lichen planus. The pustular rash resembles acne, rosacea, chicken pox, and drug eruptions due to bromides or iodides. Palmar lesions can be mistaken for pustular psoriasis, dyshidrosis, erythema multiforme, and contact dermatitis, while plantar lesions resemble tinea pedis, dyshidrosis, pustular psoriasis, and keratoderma blennorrhagica.

Condylomata lata can be mistaken for hemorrhoids, genital warts, and squamous cell carcinoma. Alopecia syphilitica resembles alopecia areata, traumatic alopecia, and ringworm of the scalp.

Mucous membrane lesions can be mistaken for aphthous ulcers, viral exanthems, strep throat, lichen planus, Steven-Johnson syndrome, leukoplakia, herpes simplex, and balanitis/balanoposthitis caused by yeasts or bacteria. Nodules and nodulo-ulcerative lesions as well as gummata in tertiary syphilis should be distinguished from cutaneous tuberculosis, sarcoidosis, leprosy, granuloma annulare, lupus erythematosus, erythema nodosum, erythema induratum, nodular vasculitis, basal cell carcinoma, and squamous cell carcinoma.

• TREATMENT AND CLINICAL COURSE •

Penicillin remains the drug of choice in the treatment of syphilis. Acquired early syphilis (primary, secondary, and latent syphilis) of less than 1 year's duration should be treated with benzathine penicillin G, 2.4 million units IM, given as a single dose or 2 doses 1 week apart. Syphilis of more than 1 year's duration (except neurosyphilis) should be treated with benzathine penicillin G, 2.4 million units IM once a week for 3 consecutive weeks for a total dose of 7.2 million units. Neurosyphilis can be treated successfully with this regimen as well, but most experts now recommend high-dose parenteral aqueous penicillin G or procaine penicillin G for 10 days.

Those allergic to penicillin should be treated with doxycycline 100 mg twice daily, or tetracycline 500 mg 4 times daily for 2 weeks in early syphilis and for 1 month in late disease. Penicillin-allergic pregnant women should be desensitized and treated with penicillin as above. Patients who cannot tolerate tetracycline may be given erythromycin 500 mg 4 times daily for the same duration as for the tetracyclines. For more detailed information on treatment see the CDCP's (Centers for Disease Control and Prevention) STD Treatment Guidelines published in the Morbidity and Mortality Weekly Report (see bibliography).

CHANCROID

• PATHOGENESIS •

Chancroid, like syphilis, is a sexually transmitted disease producing genital ulcerations. It is caused by the Gram-negative bacillus *Haemophilus ducreyi*. Chancroid is often endemic in developing countries, but, within the last 10 to 20 years, outbreaks have been observed in Europe, Canada, and the United States. The incidence of clinical disease is disproportionately low in women; however, as a group, female prostitutes have been frequently found to be important reservoirs of infection. Uncircumcised men are significantly more likely to become infected than circumcised men.

• CLINICAL FEATURES •

The incubation period is short, usually 3 to 7 days (range of 1 to 35 days), without prodromal symptoms. The typical lesion begins at the site of inoculation as a small, tender, red papule or pustule that rapidly ulcerates. The ulcer is sharply demarcated with a ragged, undermined edge and a grayish, necrotic exudate covering the base. Removal of this exudate reveals an uneven granulation tissue. As opposed to the classic syphilitic chancre, the ulcer edge is soft ("ulcus molle") and will change its shape when squeezed. Multiple ulcers are frequent, and the so-called "kissing" lesions from auto-inoculation of opposing mucous membrane surfaces are common (Fig. 8.13). Multiple ulcers sometimes merge to form one giant ulcer.

The ulcers are usually located in the genitalia at the sites most subject to sexual trauma. In men, they are found on the frenulum, coronal sulcus, internal and external surfaces of the prepuce, the glans penis, and the shaft of the penis. In women, most of the lesions are found at the introitus; however, they may

Table 8.3. Characteristics of Sexually Transmitted Genital Ulcers

	Primary Syphilis	Genital Herpes	Chancroid	Lymphogranuloma Venerum	Donovanosis
Incubation period	9–90 days; avg, 2–4 weeks	2–7 days	Range 1–35 days; avg, 3–7 days	3 days–3 weeks; avg, 10–14 days	Precise data unavailable; probably from a few days to several months
Number of lesions	Usually 1; may be multiple	Multiple; may coalesce; more with primary episodes than with recurrences	Usually 1-3, may be multiple	Usually single	Single or multiple
Description of genital ulcers	Sharply demarcated round or oval ulcer with slightly elevated edges; may be irregular, symetrical ("kissing chancre")	Small, superficial grouped vesicles and/or erosions; lesions may coalesce, forming bullae or large areas of ulceration; lesions have irregular borders	Deep, sharply demarcated ulcer; irregular, ragged, undermined edge; size from a few millimeters to 2 cm in diameter	Papule, pustule, vesicle, or ulcer; discrete and transient; frequently overlooked	Sharply defined, irregular ulcerations or hypertrophic, verrucous, necrotic or cicatrical granulomas
Base	Red, smooth, and shiny or crusted; oozing serous exudate when squeezed	Bright, red, and smooth	Rough, uneven, yellow-to-gray color	Variable	Usually friable, rough, beefy granulations; can be necrotic, verrucous, or cicatrical
Induration	Firm; does not change shape with pressure	None	Soft; changes shape with pressure	None	Firm granulation tissue
Pain	Painless, may become tender if secondarily infected	Common; more prominent with initial infection than recurrences	Common	Variable	Rare
Inguinal lymphadenopathy	Unilateral or bilateral, firm, movable, and nontender; does not suppurate	Usually bilateral, firm, and tender; more common in primary episodes than in recurrences	Unilateral (bilateral rarely occurs); overlying erythema; matted, fixed, and tender; suppuration may occur	Unilateral or bilateral; initially movable, firm, and tender; later indolent; fixed and matted; "sign of Groove" may suppurate; fistulas	Pseudobuboes; subcutaneous perilymphatic granulomatous lesions that produce inguinal swelling
Constitutional symptoms	Rare	Common in primary episode; less likely in recurrences	Rare	Frequent	Rare
Course of untreated disease	Slowly (2–6 weeks) resolves to latency	Recurrence is the rule	May progress to erosive lesions	Local lesions heal; systemic disease may progress; disfiguring; late complications	Worsens slowly
Diagnostic tests	Dark-field exam, direct immuno-fluorescence, FTA-ABS, VDRL	Tzanck smear, culture, Pap smear, direct immunofluorescence, electronmicroscopy, direct immuno-peroxidase staining, serology	Culture, biopsy (rarely used), Gram-stained smears have low specificity	LGV complement fixation test; isolation of the microorganism by culture	"Donovan bodies" in tissue smears; biopsy

also be present on the vaginal wall, the cervix, and in the perineum (Figs. 8.14, 8.15). Extragenital lesions are rare but can occur inside the mouth and on the fingers, breasts, and thighs.

In approximately half the cases, genital chancroidal ulcers are accompanied by inguinal lymphadenitis. The typical bubo of chancroid appears approximately a week after the ulcer and is characteristically unilateral, unilocular, spherical, and painful. The bubo may become fluctuant with spontaneous rupture, often oozing a thick, viscous pus. Following bubo rupture, a large inguinal ulcer may form and enlarge with time (Fig. 8.16). Mild and nonspecific constitutional symptoms only rarely accompany genital lesions.

• DIAGNOSIS AND DIFFERENTIAL DIAGNOSIS •

Although the diagnosis of chancroid often is based on the clinical presentation and/or Gram-stained smears, the demonstration of *H. ducreyi* in culture is recommended. Gram's stain lacks both sensitivity and specificity. Up to 50% of chancroid ulcers may be incorrectly diagnosed in the absence of laboratory confirmation of the etiology. Specimens for cultures are best obtained from the ulcer base, but specially prepared media and specific growth conditions are required to successfully isolate the organism. Since most clinical laboratories are not prepared to work with *H. ducreyi*, the clinician should discuss the best approach to diagnosis with the microbiologist prior to sending specimens to the laboratory. Newer diagnostic methods, including direct immunofluorescence and polymerase chain reactions, are under investigation.

Differential diagnosis includes other STDs causing genital ulceration, such as primary and secondary syphilis, genital herpes, lymphogranuloma venereum, and donovanosis (Table 8.3). Mixed infections, especially with syphilis and herpes, may occur. Other conditions that can be mistaken for chancroid include traumatic ulceration, pyogenic bacterial infections, and squamous cell carcinoma.

• TREATMENT AND CLINICAL COURSE •

The susceptibility of *H. ducreyi* to antimicrobial agents differs geographically, which may influence drug selection. The following are current CDC recommendations for treatment of chancroid in the United States: erythromycin 500 mg p.o. QID for 7 days, ceftriaxone 250 mg IM in a single dose, or azithromycin 1 gm in a single dose. The alternative regimens are ciprofloxacin 500 mg p.o. BID for 3 days or amoxicillin 500 mg plus clavulanic acid 125 mg p.o. TID for 7 days. Trimethoprim-sulfamethoxazole is no longer recommended because of rising resistance rates worldwide.

Local therapy includes topical cleansing and/or soaks and measures to reduce edema. Retraction of the foreskin is not recommended in the presence of preputial edema. Circumcision, if needed, should be postponed until therapy has been effective.

Patients with nonfluctuant buboes respond to antimicrobial therapy. Fluctuant buboes should be drained with a large-gauge needle inserted into the center of the necrotic node from the side of the lesion through normal tissue. Reaspiration may be required periodically.

GENITAL HERPES

• PATHOGENESIS •

Genital herpes is a sexually transmitted disease caused by the herpes simplex virus type 2 (HSV-2) and much less frequently by type 1 (HSV-1). The disease is the most common infection causing genital ulcerations in men and women in the United States. Both viruses produce identical clinical manifestations. However, patients with HSV-2 genital infections are more likely to experience recurrences than patients with HSV-1.

• CLINICAL FEATURES •

Cases are divided into two groups: those with first-episode disease, primary or nonprimary, and those with recurrent disease. Patients with primary, first-episode disease are those never previously exposed to the virus, while those with nonprimary, first-episode disease have been previously infected as demonstrated by the presence of specific antibody at the time of presentation.

The incubation period for primary, first-episode infection ranges from 2 to 12 days. Symptoms may be systemic (chills, fever, nausea, malaise, headache, and generalized myalgias) as well as locally severe. Occasionally, paresthesias at the site of inoculation precede the appearance of skin lesions. As the disease develops, multiple, grouped, small vesicles appear on an erythematous base, which after 3 to 5 days develop into painful shallow ulcers that subsequently crust. During this stage, sacral paresthesia, dysuria, and tender inguinal lymphadenopathy may occur. Local symptoms peak in 8 to 10 days, gradually receding over the 2nd week of illness.

In men, lesions most frequently occur on the prepuce, glans, and shaft of the penis (Fig. 8.17). Herpetic balanitis, balanoposthitis, and urethritis occasionally occur. In women, the first primary episode of genital herpes causes severe vulvovaginitis and edema of the labia with extensive vesiculation and erosions. The lesions usually involve the labia majora, labia minora, cervix, and, less often, the vagina (Fig. 8.18). In general, women seem to have more discomfort than men, which can include dysuria severe enough to result in acute urinary retention.

As a result of anal sex, HSV infection may also affect the anus and perianal area. Herpes simplex proctitis is characterized by systemic symptoms as discussed above plus severe rectal pain, tenesmus, constipation, and anal discharge. Perianal vesicles and ulcers often are absent.

Patients with nonprimary, first-episode or recurrent disease usually do not develop constitutional symptoms. The lesions tend to be unilateral and well-localized and are fewer, smaller, and quicker to heal than primary, first-episode disease with a shorter duration of viral shedding.

In immunocompromised patients, especially those with AIDS, genital herpes can be severe and prolonged, producing extensive and persistent anogenital lesions.

• DIAGNOSIS AND DIFFERENTIAL DIAGNOSIS •

The diagnosis of genital herpes often can be made by clinical characteristics, but viral isolation is necessary for confirmation. Viral isolation rates depend on the type and the age of the lesions. The optimal yield of the virus is from fluid obtained from early vesicles; in older, crusted lesions the yield may be close to zero. Alternatives to viral culture include cytologic diagnosis by Tzanck or Papanicolaou smears (Fig. 8.19), electronmicroscopy, and viral antigen or DNA detection tests. Generally, serological assays are not useful, and commercial assays do not reliably distinguish between past infections with HSV-1, which is prevalent in most populations, and HSV-2. The only utility of a single test for HSV antibodies is to rule out prior herpes infections in patients who are worried about having genital herpes. A negative test is helpful in this regard, but a single positive antibody test is of no significance.

The initial episode of genital herpes should be distinguished from other diseases causing genital vesicles, erosions, or ulcerations (Table 8.3). A history of recurrent vesicular genital lesions is strongly suggestive of genital herpes.

• TREATMENT AND CLINICAL COURSE •

Lesions of this self-limited disease heal unless secondarily infected, which is an uncommon occurrence. The only approved drug for genital herpes is acyclovir, which is available in oral, intravenous, and topical formulations. For first-episode primary genital herpes, acyclovir is recommended 200 mg p.o. 5 times daily for 10 days. A more convenient dosing regimen is 400 mg TID. Suppressive acyclovir therapy, approved for up to 1 year, is recommended for patients with severe and frequent recurrences in a dose of 200 mg 3 times a day.

In immunocompromised patients, including patients infected with HIV, acyclovir is recommended in higher daily doses. For first-episode primary herpes, the dose is 400 mg p.o. 5 times a day for 10 days. For suppressive therapy, the dose is 400 mg p.o. 3 or 4 times daily; however, as is the case with normal patients, the lowest dose necessary to suppress lesion recurrence should be sought by the physician and patient.

LYMPHOGRANULOMA VENEREUM

• PATHOGENESIS •

Lymphogranuloma venereum (LGV) is an uncommon sexually transmitted disease caused by *Chlamydia trachomatis* immunotypes L_1, L_2, and L_3, which are invasive strains that can result in severe inflammatory regional lymphadenitis along with marked systemic symptoms. LGV is most prevalent in tropical and subtropical regions, with only a few hundred cases reported annually in the U.S.

• CLINICAL FEATURES •

The average incubation period after exposure to LGV is 10 to 14 days, but ranges from 3 to 42 days. The primary lesion is usually transient, nonpainful, and, therefore, frequently unno-ticed by the patient. In fact, only 10% of cases present with a primary lesion. The lesion is a small, painless papule or herpetiform ulcer (Fig. 8. 20) usually on the coronal sulcus, prepuce, glans of the penis, and the urethral meatus in men and the vaginal wall, the vulva, and the fourchette in women. The primary lesions may also be located on the cervix or in the cervical canal as well as on the rectal mucosa.

Since the primary lesion in LGV is usually clinically inapparent, the most prominent clinical feature of this disease is enlarged, painful inguinal lymphadenopathy that is unilateral in over two-thirds of cases. Enlargement of nodes above and below the inguinal ligament produce the characteristic "groove sign" in approximately one-third of cases. This finding is said to be pathognomonic for LGV, however, we have seen the groove sign in buboes caused by *H. ducreyi.* The buboes of LGV are often very tender and eventually break down with the formation of multiple draining sinuses (Fig. 8.21). Approximately one-third of inguinal buboes become fluctuant and rupture; the remaining involute and form a hard inguinal mass without suppuration. Constitutional symptoms of fever, chills, malaise, and muscle and joint pain are common. A few patients may demonstrate systemic adenopathy in addition to inguinal lymphadenopathy.

Only 30% of women develop inguinal lymphadenopathy. Instead, most develop pelvic lymphadenopathy as a result of primary infections in the posterior portion of the vagina or in the endocervix. Pelvic pain and proctitis may also occur.

In women and homosexual men who practice passive anal intercourse, the rectal mucosa can be directly inoculated with LGV microorganisms, producing proctitis. Additionally, in women, the rectal mucosa may be involved by vaginal secretion, contamination, or by the spread of infection from the cervix or vagina through the lymphatic channels. Without treatment, proctitis or proctocolitis caused by LGV may lead to perianal abscess, and to rectovaginal, rectovesical, and anal fistulas as well as anal strictures, the latter being associated with rectal cancer.

Chronic lymphatic obstruction and lymphedema of the external genitalia frequently accompanied by draining sinuses are the cause of esthiomene, an ulcerative lesion of the vulva, in women (Fig. 8.22). In men, damage to the lymphatic system may result in obstruction of lymphatic channels, causing penile and/or scrotal edema or distortion of the penis known as "saxophone penis."

• DIAGNOSIS AND DIFFERENTIAL DIAGNOSIS •

The diagnosis of LGV is based on the clinical picture and positive laboratory tests, especially isolation of the organism in cell culture. The best results are achieved if bubo aspirates are cultured. In any case, recovery rates of chlamydia are less than 30%. Cultures of material obtained from several involved sites, such as endocervix, urethral or rectal mucosa, buboes, and primary lesions, may be more likely to produce the organism. When culture is not available, serologic testing that shows a very high antibody titer (specific cut points are not firmly established) in conjunction with appropriate clinical findings and the absence of other diseases supports the diagnosis.

The primary lesion of LGV should be distinguished from genital herpes, primary syphilis, and chancroid as well as traumatic abrasion (Table 8.3). Patients with buboes may appear to have chancroid. The key differentiating point here is that patients with LGV seldom have primary lesions whereas patients with chancroid almost always have prominent genital ulcers in conjunction with their inguinal lymphadenopathy. LGV cases with simple lymphadenopathy may be confused with primary and secondary syphilis, donovanosis, and all non-venereal causes of lymphadenopathy, such as: cat scratch disease, infectious mononucleosis, tuberculosis, tularemia, brucellosis, bubonic plague, lymphoma, or metastatic malignancies.

• TREATMENT AND CLINICAL COURSE •

Tetracycline and its congeners are the most effective treatment for LGV. Doxycycline 100 mg p.o. BID or tetracycline 500 mg tablets QID should be given for 3 weeks. In the case of tetracycline intolerance or allergy, erythromycin 500 mg QID for 3 weeks is recommended.

Fluctuant nodes should be drained by needle aspiration rather than by incision, which may produce chronic lymphocutaneous fistulae. Anatomical changes resulting from chronic infection may warrant reconstructive surgery.

DONOVANOSIS

• PATHOGENESIS •

Donovanosis is a chronic, slowly progressive disease caused by the Gram-negative bacillus *Calymmatobacterium granulomatis*. Synonyms for donovanosis are granuloma inguinale, granuloma venereum, granuloma donovani, chronic venereal sore, and granuloma inguinale tropicum. Donovanosis is very rare in Europe and North America but endemic in certain tropical and subtropical areas. The disease is not highly contagious, and repeated exposure is probably necessary for infection. Although sexual contact is an important mode of transmission, the disease also may be acquired by close, nonsexual physical contact or by autoinoculation from the rectum.

• CLINICAL FEATURES •

The incubation period is estimated to range from a few days to several months. Onset of the disease is insidious and is marked by gradual formation of a firm, painless papule or nodule that ulcerates. Clinical variants of donovanosis are classified by morphologic appearance:

1. Ulcerative or ulcerogranulomatous;
2. Hypertrophic or verrucous;
3. Necrotic;
4. Sclerotic or cicatricial.

The ulcerative or ulcerogranulomatous variant is characterized by the presence of a nontender and nonindurated ulcer with profuse granulation tissue at the base that bleeds readily. The typical lesion has a beefy-red, fleshy appearance. Older ulcers may spread slowly, developing well-demarcated, raised lesions with slightly indurated margins (Figs. 8.23, 8.24).

Hypertrophic or verrucous lesions consist of exuberant granulation tissue with an elevated irregular border and an elevated base (Fig. 8.25). It is drier than the ulcerative form and bleeds easily.

Necrotic lesions are characterized by extensive and rapid destruction of tissue, which with large ulcerations can include the genitalia. They are often painful and are covered with a gray, foul-smelling exudate.

The sclerotic or cicatricial variant, more common in women, results from extensive formation of fibrous tissue and presents as a band-like scar in the affected parts of the genitalia and perineum.

Donovanosis primarily affects the anogenital region with involvement of the inguinal area in about 10% of cases. A true bubo is generally not formed, and the inguinal swelling called a "pseudobubo" is, in fact, a subcutaneous satellite lesion. Homosexual contact often infects the perianal region, and orogenital sex may infect the oral cavity.

Complications are related to the anatomical sites involved. In men, long-lasting donovanosis may destroy the penis. In women, massive elephantiasis-like lesions (pseudoelephantiasis) of the external genitalia may occur. Scarring may cause urethral, vaginal, and anal stenosis. An association between squamous cell carcinoma and donovanosis has been postulated.

• DIAGNOSIS AND DIFFERENTIAL DIAGNOSIS •

The history and clinical appearance is reasonably specific, especially in patients with recent sexual exposure in endemic areas. However, a clinical diagnosis should be confirmed by demonstration of "Donovan bodies" in Giemsa-stained tissue smears and biopsy specimens.

Donovanosis can be misdiagnosed as genital squamous cell carcinoma or other sexually transmitted diseases producing genital lesions (Table 8.3). Other skin diseases, such as cutaneous amebiasis, filariasis, leishmaniasis, cutaneous tuberculosis, and granuloma pyogenicum can be ruled out by biopsy or other appropriate tests.

• TREATMENT AND CLINICAL COURSE •

Donovanosis usually responds to tetracycline or doxycycline. Difficult cases may require the addition of a daily intramuscular dose of an aminoglycoside such as gentamicin. Chloramphenicol may be used in patients intolerant to the above drugs.

Sexually Transmitted Diseases Primarily Affecting the Urogenital Tract

Both *Neisseria gonorrhoeae* and oculogenital serovars of *Chlamydia trachomatis* cause urethritis in men and urethritis and endocervicitis in women. Primary infection of other sites, such as the oropharynx and the anus, are less frequent. Occasionally, both infections may produce skin lesions.

GONORRHEA

• PATHOGENESIS •

The gonococcus has the capability of adhering to urethral and endocervical epithelial cells. The host response to gonococcal antigens as well as secreted extracellular products produces a polymorphonuclear cell inflammatory response. This results in a purulent urethral discharge, the major presenting complaint in men, and an endocervical exudate that may be profuse enough to result in vaginal discharge in women.

• CLINICAL FEATURES •

An example of the typical profuse yellowish discharge produced by the gonococcus is shown in Figure 8.26. Local complications of gonorrhea in men include urethral stricture, periurethral abscess, tysonitis, littritis, cowperitis, and rarely, pyoderma of the penis. A frequent local complication in women is the infection of the Bartholin's gland, causing bartholinitis or Bartholin's gland abscess.

Bartholin's gland abscess produces pain in the vulva accompanied by tenderness, redness, and swelling of the overlying skin in the lower part of the labia majora (Fig. 8.27). A bead of pus may be expressed from the duct opening, or the duct may be blocked by the inflammation.

• DIAGNOSIS AND DIFFERENTIAL DIAGNOSIS •

Diagnosis is confirmed by demonstration of *Neisseria gonorrhoeae* in pus from the abscess and/or from other sites (endocervix, urethra). Rarely, *Chlamydia trachomatis* may be the cause of bartholinitis. Treatment for gonococcal bartholinitis is the same as for uncomplicated gonorrhea, with incision and drainage sometimes necessary in Bartholin's gland abscess.

• TREATMENT AND CLINICAL COURSE •

Current CDC recommendations for the treatment of gonorrhea are ceftriaxone 125 mg IM in a single dose, or cefixime 400 mg, ofloxacin 400 mg, or ciprofloxacin 500 mg p.o. in a single dose. Infections caused by *C. trachomatis* should be treated with doxycycline 100 mg p.o. twice a day for 7 days or azithromycin 1 gm p.o. in a single dose.

DISSEMINATED GONOCOCCAL INFECTION

• PATHOGENESIS •

This syndrome occurs in up to 2% of gonorrhea cases and results from the hematogenous spread of gonococci to various extragenital parts of the body. Disseminated gonococcal infection (DGI) occurs more frequently in women than in men. Menstruation, pregnancy (especially the third trimester), and asymptomatic and pharyngeal infections are important risk factors.

• CLINICAL FEATURES •

The most common form of DGI is the "dermatitis-arthritis" syndrome, the clinical course of which consists of an early bacteremic phase and a septic joint phase. Bacteremic phase symptoms include chills and fever, malaise, and anorexia accompanied by polyarthralgia or polyarthritis in small joints with or without effusion, mainly in the hands, wrists, ankles, and feet. Tendon sheaths may be involved, resulting in tenosynovitis (Fig. 8.28). The skin lesions appear concomitantly with polyarthralgia or polyarthritis, or shortly thereafter. The lesions begin as tiny red macules, papules, or petechiae that either disappear or progress to a pustular stage. With time, many of them develop a hemorrhagic base and a necrotic center (Fig. 8.29). Hemorrhagic bullae have been reported but are uncommon. The rash most often occurs periarticularly over the distal extremities (Fig. 8.30). Lesions are few in number (usually less than 30) and are seen in various stages of development. In the septic joint phase, monoarticular arthritis is present, often in the absence of systemic symptoms. The knees and ankles are affected most frequently.

• DIAGNOSIS AND DIFFERENTIAL DIAGNOSIS •

Diagnosis of DGI is made on clinical grounds, although confirmation by culture is important. Since DGI lesions resemble those seen in endocarditis, it is important to rule out the presence of other organisms. *Neisseria gonorrhoeae* organisms normally cannot be found in skin lesions, but pustules should always be unroofed to obtain pus for Gram's stain and culture. Blood cultures are most often positive early in the course. In contrast, joint fluid cultures usually are not positive until late in the course after the septic arthritis stage has developed. Because of the difficulties in confirming the diagnosis with these specimens, urethral, endocervical, pharyngeal, and rectal specimens also should be obtained when DGI is suspected. It should be kept in mind that DGI is the most common cause of acute asymmetrical arthritis in young, sexually active persons. Patients presenting in this manner should be cultured aggressively before antibiotics are begun in order to facilitate the diagnosis.

DGI should be distinguished from other causes of septic arthritis, endocarditis, acute rheumatoid arthritis, rheumatic fever, and Reiter's syndrome.

• TREATMENT AND CLINICAL COURSE •

Hospitalization and high-dose antibiotic therapy are recommended, particularly ceftriaxone 1 gm IM or IV every 24 hours or ceftizoxime or cefotaxime 1 gm IV every 8 hours for a week. Patients allergic to ß-lactam antibiotics can be treated with spectinomycin 2 gm IM every 12 hours. Reliable patients with uncomplicated disease may be discharged in 24 to 48 hours on oral antibiotics (for a total of 1 week of antibiotic therapy). Amoxicillin 500 mg 3 times daily can be used if the organism is penicillin-sensitive. If an isolate is not available for sensitivity testing, as is often the case, better choices would be cefixime 400 mg, ofloxacin 400 mg, or ciprofloxacin 500 mg, each taken orally twice daily.

CONJUNCTIVITIS

• PATHOGENESIS •

Both gonococci and chlamydiae may infect the eye, usually by passive transmission from the genital tract to the eye, or, more commonly in newborns, by transmission during vaginal delivery. As a result of silver nitrate prophylaxis, gonococcal conjunctivitis in newborns is rare; *Chlamydia trachomatis* is the most common cause of conjunctivitis in the first month of life in the United States.

• CLINICAL FEATURES •

Chlamydial conjunctivitis develops 5 to 14 days after birth and gonococcal conjunctivitis in 2 to 4 days. A watery eye discharge rapidly becomes mucopurulent. The eyelid is swollen and the conjunctiva becomes edematous.

• DIAGNOSIS AND DIFFERENTIAL DIAGNOSIS •

The diagnosis is made by demonstration of gonococci or *C. trachomatis* in the exudate or conjunctival scrapings. Both gonococcal conjunctivitis as well as chlamydial conjunctivitis should be distinguished from the same disease caused by other bacteria or viruses (Herpes simplex virus), allergy, and irritating chemicals.

• TREATMENT AND CLINICAL COURSE •

Gonococcal conjunctivitis can be treated with ceftriaxone 25 to 50 mg/kg IV or IM in a single dose not to exceed 125 mg. Topical therapy alone is inadequate. Chlamydial infection requires oral administration of erythromycin syrup 50 mg/kg/body weight per day in 4 divided doses for 10 to 14 days.

REITER'S SYNDROME

• PATHOGENESIS •

The classic clinical triad of Reiter's syndrome consists of arthritis, conjunctivitis, and urethritis. A variety of organisms infecting mucosal surfaces act as triggering agents of the disease, which is almost always seen in persons with HLA-B27 or closely related genotypes. About half of the cases not initiated by enteric infections are associated with chlamydial urethral infections.

• CLINICAL FEATURES •

Skin and mucous membrane lesions occur in a minority of patients. Penile lesions are found in about 25% of the cases, usually on the glans and/or the inner aspect of the prepuce, and clinically and histologically resemble psoriasis. In uncircumcised men they are rounded, shallow erosions with slightly raised edges, becoming circinate in outline as adjacent lesions coalesce (balanitis circinata) (Fig. 8.31). In circumcised men, the glans penis is dry and the lesions begin as vesicles, later becoming pus-

tules with subsequent formation of keratodermic crusts. Rarely, circinate lesions may appear on the vulva in women.

Keratoderma blennorrhagica, another skin manifestation of Reiter's syndrome, is usually confined to the soles of the feet. Lesions start as dull-red macules and develop into dry, scaly pustules or nodular keratotic patches, which may form limpet-like soft masses of scales. The lesions usually heal within a couple of months, except in severe cases in which they sometimes spread to the limbs, trunk, and scalp and strongly resemble psoriasis.

• DIAGNOSIS AND DIFFERENTIAL DIAGNOSIS •

The diagnosis of Reiter's syndrome is made on clinical grounds, but Gram-negative enteric pathogens should be searched for and urethral chlamydia cultures done. Reiter's syndrome should be distinguished from secondary syphilis, other forms of arthritis (including psoriatic arthritis), pustular psoriasis, dyshidrosis, contact eczema, and tinea pedis.

• TREATMENT AND CLINICAL COURSE •

Treatment of Reiter's syndrome is empirical and directed at reducing arthritis pain, inflammation, and other symptoms. Management of arthritis consists of rest, analgesics, and nonsteroidal antiinflammatory agents. Urethritis caused by chlamydia is best treated with doxycycline 100 mg BID for a week. Conjunctivitis is self-limited and clears up without any local treatment. Skin lesions do not require treatment, although some authors recommend topical steroids.

Other Skin Lesions Produced by Sexually Transmitted Diseases

GENITAL WARTS

• PATHOGENESIS •

Genital warts are caused by the human papillomavirus (HPV). The clinical course of genital warts is not well understood. They may persist, regress, recur, or undergo malignant transformation. The potential for malignant transformation appears to be greatest for papillomavirus types 16, 18, 31, and 35 (Fig. 8.32), especially in the presence of cervical infections (1). The course of the disease appears to be influenced by cell-mediated immunity rather than humoral immunity. While HPV is undoubtedly sexually transmitted, the exact mechanism of infection is not known. The virus remains dormant in the dermal basal layer; active expression occurs as progeny cells differentiate during their migration toward the epithelial surface, where infectious viral particles are released along with the desquamated cells that normally are shed from the skin.

• CLINICAL FEATURES •

The incubation period ranges from 3 weeks to 8 months with an average of 3 months. The clinical features of genital warts range from typical exophytic lesions to clinically unapparent infections, depending on the type of the virus and the location and duration of the lesions. (Nongenital lesions caused by HPV are discussed in Chapter 17.)

Genital warts in men most commonly present as penile condylomata acuminata, usually caused by HPV-6 and HPV-11. These lesions are skin-colored to slightly pink, and may be exophytic, elongated, filiform, or pedunculated. Warts may be solitary or, more often, multiple. They are found most frequently on the margin of the corona of the glans, the frenulum, or the inner side of the prepuce, but can occur anywhere on the penile shaft, scrotum, or glans, or, occasionally, in the urethral meatus. A second common type of wart found in the male genitalia are small, discrete, flat lesions that project slightly above the normal epithelium with a rough, sometimes slightly pigmented surface. These may be the only warts present or they may occur simultaneously with the typical exophytic condylomata acuminata described above.

Subclinical infection of the penis with HPV is common and presents as diffuse foci of epithelial hyperplasia that are macroscopically invisible. These are revealed by application of 5% acetic acid and examination under magnification. Subclinical lesions are of particular importance because of the increased possibility of unwittingly infecting the sex partner.

In women, vulvar condylomata acuminata appear as soft verrucous papules frequently with fine finger-like projections. They are most common at the fourchette, the labia, and the perineum but may affect the adjacent regions as well. Small lesions may coalesce to cover large areas or form "cock's comb-like" excrescences along the labia. The other type of vulvar condylomata are small, fleshy, or pigmented papules with smooth or slightly hyperkeratotic surfaces. In nonmucosal areas, condylomata in women are morphologically similar to those in men.

Approximately one-third of women with vulvar condylomata have vaginal lesions. They may appear as macroscopically identifiable elongated vaginal papillae or, after application of acetic acid, as sharply demarcated white patches or multiple, small, acetowhite spots on the vaginal wall identified during colposcopy (Fig. 8.33).

Cervical lesions should be suspected whenever vulvar or vaginal warts are present. Cervical warts present occasionally as classical exophytic condylomata acuminata, but more commonly as macroscopically invisible lesions recognizable only during colposcopy after the application of acetic acid. These are frequently indistinguishable from cervical intraepithelial neoplasia.

As in men, subclinical HPV infections are very common in women and can be identified by application of 5% acetic acid followed by colposcopic examination. They are usually symptomless but also have been incriminated as a possible cause of vulvodynia.

Anal warts are seen more frequently in homosexual and bisexual men and in women practicing anal sex. The majority of perianal condylomata appear as papillary growths, frequently assuming a cauliflower-like appearance (Fig. 8.34). A small proportion of anal warts are flat, with slight elevations of the epidermal contour. Perianal warts frequently extend into the anal canal; therefore, anoscopy is recommended to determine the extent of infection.

Another form of genital warts, the Buschke-Löwenstein tumor, is a rare giant condyloma that grossly appears cancerlike but histologically is benign. It is distinguished from typical condylomata by its deep tissue penetration and compression of the adjacent tissues. These tumors appear mainly on the penis but may also occur on the scrotum, perineum, and groin in men and on the vulva in females. Buschke-Löwenstein tumors usually contain HPV-6 and HPV-11, the common virus types of classical condylomata acuminata.

Another rare manifestation of genital warts is bowenoid papulosis or genital intraepithelial neoplasia, presumptively caused by HPV-16 and HPV-18. The lesions of bowenoid papulosis usually appear as small, flat multicentric papules often irregular in outline that can coalesce to form one or two larger lesions. They may be translucent or red to brown in color. In men, they occur mostly on the penile shaft, but also the foreskin and the glans penis (Fig. 8.35). In women, the slightly elevated or papillomatous lesions (Fig. 8.36) are usually found on the labia majora and, less often, the labia minora where they may coalesce to form velvety plaques over the genitalia. Genital intraepithelial neoplasia only rarely progress to squamous cell carcinoma.

• DIAGNOSIS AND DIFFERENTIAL DIAGNOSIS •

Genital warts are diagnosed predominantly on clinical grounds; however, histopathology may be necessary to rule out malignancy with cervical lesions. Cytologic examination in addition to biopsy is recommended. Because only a small proportion of HPV infections are visible, application of 5% acetic acid and colposcopy is recommended to reveal discreet lesions.

The differential diagnosis includes condyloma latum, molluscum contagiosum, lichen planus, genital herpes, Bowen's disease, genital squamous cell carcinoma, and benign neoplasms such as fibroma, lipoma, and hidradenoma.

Penile warts should be distinguished from pearly penile papules, normal excrescences on the corona of the glans penis that are frequently mistaken for warts. Cervical lesions should be distinguished from intraepithelial dysplasia and cervical malignancies. Anal warts should be distinguished primarily from hemorrhoids and rectal cancer.

• TREATMENT AND CLINICAL COURSE •

Cryotherapy with liquid nitrogen is relatively effective with minimal side effects. Other treatment modalities include topical application of podophyllin, surgical excision, CO_2 laser therapy, intralesional application of interferon, and topical 5-fluorouracil cream. Despite effective treatment, genital warts frequently recur either secondary to latent HPV infection in normal-appearing skin or by reinfection from an untreated sex partner. Until treatment is completed, sexual abstinence or the use of a condom is recommended. Patients with Buschke-Löwenstein tumors, bowenoid papulosis, or other clinical forms of genital intraepithelial neoplasia should be referred to a dermatologist or gynecologist familiar with these entities.

MOLLUSCUM CONTAGIOSUM

• PATHOGENESIS •

Molluscum contagiosum is a superficial cutaneous infection of children and young adults caused by a large DNA virus, a member of the *Poxviridae* family. While the disease in children is transmitted by direct nonsexual contact, in adults, it is presumably sexually transmitted, especially in the case of anogenital lesions.

• CLINICAL FEATURES •

The incubation period ranges from 7 days to 6 months (average 2 to 3 months). The typical lesion is a smooth, firm, shiny, hemispherical papule with an umbilicated center and a diameter averaging 2 to 5 mm. Its color is usually pearly white but can also be fleshy or even yellow. Caseous material containing the virus can be expressed from the lesion. Lesions tend to occur in groups but may be solitary.

In adults, the lesions are usually found on the lower abdomen, on the genitalia, on the upper, inner aspects of the thighs, and in the perianal region (Fig. 8.37). More rarely they occur on the palms, soles, eyelids, and conjunctivae. AIDS patients may develop extensive and persistent involvement over the face and torso. Usually, lesions enlarge for a few months, persist for months unchanged, and finally resolve spontaneously.

• DIAGNOSIS AND DIFFERENTIAL DIAGNOSIS •

The typical lesion morphology suggests the diagnosis. It can be confirmed by demonstration of the characteristic intracytoplasmic inclusions in histologic preparations or in smears of the caseous material expressed from the centers of the lesions.

Differential diagnosis includes warts, condyloma latum of secondary syphilis, lichen planus, milia, basal cell epithelioma, and other benign tumors, such as epidermal cyst, keratoacanthoma, syringoma, pyoderma, and small keloids.

• TREATMENT AND CLINICAL COURSE •

The majority of lesions resolve spontaneously within a few months. However, some authors emphasize treatment because of the contagious nature of the disease and because of chronic pruritus or cosmetic concerns. Removal with a curette under local anesthesia or freezing with liquid nitrogen are both effective therapeutic approaches. Other methods include surgical excision, electrocoagulation, expression of the contents of the lesion followed by application of iodine tincture, silver nitrate, or phenol, and topical application of cauterants or irritants such as trichloroacetic acid, podophyllin, or tretinoin.

SCABIES AND PEDICULOSIS PUBIS

Chapter 19 contains a full discussion of the infections of scabies and crab lice. This chapter focuses only on clinical manifestations resulting from sexual contact, a common mode of transmission among adults.

• PATHOGENESIS •

Scabies is caused by the mite, *Scabies sarcoptei*. The mite is transmitted by any skin-to-skin contact; sexual intercourse is not necessary. Furthermore, the infestation may be acquired by sharing unwashed bedding or clothing with an infested person. Symptoms are caused by an allergic-like reaction to mite and mite egg antigens shed into the organism's interdermal burrows.

The crab louse, *Phthirus pubis*, resides on the pubic hair and feeds on the adjacent skin. In heavy infestations, crab lice and their nits can also be found in other hairy parts of the body. The incubation period is about 30 days. The patient usually presents with pruritus in the pubic region or groin, which is probably an immunologic reaction to the louse.

• CLINICAL FEATURES •

The most characteristic symptom of scabies is severe pruritus that worsens at night or when the patient gets warm. The skin lesions of sexually acquired scabies may appear not only in the anogenital region but on any part of the body except the upper face, back, and neck, which are almost never infested except in infants and immunocompromised patients. Lesions have a predilection for finger webs, elbow bends, wrists, axillae, nipples, belt line, genitals, and lower portion of the buttocks (Fig. 8.38). The characteristic signs are the burrows, inflammatory vesicles, urticarial papules, and excoriations. In chronic or secondarily infected lesions, eczematization and pyoderma may occur. Lesions located on the genitalia, in contrast to those in other sites, tend to be more edematous, nodular, and darker. Despite treatment, nodular lesions may persist on the male genitalia for months, representing an immunologic reaction to the dead mites. Nodular scabies is rare in women.

The skin lesions caused by pubic lice are small pruritic papules with central punctae that soon become excoriated and impetiginized. With severe itching, widespread excoriations and crusts may develop. A few patients develop characteristic blue-gray macules (*maculae ceruleae*) mainly on the trunk or thighs, which are asymptomatic and do not blanch upon pressure.

The infestation mainly affects the pubic region but may extend to the hair around the anus and thighs. Very hairy individuals may have lice on their chest hair, arms, beard, and even mustache. Involvement of the eyelashes, eyebrows, and periphery of the scalp occurs infrequently.

• DIAGNOSIS AND DIFFERENTIAL DIAGNOSIS •

The diagnosis of scabies is made on clinical grounds and can be confirmed by demonstration of mites in scrapings of the superficial layer of the epithelium.

Diagnosis of pubic lice is based on itching in the pubic region confirmed by the finding of motile lice or nits attached to the hair. Differential diagnosis should include seborrheic dermatitis, contact dermatitis, atopic dermatitis, eczema, dermatophytosis, and psoriasis.

(See Chapter 19 for more information.)

• TREATMENT AND CLINICAL COURSE •

Treatment of scabies begins with a warm, soapy bath, followed by application of a thin layer of lindane 1% cream or lotion to the entire body to remain for 8 hours or 5% permethrin dermal cream for 8 to 12 hours, after which a second bath follows to thoroughly remove the medication. Bedding and clothes should be thoroughly washed with hot water. Posttreatment pruritus can be controlled by medium-potency steroid creams applied 2 to 3 times a day for several days.

To treat pubic lice, permethrin 1% cream or 1% lindane (lotion, cream, shampoo) should be applied to the affected area and washed off after 10 minutes (it is not recommended for pregnant or lactating women). Alternate treatment includes over-the-counter pyrethrins and piperonyl butoxide.

REFERENCES

1. Brown DR, Fife KH. Human papillomavirus infections of the genital tract. Med Clin North Am 1990:74(6):1455.

ANNOTATED BIBLIOGRAPHY

Centers for Disease Control and Prevention. 1993 Sexually transmitted diseases treatment guidelines. MMWR 1993;42 (RR-14).

    The most recent treatment guidelines formulated by an expert committee that meets every 4 years for this purpose. A handy reference in pamphlet form that can be obtained from the CDC for personal use.

Holmes KK, et al, eds. Sexually transmitted diseases. 4th ed. Philadelphia: McGraw-Hill, 1990.

    The definitive text on this subject. Contains voluminous details on all aspects of all STDs.

Martin DH, vol ed. Sexually transmitted diseases. Med Clin North Am 1990:74(6).

    Seventeen chapters dealing with current issues in the diagnosis and management of the most important STDs and STD syndromes. Emphasis is on practical management of patients.

Mroczkowski TF. Topics in clinical dermatology: Sexually transmitted diseases. Vol 1. New York: Igaku-Shoin, 1990.

    Focuses on the skin manifestations of STDs.

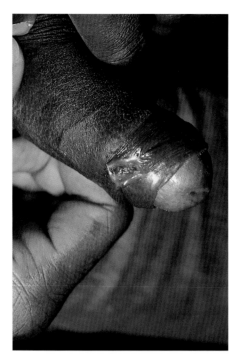

Figure 8.1.   Primary syphilis. Typical primary chancre on the penis. (Courtesy of Dr. Lee T. Nesbitt, Jr.)

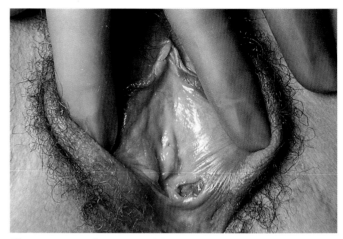

Figure 8.2.   Primary syphilis. Primary chancre on the labia majora. (Courtesy of Dr. Lee T. Nesbitt, Jr.)

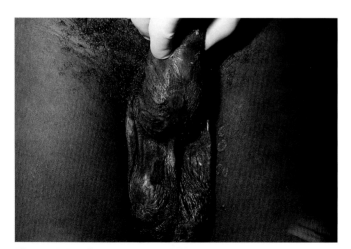

Figure 8.3.   Secondary syphilis. Extensive annular eruption on the scrotum and thigh. (Courtesy of Dr. Lee T. Nesbitt, Jr.)

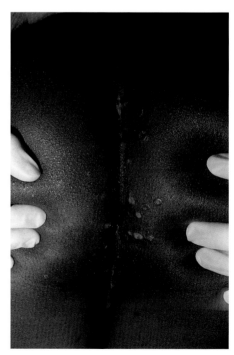

Figure 8.4.   Secondary syphilis. Maculopapular eruption on the perianal area. (Courtesy of Dr. Lee T. Nesbitt, Jr.)

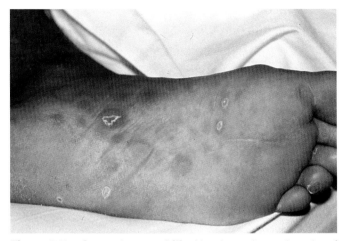

Figure 8.5.   Secondary syphilis. Maculopapules on the soles of the feet. (Courtesy of Dr. Lee T. Nesbitt, Jr.)

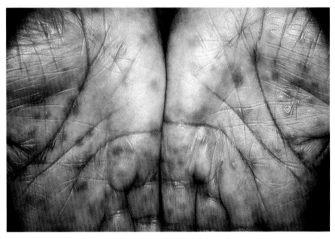

Figure 8.6.   Secondary syphilis. Maculopapular rash on the palms.

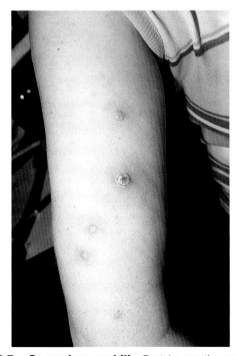

Figure 8.7.   Secondary syphilis. Pustular eruption on the upper arm in an alcoholic patient. (Courtesy of Dr. Lee T. Nesbitt, Jr.)

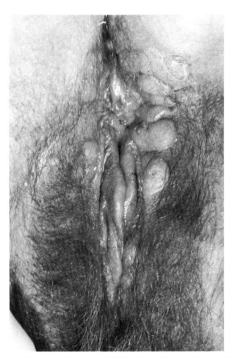

Figure 8.8.   Secondary syphilis. Condyloma latum. Flat condylomas in a woman with secondary syphilis.

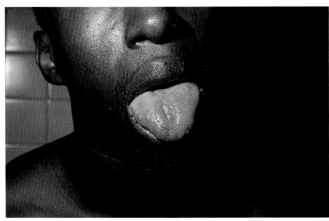

Figure 8.9. Secondary syphilis. Well-demarcated, faintly inflamed white patches on the tongue. (Courtesy of Dr. Lee T. Nesbitt, Jr.)

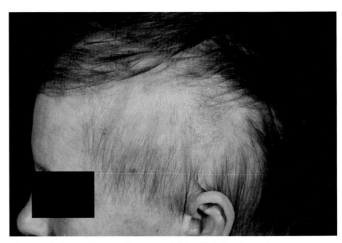

Figure 8.10. Secondary syphilis. Patchy alopecia.

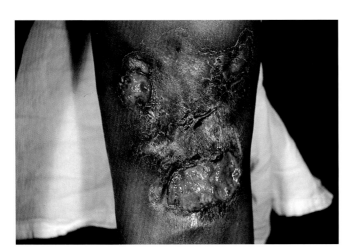

Figure 8.11. Tertiary syphilis. Noduloulcerative lesion on the posterior thigh.

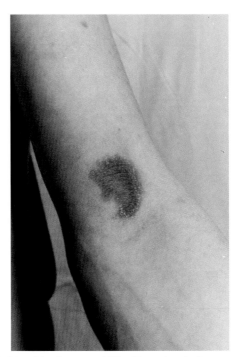

Figure 8.12. Tertiary syphilis. Horseshoe lesion.

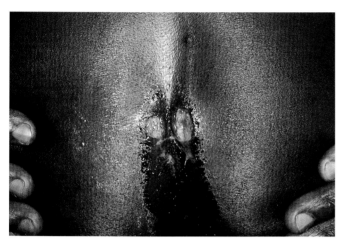

Figure 8.13. **Chancroid.** "Kissing" lesion caused by autoinoculation.

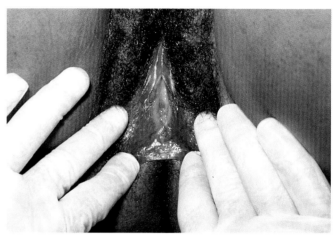

Figure 8.14. **Chancroid.** Single, painful, irregular ulceration at the introitus caused by *Haemophilus ducreyi.*

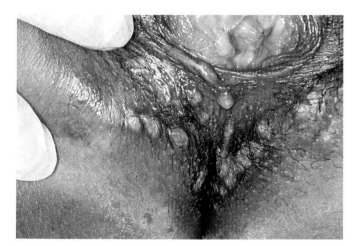

Figure 8.15. **Chancroid.** Multiple superficial ulcerations in a female caused by *Haemophilus ducreyi.* These lesions closely resemble the macerated papules of secondary syphilis. (Courtesy of Dr. Sharon Smith)

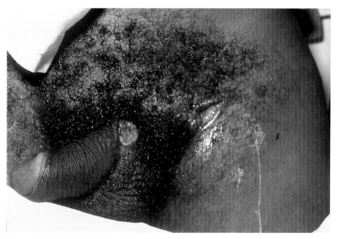

Figure 8.16. **Chancroid.** Single ulceration at the base of the penis accompanied by a ruptured bubo.

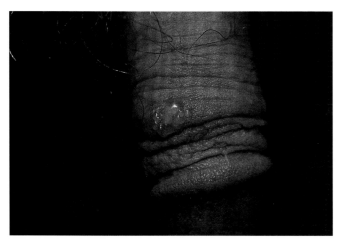

Figure 8.17.   Genital herpes. Multiple grouped vesicles on the skin of the penis. (Courtesy of Dr. Larry Millikan)

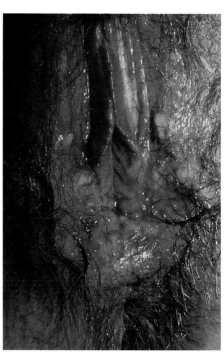

Figure 8.18.   Genital herpes in a female. Several groups of vesicles located in the vulva and the perianal area. (Courtesy of American Academy of Dermatology)

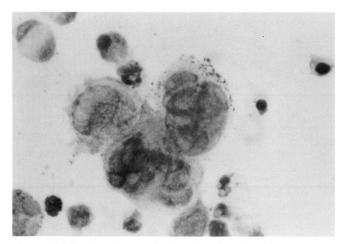

Figure 8.19.   Tzank test. Multinucleated giant cells.

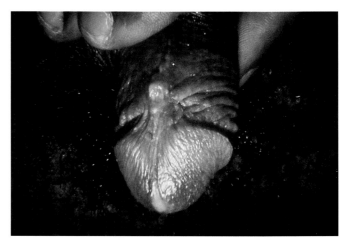

Figure 8.20.   Lymphogranuloma venereum. Primary lesion on the frenulum.

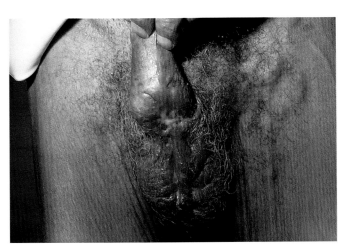

Figure 8.21.   Lymphogranuloma venereum. Lymphadenopathy and chronic draining sinuses of the scrotum and base of penis.

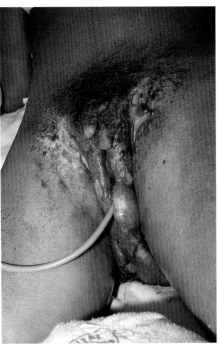

Figure 8.22.   Lymphogranuloma venereum. Esthiomene, showing edema and chronic ulcerations. (Courtesy of Dr. Lee T. Nesbitt, Jr.)

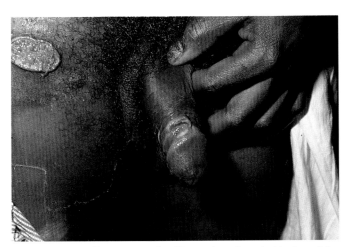

Figure 8.23.   Donovanosis. Nontender, ulcerated lesion of the penis and inguinal areas. (Courtesy of Dr. Lee T. Nesbitt, Jr.)

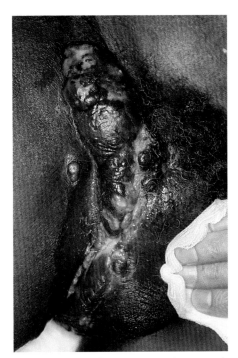

Figure 8.24.   Donovanosis. Numerous ulcerogranulomatous, friable lesions on the inguinal area and scrotum. (Courtesy of Dr. Lee T. Nesbitt, Jr.)

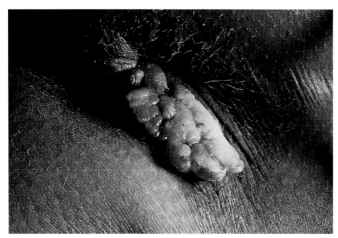

Figure 8.25.   Donovanosis. Verrucous form of the disease resembling genital warts.

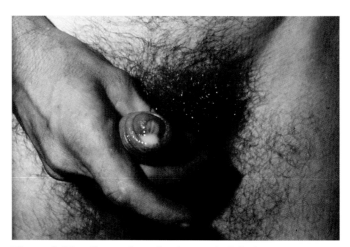

Figure 8.26.   Gonorrhea. Purulent urethral discharge.

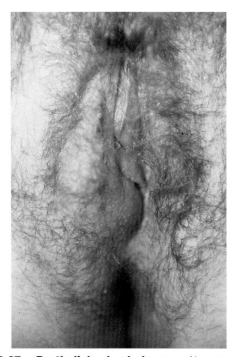

Figure 8.27.   Bartholin's gland abscess. Abscess caused by *Neisseria gonorrhoeae*.

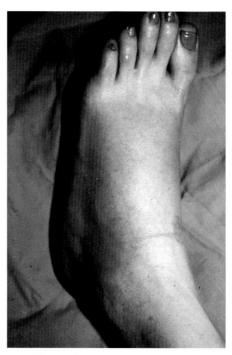

Figure 8.28.   Disseminated gonococcal infection. Tenosynovitis of the dorsal foot. (Courtesy of Dr. Charles V. Sanders)

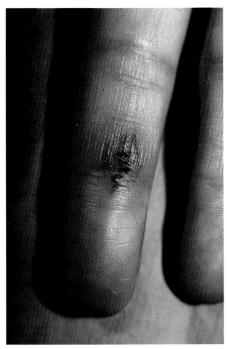

Figure 8.29.   Disseminated gonococcal infection. Necrotic vesiculopustule with hemorrhagic base on the fingers. (Courtesy of Dr. Charles V. Sanders)

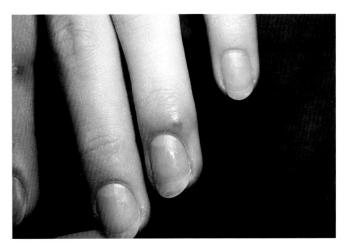

Figure 8.30.   Disseminated gonococcal infection. Pustule on the fingers. (Courtesy of Dr. Lee T. Nesbitt, Jr.)

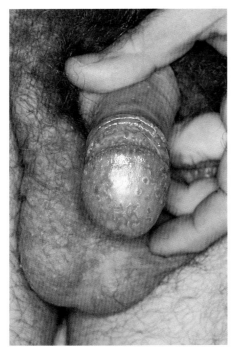

Figure 8.31.   Reiter's syndrome. Balanitis circinata.

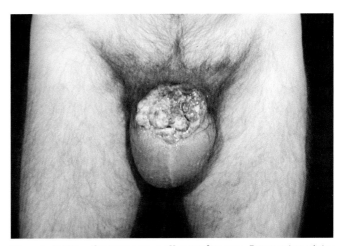

Figure 8.32.   Squamous cell carcinoma. Destruction of the penis caused by squamous cell carcinoma now recognized as a possible complication of human papillomavirus.

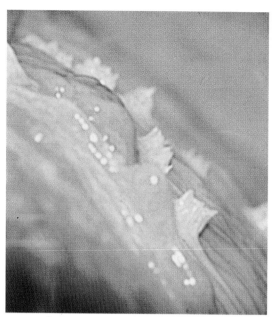

Figure 8.33.   Vulvar warts. Vulvar warts after application of 5% acetic acid. (Courtesy of Dr. Paul Summer)

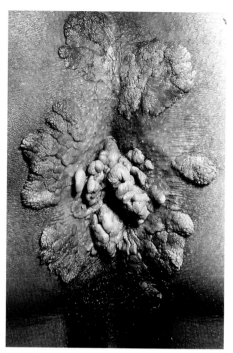

Figure 8.34.   Condylomata acuminata. Large mass of hyperpigmented condylomata acuminata affecting the perianal area in a male homosexual. (Courtesy of Dr. Lee T. Nesbitt, Jr.)

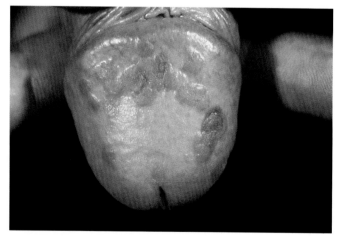

Figure 8.35.   Bowenoid papulosis. Bowenoid papulosis on the glans of the penis. The disease is presumably caused by HPV-16 and HPV-18. (Courtesy of Prof. S. Obalek)

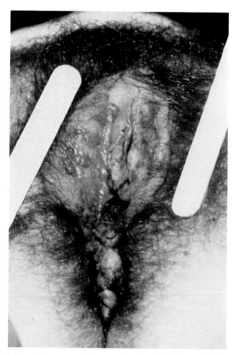

Figure 8.36.   Bowenoid papulosis. Multicentric flat, hyperpigmented papules in the vulva. (Courtesy of Prof. S. Jablonska)

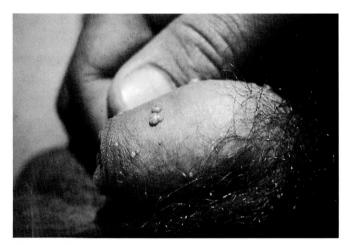

Figure 8.37.   Molluscum contagiosum. Pearly nodules on the skin of the penis. (Courtesy of Dr. Larry Millikan)

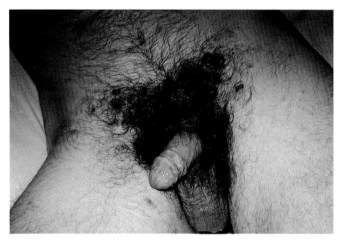

Figure 8.38.   Scabies. Widespread pruritic papular nodules, including genitalia. (Courtesy of Dr. Lee T. Nesbitt, Jr.)

CHAPTER 9

Lyme Disease

BERNARD W. BERGER

Lyme disease is a multisystem disorder caused by the spiro-chete *Borrelia burgdorferi* and transmitted by ticks of the *Ixodes ricinus* complex. Lyme disease has a world-wide distribution. In 1992 alone, 9,677 cases were reported in the United States. Although 48 states have reported the disease, more than 90% of the cases have occurred in the Eastern, Midatlantic, North Central, and Pacific coastal regions, most commonly during the months of May through August.

• PATHOGENESIS •

Ticks of the *Ixodes ricinus* complex begin their life cycle of 2 to 3 years in the early spring, when engorged females deposit several thousand eggs from which larvae emerge 6 to 8 weeks later. During the summer, the larval ticks feed once on a small rodent and develop into nymphs. Then, in the early spring or summer of the next year, they feed again on a small rodent, bird, or medium-sized vertebrate for 3 to 5 days, then molt and become adults in the early fall. Adult ticks attach to a larger host (deer or cattle) for feeding and mating. The female drops to the ground and awaits early spring, when she begins laying eggs.

The tick acquires *Borrelia burgdorferi* from an infected host while feeding. The spirochete remains in the tick's midgut and multiplies when the tick feeds again. Spirochetes then penetrate the gut epithelium and enter the tick's circulation, where they invade the salivary gland and subsequently enter the host via the saliva. Laboratory studies indicate that spirochete transmission from the infected tick to the host takes an average of 48 hours of attachment (range: 24 to 72 hours) because of the time required for the spirochete to travel from the tick's midgut into its salivary glands.

Much of the basic information about pathogenesis was provided by Willy Burgdorfer, who also discovered the etiologic agent of Lyme Disease.

• CLINICAL FEATURES •

Lyme disease has been divided into three overlapping clinical stages—early localized Lyme disease (onset of days to weeks after infection), early disseminated Lyme disease (days to months), and late Lyme disease (months to years). The early stage of Lyme disease usually begins with a characteristic skin lesion, erythema migrans. A viral-like illness may precede, follow, or appear in concert with erythema migrans. Cardiac, neurologic, and skeletal abnormalities may occur early in the course of the illness but more often appear weeks to months after the initial infection. Less frequently reported complications may involve the eye, heart, liver, and spleen. Lyme disease occurring during pregnancy may result in fetal abnormalities and, rarely, fetal death.

Cutaneous Manifestations

Three cutaneous entities firmly associated with Lyme disease are erythema migrans, borrelial lymphocytoma (benign lymphocytoma cutis), and acrodermatitis chronica atrophicans. This was based on the isolation of *Borrelia burgdorferi* from skin biopsy specimens of these lesions. Erythema migrans and borrelial lymphocytoma are associated with early Lyme disease, and acrodermatitis chronica atrophicans is associated with late Lyme disease. Whereas erythema migrans is seen in patients from all locales, *Borrelia* lymphocytoma and acrodermatitis chronica atrophicans are primarily seen in Europe.

ERYTHEMA MIGRANS

The distinctive cutaneous marker of Lyme disease is erythema migrans, which begins as a red macule that becomes papular, and then expands into a red, annular plaque. Two general forms have been described: an expanding, red, annular plaque with varying intensities of erythema within the plaque (Figs. 9.1, 9.2), or, less commonly, a central red plaque surrounded by normal-appearing skin that is, in turn, surrounded by an expanding, red band resembling a target (a ring-within-a-ring configuration) (Figs. 9.3, 9.4). Although circular shapes predominate, triangular or elongated oval lesions can occur. Lesions may be solitary or multiple (Fig. 9.5).

Most erythema migrans lesions are reddish, but some, particularly those appearing on the lower extremities, may have a bluish-red hue (Fig. 9.6). The central portion of the lesion can vary greatly in appearance, being erythematous, clear, edematous (Fig. 9.7), vesicular (Fig. 9.8), or crusted. Lesions are usually asymptomatic but have been described as being pruritic or painful. They are often warmer than the surrounding uninvolved skin.

The lesions appear 7 to 8 days (range: 2 to 28 days) after the bite of an infected ixodid tick. The size and rate of expansion of these lesions are variable. Most lesions show gradual centrifugal enlargement (median size in 7 days: 4 x 8 cm) or may expand rapidly to as much as 25 x 25 cm in just 7 days (Fig. 9.9). Approximately 9% of Lyme disease patients evaluated 1 week after the onset of illness have multiple lesions. An estimated 20% of Lyme disease patients do not experience erythema migrans.

Erythema migrans may be the only clinical manifestation of Lyme disease in patients evaluated 1 week after the onset of the disease, but approximately 50% of the patients will have extracutaneous signs and symptoms of major intensity. The most frequently experienced are fever, fatigue, musculoskeletal pain, headache, chills, and regional lymphadenopathy. Also described are heart rate and rhythm abnormalities, irritability, gastrointestinal complaints, peripheral neuropathies, diaphoresis, sore throat, nonexertional shortness of breath, and short-term memory loss. These signs and symptoms can occur before, after, or in concert with the appearance of erythema migrans.

BORRELIAL LYMPHOCYTOMA

Borrelial lymphocytoma is a bluish-red, tumor-like lesion that has a predilection for the ear lobes, particularly in children, and the nipple/areola region in adults. This lesion is also a cutaneous manifestation of early Lyme disease. Extracutaneous signs and symptoms of the neurologic and skeletal systems, similar to those associated with erythema migrans, may accompany borrelial lymphocytoma.

ACRODERMATITIS CHRONICA ATROPHICANS

Acrodermatitis chronica atrophicans is considered a late cutaneous manifestation of Lyme disease (Fig. 9.10). It occurs predominately in women 40 to 70 years of age. The initial lesion consists of erythema and edema affecting one extremity, usually the leg or foot. Eventually, the lesions become atrophic. Subluxations of the small joints of the feet or hands, as well as peripheral polyneuropathies, may be seen in patients whose lesions have been present for more than 3 years.

MORPHEA AND LICHEN SCLEROSUS ET ATROPHICUS

The European literature has provided evidence that *Borrelia burgdorferi* may be involved in the pathogenesis of morphea and of lichen sclerosus et atrophicus, but there is little evidence to support this conclusion in cases as seen in the United States. This controversy can be explained in part by the observation in Europe that sclerotic lesions can develop in up to 10% of patients with acrodermatitis chronica atrophicans, and that these lesions may be indistinguishable from morphea and lichen sclerosus et atrophicus seen in nonacrodermatitis chronica atrophi-

cans patients. In addition, European investigators have isolated phenotypically heterogenous strains of *Borrelia* that are different from the North American strain of *Borrelia burgdorferi*. These strain variants are probably the basis for the almost exclusive incidence of acrodermatitis chronica atrophicans and borrelial lymphocytoma in Europe compared to the United States, and to the borrelial-associated sclerotic lesions.

Extracutaneous Complications of Lyme Disease

Peripheral neuropathies, cranial neuropathies, and disorders of the central nervous system can complicate Lyme disease. Peripheral neuropathies include painful radiculitis, brachial neuritis, intermittent paresthesias, and carpal tunnel syndrome. The most common cranial neuropathy is that of cranial nerve VII (Bell's palsy), which usually occurs in early Lyme disease. Central nervous system complications include meningitis, encephalitis, and encephalopathy.

Varying degrees of atrioventricular block (occasionally requiring the insertion of a temporary pacemaker) may occur in early Lyme disease. Myocarditis and pericarditis are relatively uncommon complications.

Oligoarticular arthritis occurs a mean of 6 months following early infection. The attacks of arthritis are brief and intermittent and usually involve the large joints, especially the knee. Immunogenic factors are thought to be involved in patients with chronic Lyme arthritis because these patients have an increased frequency of haplotype HLA-DR4 and respond poorly to antibiotic treatment.

• DIAGNOSIS AND DIFFERENTIAL DIAGNOSIS •

LABORATORY

The laboratory diagnosis of Lyme disease in the United States has been problematic because of the lack of sufficient sensitivity and specificity of relevant tests and the lack of inter-laboratory standardization in their utilization. Although helpful, laboratory tests can only serve to support the clinical findings in making the diagnosis of active Lyme disease, the exception being a positive culture for *Borrelia burgdorferi*.

MICROBIOLOGY

The cultivation of *Borrelia burgdorferi* from a patient is currently the only unequivocal laboratory means of confirming the diagnosis of Lyme disease. The spirochete has been isolated and successfully subcultured from the blood, cerebrospinal fluid, cutaneous lesions, synovial fluid, and myocardium of Lyme disease patients (Fig. 9.11). This has generally been a low-yield procedure; however, improvements in culture media and culture techniques have greatly increased the frequency of isolation and shortened the time in which the organism can be identified.

HISTOPATHOLOGY

The histologic picture of erythema migrans is variable. The most common and characteristic pattern—superficial and deep perivascular and interstitial lymphocytic infiltrate with plasma cells—is seen more frequently in specimens obtained from the periphery of the lesion. A second histologic pattern—a superficial and deep perivascular and interstitial lymphocytic infiltrate with eosinophils but devoid of plasma cells—is seen in specimens obtained from the center of the lesion. This pattern is indistinguishable from the histologic reaction to an insect bite.

With silver staining, spirochetes can be found in erythema migrans lesions. They are situated in the epidermis and the upper dermis and are most detectable in biopsy specimens taken from the periphery of a lesion and in specimens containing plasma cells.

TESTING FOR ANTIBODIES TO *BORRELIA BURGDORFERI*

The antibody response in Lyme disease was initially evaluated by immunofluorescence assay but is now done by enzyme assay, which is more easily performed and more objectively interpreted. However, some problems persist with serologic antibody tests. False negative results occur primarily during the first few weeks of the illness when a patient may present with clinical evidence of Lyme disease (erythema migrans) but without a detectable serologic antibody response. False-positive reactions have occurred both in healthy patients and in patients with other diseases, such as other spirochetosis, systemic lupus erythematosis, subacute bacterial endocarditis, infectious mononucleosis, and rheumatoid arthritis.

Western blot analysis may be useful in late Lyme disease for confirming borderline-positive serology and evaluating suspected false-positive serology by detecting bands specific for *Borrelia burgdorferi* (the 31 kD outer surface protein A and the 34 kD outer surface protein B). In early Lyme disease, however, Western blotting provides equivocal results because it usually detects only nonspecific polypeptides.

Current serologic tests are not sufficiently reliable to make a definitive diagnosis of Lyme disease. They should be considered supportive only when careful clinical evaluation suggests the diagnosis of Lyme disease. Demonstration of local antibody production to *Borrelia burgdorferi* in the cerebrospinal fluid, however, is considered to be useful in the diagnosis of central nervous system Lyme disease.

POLYMERASE CHAIN REACTION

The amplification of DNA with polymerase chain reaction (PCR) has impacted on infectious disease epidemiology and on the detection of pathogens for which in vitro cultivation has been difficult or unsuccessful. While PCR's use in Lyme dis-

ease remains experimental, the test has been successful in detecting *Borrelia burgdorferi* in the skin, blood, cerebrospinal fluid, and urine of patients with Lyme disease.

• TREATMENT AND CLINICAL COURSE •

Years prior to the establishment of Lyme disease as a distinct clinical entity, the usefulness of antibiotic treatment for certain cutaneous manifestations seen with this disorder had been described. Currently, antimicrobial agents still remain effective in the treatment of most cases of Lyme disease, but a universally efficacious drug has not been identified.

Early localized disease responds readily to a 2- to 3-week course of doxycycline or amoxicillin. When disseminated infection does not respond to oral agents or when a patient presents with one of the major complications of Lyme disease (e.g., meningitis or complete heart block) intravenous therapy with ceftriaxone or penicillin G is instituted. The choice of drugs and the duration of treatment for disseminated or late infection remains controversial. Controlled clinical trials in progress will help to define optimal treatment.

In regions where tick exposure is likely, prevention should be attempted with protective garments and tick repellent. Embedded ticks should be removed promptly to decrease the chance of transmission of the organism. Although the risk of acquiring an infection appears to be low, if a tick has been attached for at least 24 hours and is engorged, some clinicians favor the use of prophylactic antimicrobial agents. This remains controversial in asymptomatic *Ixodes* tick bites.

Clinical trials of a vaccine using recombinant outer surface protein A are currently being evaluated.

ANNOTATED BIBLIOGRAPHY

Asbrink E, Hovmark A, eds. Lyme Borreliosis. Clinics in Dermatology 1993;11:329.
> Fifteen papers by international experts present a balanced view of the current knowledge of Lyme disease.

Coyle PK, ed. Lyme Disease. St. Louis: Mosby-Year Book, 1993.
> Basic science, clinical aspects, diagnosis, therapy, and special topics regarding Lyme disease are presented in detail by 28 clinical and basic science researchers.

Rahn DW, Malawista SE. Lyme disease: Recommendations for diagnosis and treatment. Ann Intern Med 1991;114:472.
> Diagnosis and treatment recommendations.

Spach DH, Liles WC, Campbell GL, et al. Tick-borne diseases in the United States. N Engl J Med 1993;329:936.
> A review of the major tick-borne diseases in the United States, with an emphasis on Lyme disease.

Steere AC. Lyme disease. N Engl J Med 1989;321:586.
> A review of Lyme disease.

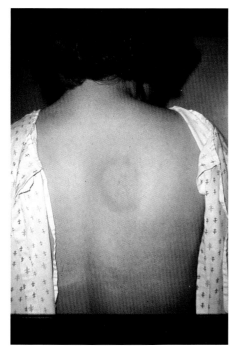

Figure 9.1.   Lyme disease. Expanding red annular plaque of Lyme disease. (Courtesy of Dr. Lee T. Nesbitt, Jr.)

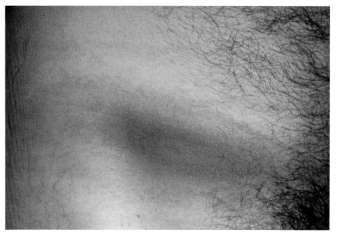

Figure 9.2.   Lyme disease. Solitary erythema migrans demonstrating varying intensities of erythema within the lesion.

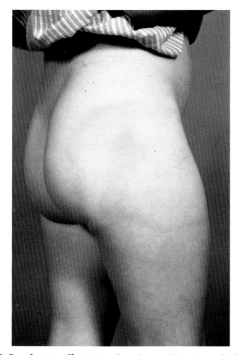

Figure 9.3.   Lyme disease. Annular erythematous lesions of the thigh and buttocks. (Courtesy of Dr. Lee T. Nesbitt, Jr.)

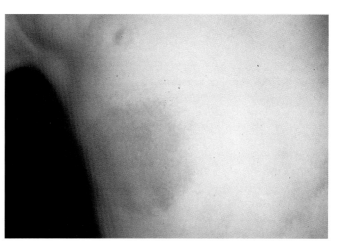

Figure 9.4.   Lyme disease. Erythema migrans presenting as a ring-within-a-ring configuration. (From Berger BW. Dermatologic manifestations of Lyme disease. Rev Infect Dis 1989;11:S1475–S1481)

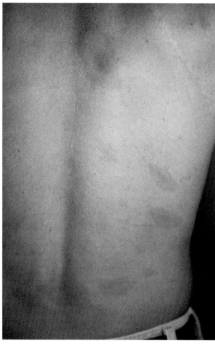

Figure 9.5.   Lyme disease. Erythema migrans lesions appearing in multiplicity.

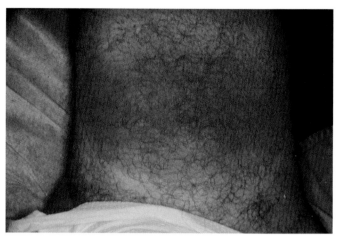

Figure 9.6.   Lyme disease. Bluish annular band situated between two erythematous areas. Bluish erythema migrans lesions appear most commonly on the lower extremities.

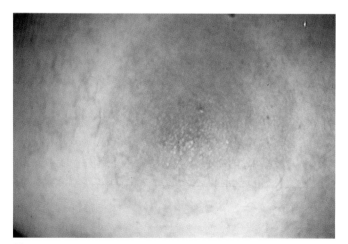

Figure 9.7.   Lyme disease. Annular plaque of erythema migrans lesions with edematous center. (From Berger BW. Erythema chronicum migrans of Lyme disease. Arch Dermatol 1984;120:1017–1021)

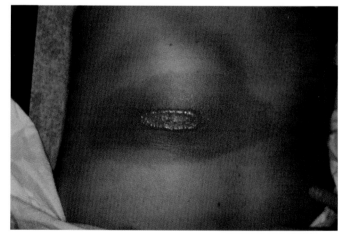

Figure 9.8.   Lyme disease. Erythema migrans with an annular vesicular center. This is in contrast to some erythema migrans lesions having clear centers.

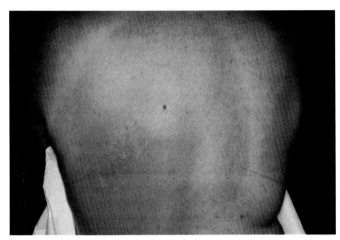

Figure 9.9. Lyme disease. Large, rapidly expanding erythema migrans lesion. It had been present for 21 days and measured 30 x 33 cm. (From Berger BW, MacDonald AB, Benach, JL. Use of an autologous antigen in serologic testing. J Am Acad Dermatol 1988;18:1243–1246)

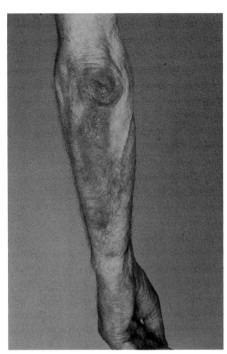

Figure 9.10. Lyme disease. A sclerotic acrodermatitis chronica atrophicans lesion.

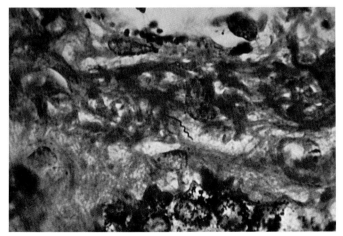

Figure 9.11. Lyme disease. The Lyme disease spirochete, *Borrelia burgdorferi,* appearing in the papillary dermis. (From Berger BW, Kaplan MH, Rothenberg IR, Barbour AG. Isolation and characterization of the Lyme disease spirochete from the skin of patients with erythema chronicum migrans. J Am Acad Dermatol 1985;13:444)

CHAPTER 10

The Rickettsioses

DOUGLAS P. FINE

Most rickettsiae exist primarily as zoonotic organisms and involve humans only incidentally. Spread is by insect vectors, particularly ticks and lice. Exanthems are characteristic of most of the rickettsioses; exceptions include Q fever (which will not be further discussed in this chapter) and trench fever (which uncommonly has a skin eruption but will be discussed). *Rochalimaea quintana*, the agent of trench fever, and *Rochalimaea henselae*, the agent of bacillary angiomatosis, may soon be reclassified as *Bartonella* species but will be considered with the rickettsiae for purposes of this chapter.

The rickettsioses considered in this chapter all appear to share the cardinal pathogenetic mechanism of vasculitis, caused by replication of organisms in endothelial cells in capillaries and small arteries and veins. This mechanism underlies the exanthems, although clinical presentation varies among the diseases.

Spotted Fever Group

ROCKY MOUNTAIN SPOTTED FEVER (*RICKETTSIA RICKETTSII*)

• PATHOGENESIS •

The primary reservoir, as well as vector, for *Rickettsia rickettsii* is the tick: *Dermacentor variabilis* (the American dog tick) in the eastern United States, *D. andersoni* (the Rocky Mountain wood tick) in the western states, *Amblyomma americanum* (the Lone Star tick) in the southern states, *A. cajennese* in Central and South America, and *Rhipicephalus sanguineus* in Mexico. The organisms are spread from ticks to humans during prolonged feeding, principally through infected tick salivary secretions. Thus, for human infection to occur, there must be a focus of infected ticks, exposure must occur during a time of year when ticks are active and feeding (generally the warmer months of the year), and attachment and feeding must proceed long enough for rickettsiae to be released into the tick's saliva (usually several hours).

Rickettsiae are introduced into the skin where local replication occurs, followed by systemic vascular dissemination. Organisms attach to and invade vascular endothelial cells (Fig. 10.1). Damage to these cells underlies the clinical findings of rash, edema, hypovolemia, and specific organ dysfunction.

• CLINICAL FEATURES •

Between 1 day and 2 weeks after the bite of an infected tick, the patient acutely develops fever and some neurological manifestation, usually severe headache and often altered mentation or consciousness. Rash may present simultaneously or be delayed, rarely more than a week after initial onset.

The eruption of Rocky Mountain spotted fever characteristically begins on the ankles and wrists and spreads centripetally to arms, legs, trunk, and face (Fig. 10.2). Palms and soles are often involved as well, a useful though not diagnostic feature (Figs. 10.3, 10.4). Earliest lesions tend to be erythematous macules or papules and may be subtle. Perhaps in a majority of cases, lesions eventually become petechial (Figs. 10.5–10.9). In more severe infections, often with laboratory evidence of disseminated intravascular coagulation, purpura and even dermal necrosis may develop (Figs. 10.10, 10.11). Petechiae can also be seen on mucous membranes and conjunctivae.

Rarely, an eschar may be seen at the site of the original tick bite, with rickettsiae demonstrable by histologic and immunofluorescent techniques. This lesion resembles the characteristic skin lesion of the eastern tick-borne rickettsioses (see below).

Other manifestations of Rocky Mountain spotted fever reflect the organs with the greatest vasculitic involvement in the patient. Neurologic dysfunction, including central and peripheral nervous system disease, is extremely common. Other systems prominently involved include the gastrointestinal tract, the muscular system, and the lungs.

• DIAGNOSIS AND DIFFERENTIAL DIAGNOSIS •

Because prompt therapy is critical, the diagnosis of Rocky Mountain spotted fever must be based on a clinical picture compatible with possible tick exposure in an endemic area at the right time of year in the absence of a likely alternative diagnosis. All patients have fever, most have some neurologic dysfunction, and most have rash. But only about two-thirds have the characteristic triad of fever, severe headache, and rash. Most patients with documented Rocky Mountain spotted fever report exposure to dogs or to the outdoors, even though only about half will report definite tick bite. Empiric therapy should be initiated on clinical grounds alone.

Diagnosis can be established by biopsy of skin involved with the eruption and demonstration of organisms in endothelial cells by direct immunofluorescence. The procedure must be accomplished rapidly, but relatively few hospitals are prepared to carry it out. Otherwise, definitive diagnosis can only be made in retrospect with serological studies, generally by a 4-fold or greater rise in antibody titers measured by complement fixation or immunofluorescent methods. Less satisfactory is the somewhat nonspecific Weil-Felix agglutination reaction to Proteus OX-19, signifying the presence of a common antigen.

The differential diagnosis of Rocky Mountain spotted fever is rather broad. In the absence of rash, one must consider meningitis (both bacterial and viral), leptospirosis, typhoid fever, ehrlichiosis, infectious mononucleosis, and a host of other febrile diseases. With onset of rash, the differential diagnosis includes the viral exanthems (e.g., measles, rubella), ehrlichiosis, *Staphylococcus aureus* endocarditis, meningococcemia, syphilis, and drug reactions.

• TREATMENT AND CLINICAL COURSE •

The treatment of choice is doxycycline (or some other tetracycline) or chloramphenicol. Oral treatment can be administered if the patient is reasonably stable and can tolerate oral medicines. Otherwise, intravenous therapy should be used. Prepubescent children generally should not receive tetracyclines if possible. Adjunctive therapy includes maintenance of adequate intravascular volume and pressure. There are no data on which to recommend corticosteroids or anticoagulation.

Defervescence and improvement are usually seen 24 to 72 hours after beginning therapy. Most patients recover satisfactorily and without sequelae. In severe cases, patients may have a stormy course and prolonged recovery. Serious sequelae, including cognitive, sensory, or motor/neurologic dysfunction, are well documented. Death occurs in relatively few cases and usually relates to shock and multi-organ-system failure, often with disseminated intravascular coagulation.

EASTERN TICK-BORNE RICKETTSIOSES

• PATHOGENESIS •

Several rickettsioses occur in the eastern hemisphere that share similar clinical characteristics and are caused by closely related organisms. The prototype illness is Mediterranean spotted fever (African tick typhus, boutonneuse fever) caused by *Rickettsia conorii*. Other variants are Queensland tick typhus (*R. australis*) and North Asian tick typhus (*R. sibirica*).

Wild animals, particularly rodents, and tick vectors maintain the disease—with humans incidentally infected, as occurs with Rocky Mountain spotted fever. Invasion of endothelial cells of

dermal vessels occurs at the initial site of inoculation with local ischemic necrosis, regional spread, and finally systemic vascular spread, as with *R. rickettsii*.

• CLINICAL FEATURES •

The mean incubation period is about 1 week, at which time fever, headache, and myalgia develop. Conjunctival injection may be prominent. At that same time, a lesion is often evident at the site of the original tick bite: a small (less than 1 cm) erythematous lesion with a necrotic center, usually not painful. This is the "tache noire" (black macule), or eschar, that can be useful in diagnosis (Fig. 10.12). Regional nodes may be palpable and tender. Several days later, a generalized erythematous macular eruption develops, including the palms and soles. It may begin distally and spread to the trunk or appear first on the trunk. The eruption may become petechial or purpuric. Systemic disease may involve any organ but is usually milder than Rocky Mountain spotted fever.

• DIAGNOSIS AND DIFFERENTIAL DIAGNOSIS •

Diagnosis is clinically established based on a compatible syndrome and confirmed either by immunofluorescent stains of skin biopsy specimens (including the eschar) or serology. Weil-Felix reactions (Proteus OX-19, OX-K, and OX-2) may be positive but in variable patterns. Both complement fixation and immunofluorescence tests are available.

Differential diagnosis is similar to that of Rocky Mountain spotted fever. One may also consider ulceroglandular tularemia.

• TREATMENT AND CLINICAL COURSE •

Treatment is with tetracyclines or chloramphenicol. The eastern tick-borne rickettsioses are generally milder than Rocky Mountain spotted fever except in the case of compromised hosts, including the elderly. Severe disease, serious sequelae, and death are rare, but skin manifestations, particularly the eschar, may persist for up to 3 weeks after recovery.

RICKETTSIALPOX (*RICKETTSIA AKARI*)

• PATHOGENESIS •

The reservoir for *R. akari* is the house mouse and the vector is the mouse mite (*Allodermanyssus sanguineus*). The infection has been recognized worldwide in widely scattered locales, including New York City and other sites in the United States, Russia, Korea, and South Africa. The mite is almost invisible, and its bite goes unnoticed.

Like the eastern rickettsioses, local proliferation in endothelial cells is followed by dissemination and widespread vascular involvement.

• CLINICAL FEATURES •

Several days to a week after the bite, a small, painless papulovesicular lesion develops, associated with mild regional adenopathy and eventually forming a characteristic eschar. About 1 to 2 weeks later, the systemic syndrome develops suddenly with chills, fever, and headache. Myalgias and photophobia may be prominent. An eruption develops in about 3 days, beginning as erythematous indurated macules or papules, which may form central vesicles that heal by crusting. The rash usually spares the palms, soles, and mucous membranes.

• DIAGNOSIS AND DIFFERENTIAL DIAGNOSIS •

Diagnosis is established retrospectively by serology, primarily by complement fixation or indirect immunofluorescence.

Differential diagnosis includes not only the other rickettsioses and exanthems but also vesiculating diseases. Chickenpox, disseminated zoster, and disseminated herpes simplex should be considered. The vesicles of rickettsialpox tend to be smaller than those of chickenpox. Enteroviral infections might produce similar lesions.

• TREATMENT AND CLINICAL COURSE •

Tetracyclines are the drugs of choice. Chloramphenicol is an alternative. Healing of the rash occurs within 2 weeks. Malaise and headache may persist for a few weeks, but serious sequelae or death are rare.

Typhus Group

EPIDEMIC TYPHUS AND BRILL-ZINSSER DISEASE (*RICKETTSIA PROWAZEKII*)

• PATHOGENESIS •

The principal reservoir of *Rickettsia prowazekii* is thought to be human, although the southern flying squirrel has been shown to be a reservoir in the eastern United States. Other zoonotic reservoirs may exist. Transmission occurs by the bite of the human body louse, *Pediculus humanus*. Historically, epidemic typhus has been a disease of crowding and war, spread by close contact and poor hygiene. The louse moves from one person to another, carrying rickettsiae in its gut to spread during a blood meal. After the local invasion, bloodstream dissemination and widespread vascular endothelial infection occur.

• CLINICAL FEATURES •

The incubation is about 1 week. The illness is similar to other rickettsioses: abrupt onset with fever, chills, severe headache, and myalgia. The fever tends to spike and remain high, and the patient may be prostrated. Disease may be less severe in persons who acquire infection from flying squirrels.

The rash of epidemic typhus begins centrally and spreads centrifugally, originally as blanching erythematous macules, later turning confluent, maculopapular, and often petechial. Unlike Rocky Mountain spotted fever, the palms and soles are spared, as is the face.

Volume depletion and vascular collapse may occur. Specific tissue involvement reflects the distribution of the vasculitis.

• DIAGNOSIS AND DIFFERENTIAL DIAGNOSIS •

The diagnosis is established clinically, based particularly on a proper epidemiologic history and a compatible syndrome. Confirmation by serology is possible. A complement fixation test uses antigens cross-reactive with those of *Rickettsia typhi*, the agent of endemic or murine typhus (see below). Weil-Felix reactions (OX-19, variably OX-2, not OX-K) may be helpful.

The differential diagnosis is, like most rickettsial diseases, rather broad. Leptospirosis, meningococcemia, bacterial meningitis, infectious mononucleosis, syphilis, and rubella should be considered in addition to endemic typhus.

• TREATMENT AND CLINICAL COURSE •

Tetracyclines and chloramphenicol are the drugs of choice and effect a cure in most patients. In debilitated populations and the elderly, however, fatalities may be high.

In some persons, infection may remit spontaneously but remain dormant. Years later, infection may relapse, usually presenting as a milder disease (Brill-Zinsser disease). Diagnosis is problematic. Distinction from endemic typhus, which it resembles clinically, may be particularly difficult but is based on demonstration that complement-fixation antibodies are IgG (Brill-Zinsser disease), rather than IgM (endemic typhus).

ENDEMIC (MURINE) TYPHUS (*RICKETTSIA TYPHI*)

• PATHOGENESIS •

Endemic typhus occurs world-wide, including many parts of the United States. The reservoir of *Rickettsia typhi* is the common rat and the vector is the rat flea, *Xenopsylla cheopis*. Transmission to humans is favored by poor living conditions and by occupational exposure to rats.

The pathophysiology is less well studied than that of other rickettsioses, in part because endemic typhus is a milder disease. It resembles epidemic typhus closely, with systemic rickettsial endothelial cell infection.

• CLINICAL FEATURES •

Unlike most other rickettsioses, the onset of endemic typhus tends to be gradual, occuring about 2 weeks after infection. Headache, fever, myalgia, and malaise are predominant symptoms, although not usually as severe as with other rickettsioses. A rash is usual but may be subtle. It is macular, blanching, sometimes confluent, and usually limited to the trunk. It may become maculopapular or fade quickly.

• DIAGNOSIS AND DIFFERENTIAL DIAGNOSIS •

Serology suggests the diagnosis, as in epidemic typhus, but cannot distinguish epidemic from endemic typhus. The differential diagnosis is similar to that of epidemic typhus but includes, especially, Brill-Zinsser disease.

• TREATMENT AND CLINICAL COURSE •

The disease is mild, even in the absence of therapy. Death is extremely rare. Treatment is with tetracyclines or chloramphenicol.

SCRUB TYPHUS (*RICKETTSIA TSUTSUGAMUSHI*)

• PATHOGENESIS •

The vector and primary reservoir is the trombiculid mite, whose larval stage infects humans during feeding. Rodents are a secondary reservoir. *R. tsutsugamushi* is found throughout eastern Asia and the western rim of the Pacific Basin. Local infection is followed by endothelial cell invasion and proliferation with a local lesion and, later, systemic disease.

• CLINICAL FEATURES •

About 2 weeks after infection, an eschar usually develops at the inoculation site, with regional lymphadenopathy. The eschar, however, may be unnoticed. A generalized maculopapular rash develops in a small percentage of patients. Dissemination quickly occurs with acute onset of fever, chills, headache, and myalgia. Other systemic symptoms and signs reflect organ involvement, which may be severe. Neurological signs may be dominant, reminiscent of Rocky Mountain spotted fever.

• DIAGNOSIS AND DIFFERENTIAL DIAGNOSIS •

As with other rickettsioses, diagnosis is clinical, based on appropriate exposure history and a compatible clinical syndrome. Serologic studies (Proteus OX-K and fluorescent antibody tests) are helpful only in retrospect or well into the course and are often negative even then. The differential includes other rickettsioses, leptospirosis, *Flavivirus* infections (particularly dengue), typhoid fever, and, perhaps, infectious mononucleosis.

• TREATMENT AND CLINICAL COURSE •

Scrub typhus can be treated with either tetracyclines or chloramphenicol. Most cases of scrub typhus are benign, even if untreated, although recovery may require 2 to 3 weeks. Death may occur, usually as the result of volume depletion. With treatment, the course is shortened and mortality is extremely rare.

Rochalimaea Group

TRENCH FEVER (*ROCHALIMAEA QUINTANA*)

• PATHOGENESIS •

The principal reservoir of *R. quintana* is human. The disease has been seen chiefly in military populations during World Wars I and II, hence the name, trench fever. It is also endemic in Mexico, Eastern Europe, and parts of North Africa. Pockets of disease have been reported worldwide, usually in association with poverty and crowding. Transmission occurs when the infected vector, the body louse, defecates during feeding and organisms in the feces enter through abraded skin.

The disease is characterized by repeated or persistent bacteremia occurring for several weeks or months. Pathological studies are few, but the pathophysiology is thought to involve endothelial cell infection and damage, as in other rickettsioses.

• CLINICAL FEATURES •

Onset is sudden and the syndrome nonspecific: fever, myalgia (sometimes severe), headache, and malaise. These symptoms may last several days, after which the course is characterized by relapses of a similar syndrome occurring at about 5-day intervals.

Rash is not a prominent feature of this disease but may occur. Eruptions tend to be transient with faint erythematous macules, which can be easily missed.

• DIAGNOSIS AND DIFFERENTIAL DIAGNOSIS •

Unlike other rickettsiae, *Rochalimaea* can be cultured in vitro on artificial media. Thus, blood culture is an approach to diagnosis, particularly with newer culture methods, such as lysis-centrifugation. Serological studies include complement fixation and fluorescent antibody tests.

Differential diagnosis is broad and includes other rickettsioses, influenza, leptospirosis, tularemia, brucellosis, infectious mononucleosis, and typhoid fever. Malaria and relapsing fever are particularly suggested by the relapses of trench fever.

• TREATMENT AND CLINICAL COURSE •

Too few cases have been seen since World War II for definitive studies of antimicrobial therapy. Based on analogy to other rickettsioses and in vitro studies, both tetracyclines and chloramphenicol can be predicted to be effective clinically. The course is almost always benign, albeit temporarily debilitating, even if untreated. There are, however, reports of relapse years later in untreated patients.

BACILLARY ANGIOMATOSIS
(*ROCHALIMAEA HENSELAE* and *QUINTANA*)

• PATHOGENESIS •

For this syndrome, reservoirs and modes of transmission remain unclear. Cats have been implicated, but their relative importance is not fully established; nor is it known whether an insect vector plays any role. Distribution of the organisms is probably worldwide. At this time, *Rochalimaea henselae* is thought to be the predominant cause of bacillary angiomatosis, although *R. quintana* may cause the same syndrome.

These organisms produce a wide spectrum of diseases, including transient or persistent bacteremia, bacillary angiomatosis, peliosis, and cat-scratch fever. Bacillary angiomatosis is primarily a disease of immunocompromised hosts, particularly patients with AIDS. How the status of the immune system modulates clinical manifestations of the infection is unclear.

Lesions are characterized by proliferation of capillary-like vessels, which are lined by prominent and, sometimes, atypical endothelial cells. Inflammatory cells, principally neutrophils and lymphocytes, surround the vessels. Interstitial tissues contain granular material (on hematoxylin and eosin staining) which are revealed to be clumps of organisms by methenamine-silver or Warthin-Starry staining or electron microscopy.

• CLINICAL FEATURES •

Bacillary angiomatosis is typically seen in patients with AIDS. Lesions present abruptly or evolve slowly as cutaneous or subcutaneous lesions, singly or in large numbers. A typical lesion is an obviously vascular, reddish, glistening, superficial nodule less than 1 cm in diameter. However, varied appearances have been described: dry, scaly, plaque-like, pedunculated, large, flesh-colored, purple, or black (Fig. 10.13). The patient is usually febrile.

• DIAGNOSIS AND DIFFERENTIAL DIAGNOSIS •

Diagnosis is based on histopathology, including special stains (Warthin-Starry, methenamine-silver) or electron microscopy. Immunocytochemical and immunofluorescent techniques are being developed, as are serological methods. Organisms can be cultured from blood and tissue with special techniques, particularly lysis-centrifugation methods. Polymerase chain reaction amplification of bacterial DNA may be clinically useful.

Bacillary angiomatosis must be differentiated from Kaposi's sarcoma, from which it may be clinically indistinguishable. Bacillary angiomatosis also can resemble the cutaneous lesions of disseminated fungal infections (e.g., *Cryptococcus neoformans, Sporothrix schenckii, Histoplasma capsulatum*) and mycobacterial infections (e.g., *Mycobacterium avium* complex). *Bartonella bacilliformis* causes a very similar lesion, verruga peruana, that would only be encountered at certain altitudes in the Andes Mountains.

• TREATMENT AND CLINICAL COURSE •

Organisms are susceptible in vitro to many antimicrobials, but clinical experience is greatest with erythromycins and tetracyclines, which are the recommended agents. Oral therapy is usually successful but should be continued for 2 to 3 months, because relapse rates are otherwise high. Most patients respond quickly and satisfactorily.

Ehrlichiosis (*Ehrlichia chaffeensis*)

• PATHOGENESIS •

Ehrlichia species in humans cause a mononucleosis syndrome thus far recognized only in Japan (Sennetsu fever, *E. sennetsu*) and human ehrlichiosis primarily identified in the southeastern and south central parts of the United States (*E. chaffeensis*). It is presumed that ticks are the vector in human ehrlichiosis; whether there are other hosts is unknown.

Organisms infect neutrophils and lymphocytes, proliferate intracellularly, and then are released by rupture into the circulation. This alteration and destruction of leukocytes is the principal cause of the clinical syndrome. Pathologic studies are sparse.

• CLINICAL FEATURES •

Ehrlichiosis presents a syndrome practically indistinguishable from Rocky Mountain spotted fever, except in the nature of the rash. Patients develop fever, neurological symptoms (headache, confusion), gastrointestinal symptoms, myalgia, and arthralgia. Symptoms generally are milder than in Rocky Mountain spotted fever. The physical exam is usually remarkable only for fever and altered sensorium. Lymphopenia, neutropenia, thrombocytopenia, and anemia are prominent laboratory abnormalities.

A rash is present in no more than half the patients, occurs late in the course, and is usually subtle. Although petechiae can occur, lesions are typically maculopapular. In contrast to Rocky Mountain spotted fever, palms and soles are usually spared and the trunk is the predominant site involved.

• DIAGNOSIS AND DIFFERENTIAL DIAGNOSIS •

As with Rocky Mountain spotted fever, diagnosis is presumptive and based on the clinical syndrome, time of year, and history of potential exposure. Serologic confirmation can be obtained retrospectively. The differential diagnosis is identical to that of Rocky Mountain spotted fever.

• TREATMENT AND CLINICAL COURSE •

Ehrlichiosis is treated with doxycycline or another tetracycline for at least 1 week. Chloramphenicol is probably an acceptable alternative. The course is milder than Rocky Mountain spotted fever and prognosis is usually excellent. With treatment, symptoms resolve promptly. Some patients have had more severe courses, including renal and respiratory failure and disseminated intravascular coagulation.

ANNOTATED BIBLIOGRAPHY

Berman SJ, Kundin WD. Scrub typhus in South Vietnam: A study of 87 cases. Ann Intern Med 1973;79:26.
    Serologically identified cases in United States soldiers in Vietnam, many of whom were thought to have infectious mononucleosis.
Brettman LR, et al. Rickettsialpox: Report of an outbreak and a contemporary review. Medicine 1981;60:363.
    A report of five cases from New York City and a review of the literature.
Duma RJ, et al. Epidemic typhus in the United States associated with flying squirrels. JAMA 1981;245:2318.
    A report of seven sporadic cases in which the southern flying squirrel seemed to be the reservoir.
Font-Creus B, et al. Mediterranean spotted fever: A cooperative study of 227 cases. Rev Infect Dis 1985;7:635.
    A thorough review of many cases and a comprehensive view of the spectrum of disease.
Harkess J. Ehrlichiosis. Infect Dis Clin North Am 1991;5:37.
    A comprehensive review of the history and clinical features of this infection.

Harris RL, Kaplan SL, Bradshaw MW, Williams TW, Jr. Boutonneuse fever in American travelers. J Infect Dis 1986;153:126.

A reminder that modern travel allows patients to present with distantly acquired "exotic" diseases. African guide scoops United States infectious disease consultant (over the telephone, yet).

Helmick CG, Bernard KW, D'Angelo LJ. Rocky Mountain spotted fever: Clinical, laboratory, and epidemiologic features of 262 cases. J Infect Dis 1984;150:480.

A comprehensive review based on case reports submitted to the Centers for Disease Control and Prevention (CDCP).

Kirk JL, Fine DP, Sexton DJ, Muchmore HG. Rocky Mountain spotted fever: A clinical review based on 48 confirmed cases, 1943–1986. Medicine 1990;69:35.

Retrospective review focusing on clinical features of confirmed cases seen at a university medical center during 4 decades. Most patients were seen personally by the authors.

Koehler JE, Tappero JW. Bacillary angiomatosis and bacillary peliosis in patients infected with human immunodeficiency virus. Clin Infect Dis 1993;17:612.

A thorough review, including clear photographs of the varied presentations of cutaneous and internal lesions caused by *R. henselae* and *R. quintana* in patients with AIDS.

Stasko T, DeVillez RL. Murine typhus: A case report and review. J Am Acad Dermatol 1982;7:377.

A focus on dermatologic features.

Walker DH. Rickettsioses of the spotted fever group around the world. J Dermatol 1989;16:169.

Reviews of the rickettsioses with particular focus on skin manifestations.

Walker DH, Gay RM, Valdes-Dapena M. The occurrence of eschars in Rocky Mountain spotted fever. J Am Acad Dermatol 1981;4:571.

A report of two patients with the rare occurrence of eschar at the primary site of tick bite similar to the characteristic lesion (tache noire) of Mediterranean spotted fever.

Wei-tung L. Trench fever: A resume of literature and a note on some obscure phases of the disease. Chinese Med J 1984;97:179.

A thorough review of historical and clinical aspects. Speculations on the relationship of *R. quintana* to other rickettsiae.

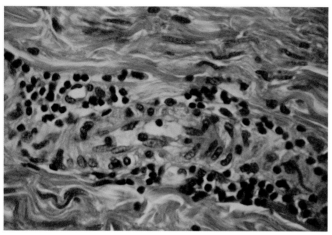

Figure 10.1. Rocky Mountain spotted fever. Histologic section of a skin biopsy showing perivascular inflammatory infiltrates and endothelial injury. (Courtesy of Dr. Harold G. Muchmore)

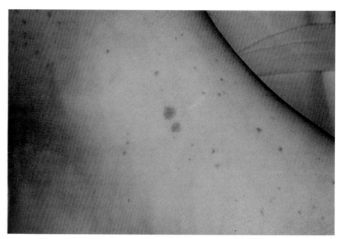

Figure 10.2. Rocky Mountain spotted fever. Early macular and petechial lesions. (Courtesy of Dr. Harold G. Muchmore)

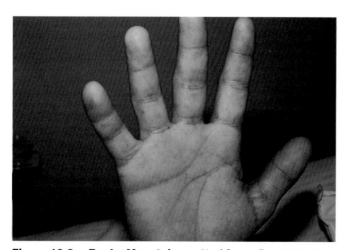

Figure 10.3. Rocky Mountain spotted fever. Petechial lesions of the palm. (Courtesy of Dr. Harold G. Muchmore)

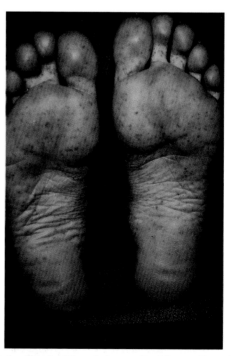

Figure 10.4. Rocky Mountain spotted fever. Purpuric macular lesions of the soles of the feet. (Courtesy of Dr. Harold E. Dascomb)

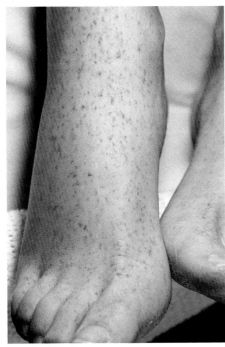

Figure 10.5. Rocky Mountain spotted fever. Petechial and reticular rash on the dorsum of the foot. (Courtesy of Dr. Gene Beyt)

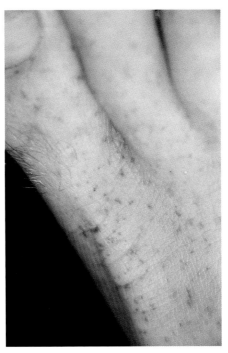

Figure 10.6. Rocky Mountain spotted fever. Close-up view of petechial eruption on the dorsum of the foot and toes. (Courtesy of Dr. Gene Beyt)

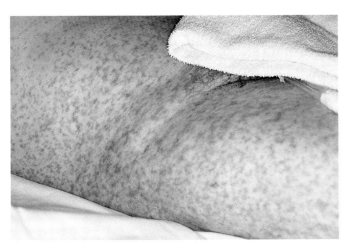

Figure 10.7. Rocky Mountain spotted fever. More extensive maculopapular and petechial lesions of the trunk and thigh. (Courtesy of Dr. Harold G. Muchmore)

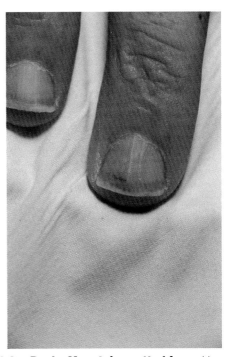

Figure 10.8. Rocky Mountain spotted fever. Linear petechial lesions of the nail bed. (Courtesy of Dr. Gene Beyt)

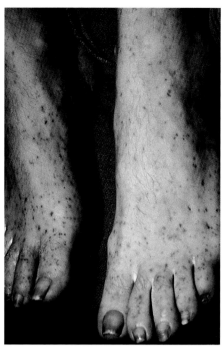

Figure 10.9.   Rocky Mountain spotted fever. Purpuric macu-lopapules of the dorsal aspect of the feet. (Courtesy of Dr. Harold E. Dascomb)

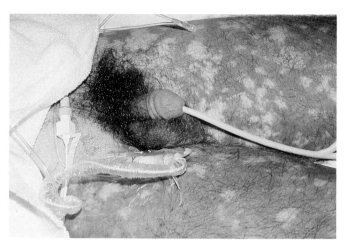

Figure 10.10.   Rocky Mountain spotted fever. Disseminated intravascular coagulopathy on the thighs.

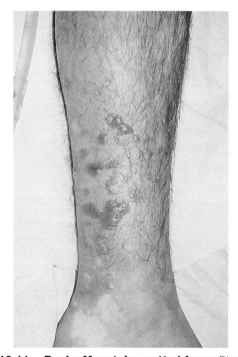

Figure 10.11.   Rocky Mountain spotted fever. Disseminated intravascular coagulopathy with bullous lesions on the leg.

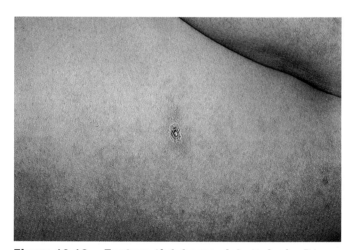

Figure 10.12.   Eastern tick-borne rickettsiosis. Primary eschar at the site of tick bite, more typical of eastern tick-borne rick-ettsioses than of Rocky Mountain spotted fever. (Courtesy of Dr. Harold G. Muchmore)

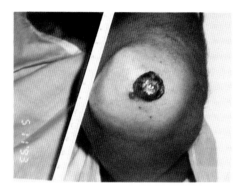

Figure 10.13. Bacillary angiomatous lesions on the elbow. The smaller lesion is more typical, a smooth, reddish, glistening, obviously vascular papule. The larger lesion is hyperkeratotic, drier, and polypoid. (Courtesy of Dr. Leonard N. Slater)

CHAPTER 11

Cutaneous Tuberculosis

DAVID S. FEINGOLD

Mycobacterium tuberculosis infection of the skin produces a variety of lesions which, unfortunately, are described and classified by many confusing terms. A far better way to classify cutaneous tuberculosis is based on the inoculation route, as shown in Table 11.1.

Effective prevention and therapy once suppressed the cutaneous manifestations of tuberculosis in the United States, but, in the era of AIDS, cutaneous tuberculosis is being seen again.

• PATHOGENESIS •

Exogenous Source

The findings of inoculation tuberculosis vary, depending on whether the host has or has not been infected previously with *M. tuberculosis.*

Primary inoculation tuberculosis (tuberculous chancre) occurs in patients who have not been infected previously. For infection to occur, the integrity of the epidermis must be violated, after which, the organisms multiply locally, and a lesion forms in 2 to 4 weeks. Regional lymphadenopathy is common. As tuberculin positivity develops, the process becomes more localized, akin to the development of a primary (Ghon) complex in pulmonary infection.

Healthcare workers and children exposed to tuberculous adults are especially susceptible to primary cutaneous tuberculosis, usually with involvement of the face or the distal parts of the extremities after trauma. As with pulmonary tuberculosis, most cases of primary inoculation tuberculosis are controlled by the host, with healing of the lesions. Progressive local disease or hematogenous spread is extremely unusual.

Exogenous postprimary inoculation tuberculosis (tuberculosis verrucosa cutis) occurs in persons who have been infected previously. Members of various occupational groups, such as pathologists and butchers, may be exposed to large numbers of *M. tuberculosis*, which may enter the skin after the person has developed hypersensitivity from primary exposure. These lesions demonstrate a verrucous skin growth and are rarely associated with regional adenopathy.

Table 11.1. Classification of Cutaneous Tuberculosis

Classification	Synonyms
A. Cutaneous tuberculosis from an exogenous source	
1. Primary inoculation	Tuberculosis chancre
	Tuberculosis primary complex
2. Post-primary inoculation	Tuberculosis verrucosa cutis
	Warty tuberculosis
	Verruca necrogenica
	Prosector's wart
B. Cutaneous tuberculosis from an endogenous source	
1. Contiguous spread	Scrofuloderma
	Tuberculosis colliquativa cutis
2. Autoinoculation	Orificial tuberculosis
	Tuberculosis cutis orificialis
	Tuberculosis ulcerosa cutis et
	mucosae
C. Cutaneous tuberculosis from hematogenous spread	
1. Lupus vulgaris	Tuberculosis luposa cutis
2. Acute hematogenous dissemination	Acute miliary tuberculosis of the skin
	Tuberculosis cutis miliaris disseminata
	Tuberculosis cutis acuta generalista
3. Nodules or abscesses	Metastatic tuberculosis abscess
	Tuberculous gumma

Adapted from Beyt BE, et al. Cutaneous mycobacteriosis. Medicine 1981;60:95.

Endogenous Source

Tuberculosis can spread directly to the skin from an adjacent focus, such as lymph nodes, bone, or even the epididymis, and is known in this form as scrofuloderma. Cervical lymphadenitis is by far the most common endogenous source for cutaneous spread. An uncommon endogenous form, orificial tuberculosis, occurs on mucous membranes or periorificial skin. Affected persons usually have advanced tuberculosis and shed large numbers of organisms onto the mucous membranes and skin of the oral, anal, or urethral regions.

Hematogenous Spread

Lupus vulgaris, the most common type of cutaneous tuberculosis, is clearly a postprimary form of skin tuberculosis, but the exact origin of the organism at that site remains less clear. It may follow tuberculous lymphadenitis or involvement of upper respiratory tract mucous membranes. From this author's experience and interpretation of the literature, however, the underlying focus of lupus vulgaris is not usually local; therefore, silent hematogenous spread must be assumed. In the course of primary pulmonary tuberculosis, organisms often disseminate hematogenously, with resultant widely scattered microscopic and macroscopic tuberculomas. Activation of these tuberculomas can produce many of the postprimary tuberculous infections, such as tuberculous meningitis, and probably lupus vulgaris as well.

Other hematogenous lesions are those of acute miliary tuberculosis, seen in infants and children with primary disease and in patients with various causes of immune deficiency. In another form of hematogenous dissemination, multiple tuberculous abscesses or nodules may form at the site of previous trauma.

• CLINICAL FEATURES •

Primary Inoculation (Tuberculous Chancre)

The initial lesion of primary inoculation cutaneous tuberculosis is a papule or nodule, usually in an exposed area at the site of trauma or another cutaneous disease. The lesion may evolve into a shallow, indolent, and usually painless ulcer (tuberculosis chancre) that can remain small or grow to several centimeters in diameter (Fig. 11.1). The base of the ulcer is sometimes studded with small abscesses and covered with a necrotic membrane resembling ecthyma. The edges become undermined and indurated. Prominent regional adenopathy occurs subsequently and is often the patient's presenting complaint.

This primary complex usually evolves slowly without systemic manifestations, but it may also develop rapidly, simulating pyogenic infection. If the skin papule or ulcer heals, adenopathy is left as the only sign of the infection. When adenopathy develops rapidly, the nodes may be tender, although ordinarily they are firm and painless. After months, the lymph nodes sometimes soften and form cold abscesses that may drain.

Postprimary Inoculation (Tuberculosis Verrucosa Cutis)

Postprimary exogenous infection, tuberculosis verrucosa cutis, most often occurs on the hands. The lesions begin as single or multiple small verrucous papules (Fig. 11.2). Slow peripheral extension results in red-brown hyperkeratotic plaques that may become deeply fissured, soften in the center, and drain purulent material. Regional adenopathy, prominent in primary inoculation disease, is not a feature of postprimary exogenous infection.

Contiguous Spread (Scrofuloderma)

Contiguous-spread cutaneous tuberculosis, or scrofuloderma, is often a bilateral process involving the lymph nodes of the neck. The firm, infected nodes often soften and liquefy, and they may drain watery or caseous material. Undermined ulcers often form along the chain of nodes. The lesions heal with scarring and hyperpigmentation; core-like keloidal scars may develop (Figs. 11.3–5).

Autoinoculation (Tuberculosis Cutis Orificialis)

This form is manifested clinically as papules that break down to yield irregular, painful, punched-out ulcers on mucous membranes or on skin adjacent to orifices. Traumatized areas are most susceptible, particularly the tip and lateral margins of the tongue, and occasionally the lips and palate, which can ulcerate. The lesions may be single or multiple; tenderness may result in dysphagia. Although it can occur secondary to gastrointestinal or urinary tract tuberculosis (Fig. 11.6), the lesion usually occurs during the course of severe pulmonary tuberculosis.

Lupus Vulgaris

The various clinical manifestations of lupus vulgaris include asymptomatic plaques, nodules, ulcers, scars, atrophy, and hypertrophic lesions. About 90% of cases occur on the head and neck. Lesions often begin as reddish-brown papules that evolve into plaques with elevated borders (Fig. 11.7). When blood is pressed out of a lesion with a glass slide (called "diascopy"), one may see small, yellow-brown "apple jelly" nodules (Figs. 11.8, 11.9). The center of the plaque often becomes atrophic or ulcerates and later heals with scarring, contractures, and mottled pigmentation (Fig. 11.10). Healing and extension occur simultaneously, resulting in plaques with a polycyclic configuration. Hypertrophic forms of the infection are marked by soft tumorous growths and hyperkeratotic changes. Ulceration and necrosis, destruction of mucous membranes and cartilage, and severe deformity occur (Figs. 11.11–13). In long-standing lesions, squamous-cell carcinoma may be a complication.

Acute Hematogenous Spread (Miliary Tuberculosis)

The various cutaneous lesions of acute miliary tuberculosis include disseminated papules, macules, and/or purpuric lesions. Hemorrhagic or necrotic vesicles may also occur when necrotizing vasculitis accompanies miliary tuberculosis. Nodules and subcutaneous abscesses may also arise from hematogenous dissemination. These lesions are generally nontender and fluctuant but may resemble an acute pyogenic infection (Fig. 11.14).

• DIAGNOSIS AND DIFFERENTIAL DIAGNOSIS •

Diagnosis of cutaneous tuberculosis is facilitated by the availability of tissue for direct examination by smear, culture, and biopsy. The presence of acid-fast bacilli in drainage or tissue is highly suggestive. In patients with good cellular immunity, such as those with lupus vulgaris, organisms are usually too sparse to identify by direct examination; therefore, culture is required to confirm *M. tuberculosis*. Several approaches to rapid and specific diagnosis of *M. tuberculosis* infection using cDNA probes with amplification by polymerase chain reaction have been used recently. In the near future, these molecular genetic methods will be important diagnostic procedures for cutaneous tuberculosis.

Early in primary infections, histology may reveal only banal inflammation, but as delayed hypersensitivity develops, the typical picture of granulomatous inflammation evolves.

The primary complex of inoculation tuberculosis must be distinguished from other chronic infectious inoculation syndromes, including nontuberculous mycobacterial disease, syphilis, cat-scratch disease, and tularemia. Cutaneous nontuberculous mycobacterial disease or sporotrichosis can be confused microscopically with primary cutaneous tuberculosis, but special stains and cultures for organism identification will be definitive. A syphilitic chancre can be confirmed by dark-field identification of spirochetes, serologic studies, and a prominence of plasma cells in the biopsy specimen. Cat-scratch disease and tularemia cause impressive overt systemic signs and symptoms not seen with cutaneous tuberculosis. Additionally, in cat-scratch disease, the primary lesion is rarely impressive; adenopathy may be more generalized; and the Warthin-Starry silver stain may reveal causative bacteria in lymph node biopsy specimens. The primary lesions of tularemia develop more rapidly than those of tuberculosis, and the history and serological test will identify tularemia.

Postprimary inoculation cutaneous tuberculosis (tuberculosis verrucosa cutis) may be confused with verruca vulgaris, keratoses (seborrheic and actinic), infections (blastomycosis, chromomycosis, and chronic pyoderma), and some skin diseases (hypertrophic lichen planus and hypertrophic lupus erythematosus). Unfortunately, biopsy may show only pseudoepitheliomatous hyperplasia, hyperkeratosis, and dense mononuclear inflammation, often without typical tubercles or acid-fast organisms. If the location of the lesion, the history, or the histological test does not suggest the diagnosis, then fungal, bacterial, and mycobacterial cultures will be pivotal.

If tuberculous lymphadenitis is present, then scrofuloderma (tuberculosis spread from a contiguous source) can occur in the overlying skin. The differential diagnosis includes nontuberculous mycobacterial infection, cervical actinomycosis, sporotrichosis or blastomycosis, acne conglobata, hidradenitis suppurativa, and subacute pyogenic lymphadenitis with sinus tract formation. Appropriate cultures are essential to differentiate these disorders.

In patients with pulmonary tuberculosis, painful oral or circumoral ulcers are suggestive of orificial tuberculosis. The finding of acid-fast bacilli in biopsy specimens supports the diagnosis, which should then be confirmed by culture. Aphthae, herpes simplex stomatitis, mucous patches of secondary syphilis, and neoplastic ulcers may be confused with orificial tuberculosis.

Because the clinical picture of lupus vulgaris is so variable, many entities are included in the differential diagnosis. The following conditions may look similar to lupus vulgaris, but they have distinctive histologic appearances: discoid lupus erythematosus, granuloma faciale, benign lymphocytic infiltrate, radiodermatitis, and Bowen's disease. The following may occur on the face and resemble lupus vulgaris both clinically and histologically: sarcoidosis, blastomycosis, tertiary cutaneous syphilis (gumma), and chronic vegetating pyoderma. Sarcoidosis is probably the most difficult to differentiate from lupus vulgaris. A positive culture for *M. tuberculosis* or a therapeutic response to antituberculous therapy is definitive. A negative tuberculin test in the absence of anergy effectively rules out lupus vulgaris. For a complete differential diagnosis of all clinical types, see Table 11.2.

Several cutaneous syndromes called tuberculids have been considered to be "tuberculous-associated." The best described of these are erythema induratum, papulonecrotic tuberculid, and lichen scrofulosorum. They will not be considered in this chapter.

• TREATMENT AND CLINICAL COURSE •

Standard antituberculous therapy is effective for cutaneous tuberculosis. Prolonged therapy with a least two agents is always indicated. Excision of caseous foci, such as may occur in a cluster of submandibular nodes, can be helpful. Plastic surgery may ameliorate disfigurements, such as the scarring seen in lupus vulgaris.

The course of cutaneous tuberculosis varies according to clinical type, amount of inoculum, extent of infection elsewhere, age of the patient, host immunity, and appropriateness of therapy. Primary inoculation lesions usually heal within 1 year, but they may proceed to lupus vulgaris, or, rarely, to miliary tuberculosis. Postprimary inoculation lesions usually extend slowly without treatment, but they may also remain relatively stable or heal spontaneously. These lesions usually respond well to antituberculous therapy. Although healing slowly and with scarring, scrofuloderma also responds well to therapy. Orificial tuberculosis usually is a symptom of advanced internal disease having an unfavorable prognosis. The same is true in hematogenous spread, especially in children, although some cases are successfully treated. Lupus vulgaris, unless treated continuously, is likely to recur for years. Despite periods of relative inactivity, this chronic disease leads to considerable scarring and disfigurement.

ANNOTATED BIBLIOGRAPHY

Beyt BE, Jr, et al. Cutaneous mycobacteriosis: Analysis of 34 cases with a new classification of the disease. Medicine 1981;60:95.
  Review of a 10-year experience at a large teaching hospital (includes nontuberculous mycobacteria), and presentation of a classification of the disease.
Brown FS, Anderson RH, Burnett JW. Cutaneous tuberculosis. J Am Acad Dematol 1982;6:101.
  A case of disseminated tuberculosis with cutaneous and pulmonary involvement in an immunocompetent patient.
Kakahel KU, Fritsch P. Cutaneous tuberculosis, Review. Int J Dermatol 1989;28:355.
  Brief review of diagnosis, histopathology, clinical manifestations, and treatment of cutaneous tuberculosis with a discussion of associated complications and problems in classification.

Table 11.2. Differential Diagnosis of Cutaneous Tuberculosis

Classification	Differential Diagnosis	Diagnosis
Primary inoculation	Nontuberculous mycobacterial infections	Biopsy, special stains and culture
Postprimary inoculation	Primary syphilis	Dark-field microscopy, serologic tests for syphilis
	Sporotrichosis	Biopsy, special stains and culture
	North American blastomycosis	Biopsy, special stains and culture
	Histoplasmosis	Biopsy, special stains and culture
	Coccidiodomycosis	Biopsy, special stains and culture
	Mycetoma	Biopsy, special stains and culture
	Leishmaniasis	Travel history, biopsy, special stains and culture
	Vegetating pyoderma	Gram's stain and culture
	Cat-scratch disease	History, biopsy, Warthin-Starry stain and culture
	Tularemia	History, biopsy, serum agglutinins for *Francisella tularensis*
	Chromomycosis	Biopsy, culture
	Bromoderma and iododerma	History, biopsy
	Verruca vulgaris	Biopsy
	Actinic or seborrheic keratosis	Biopsy
	Keratoacanthoma	Biopsy
	Squamous-cell carcinoma	Biopsy
Contiguous spread	Actinomycosis	Biopsy, special stains and culture
	Nocardiosis	Biopsy, special stains and culture
	Sporotrichosis	Biopsy, special stains and culture
	Blastomycosis	Biopsy, special stains and culture
	Tertiary syphilis	Biopsy, silver stain, serologic test for syphilis
	Lymphogranuloma venereum	Biopsy, serologic test (complement fixation)
	Tularemia	History, serum agglutinins for *Francisella tularensis*
	Hidradenitis suppurativa	Clinical presentation, negative culture
Autoinoculation	Secondary syphilis	Biopsy, serologic test for syphilis
	Tertiary syphilis	Biopsy, serologic test for syphilis
	Chancroid	Biopsy, culture
	Lymphogranuloma venereum	Biopsy, serologic test (complement fixation)
	Herpes simplex	Direct fluorescent antibody test, culture
	Aphthous stomatitis	Clinical presentation, negative cultures
	Squamous-cell carcinoma	Biopsy
	Histoplasmosis	Biopsy, special stains and culture
Lupus vulgaris	Lupus erythematosus	Biopsy, immunofluorescence, ANA[a] profile
	Secondary syphilis	Biopsy, serologic test for syphilis
	Acne vulgaris	Clinical presentation
	Rosacea	Clinical presentation
	Seborrheic dermatitis	Clinical presentation
	Tinea corporis	Wet preparation, fungal culture
	Leprosy	Biopsy
	Sarcoidosis	Biopsy
	North American blastomycosis	Biopsy, special stains and culture
	Bromoderma & iododerma	History, biopsy
	Vegetating pyoderma	Gram's stain and culture
Acute hematogenous dissemination	Any septic process	Biopsy and culture
Nodules or abscesses	Bacterial infection	Gram's stain and culture
	Fungal infection	Biopsy, special stain and culture
	Infected epidermal cysts	Biopsy
	Ecthyma	Gram's stain and culture
	Nodulocystic acne	Clinical presentation, negative cultures
	Tertiary syphilis	Biopsy, serologic test for syphilis
	Sporotrichosis	Biopsy, special stains and culture
	Nontuberculous mycobacterial infection	Biopsy, special stains and culture
	Hidradenitis suppurativa	Clinical presentation, negative cultures

[a]ANA, antinuclear antibody

Savin JA. Mycobacterial infections. In: Champion RN, Burton JL, Ebling FJG, eds. Textbook of Dermatology. Vol 1. 5th ed. London: Blackwell Scientific Publications, 1992:1033.

Review of epidemiology, necrotic reactions, histopathology, clinical manifestations, diagnosis, and treatment of tuberculosis of the skin, and the implications of BCG vaccination, tuberculin testing, and ethnicity.

Sehgal V, Wagh SA. Cutaneous tuberculosis: Current concepts. Int J Dermatol 1990;29:237.

An excellent review.

Tomecki KJ, Hall GS. Tuberculosis of the skin. In: Demis DJ, ed. Clinical Dermatology. Vol 3; Section 16-26. Philadelphia: JB Lippincott, 1989:1.

Review of and update on the history, classification, pathogenesis, epidemiology, clinical manifestations, histology, microbiology, immunology, and treatment of cutaneous tuberculosis.

Weissler JC. Southwestern Internal Medicine Conference: Tuberculosis—Immunopathogenesis and Therapy. Tuberculosis 1993;305(1):52.

General discussion of the "new" epidemiology of tuberculosis and therapeutic issues.

Wolff K, Tappeinen G. Mycobacterial diseases: Tuberculosis and atypical mycobacterial infections. In: Fitzpatrick TB, et al. Dermatology in general medicine. 3rd ed. New York: McGraw-Hill, 1987:2152.

Extensive review that includes clinical manifestations, pathogenesis, histopathology, and diagnostic aspects, and a discussion of tuberculoids. Large bibliography includes older literature and historical aspects.

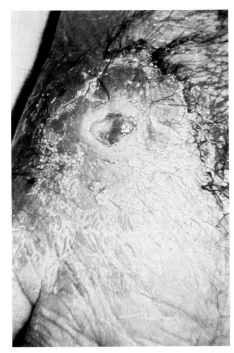

Figure 11.1.   Primary inoculation tuberculosis (tuberculosis chancre). Ulceration on the dorsum of the hand as a result of primary exposure and infection from *M. tuberculosis.* No progressive disease occurred.

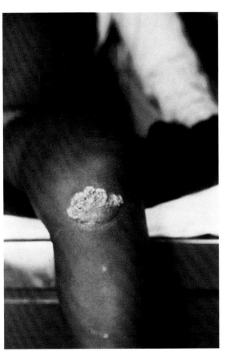

Figure 11.2.   Postprimary inoculation tuberculosis (tuberculosis verrucosa cutis). Verrucous papules and plaques on the knee of a child with previous primary tuberculosis infection.

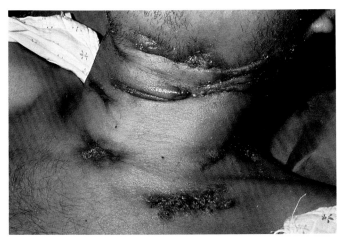

Figure 11.3.   Contiguous spread tuberculosis (scrofuloderma). Chronic sinus tracts of the neck from infected lymph nodes and subsequent cord-like keloidal scarring. (Courtesy of Dr. Lee T. Nesbitt, Jr.)

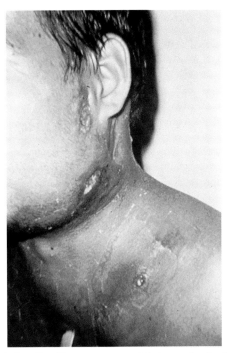

Figure 11.4.   Contiguous spread tuberculosis (scrofuloderma). Swollen cervical lymph nodes with draining sinus tracts and ulceration.

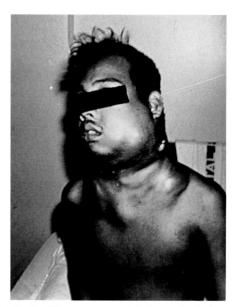

Figure 11.5. Contiguous spread tuberculosis (scrofuloder-ma). Tremendous cervical lymphadenopathy with impending sinus tract formation.

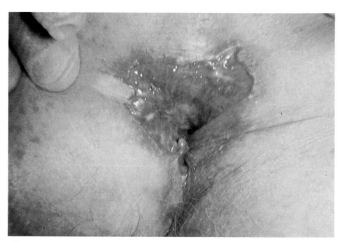

Figure 11.6.   Autoinoculation tuberculosis (tuberculosis cutis orificialis). Ulceration of perianal area secondary to gastrointestinal tract involvement. Similar lesions can occur in or around the oral cavity.

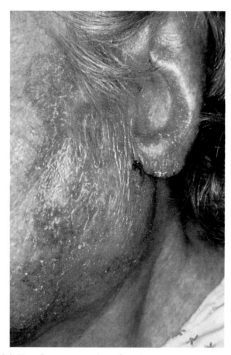

Figure 11.7.   Lupus vulgaris. Erythematous and indurated plaques on the ear and cheek. Note the reddish-brown color of the lesion.

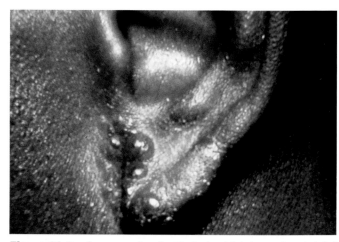

Figure 11.8.   Lupus vulgaris. Typical reddish-brown "apple jelly" papules on the earlobe of patient with early lupus vulgaris.

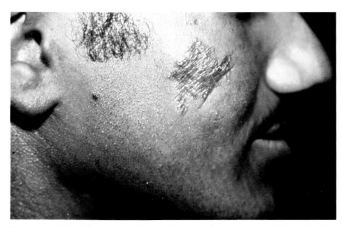

Figure 11.9. Lupus vulgaris. Early lesion on cheek with yellowish-brown "apple jelly" plaques.

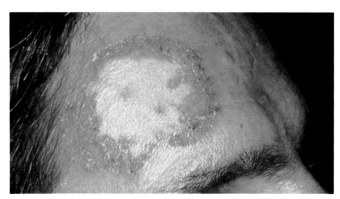

Figure 11.10. Lupus vulgaris. Atrophic, scarred plaque on forehead with active involvement at margins of lesion.

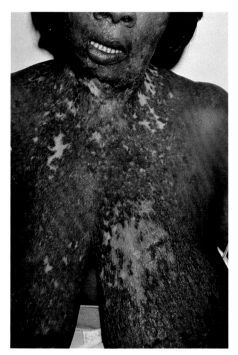

Figure 11.11. Lupus vulgaris. Extensive involvement of neck and chest with erythema, pigmentary changes, and atrophic scarring. The changes resemble disseminated discoid lupus erythematosus. (Courtesy of Dr. Lee T. Nesbitt, Jr.)

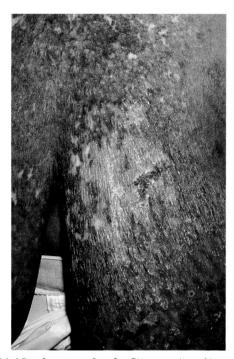

Figure 11.12. Lupus vulgaris. Close-up view of breast lesion in Figure 11.11, showing erythema and atrophic scarring along with pigmentary abnormalities. (Courtesy of Dr. Lee T. Nesbitt, Jr.)

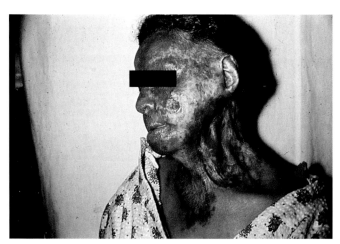

Figure 11.13.   Lupus vulgaris. Extensive scarring of neck and face in a long-standing recurrent lesion.

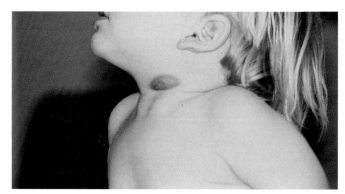

Figure 11.14.   Miliary tuberculosis. Lesion of neck from hematogenous dissemination in child with primary tuberculosis.

CHAPTER 12

Cutaneous Signs of Nontuberculous Mycobacteria

BRIAN D. LEE and DONALD L. GREER

Species of mycobacteria have been classified in the order Actinomycetales, family Mycobacteriaceae, and genus *Mycobacterium*. They are environmental saprophytes that are nonmotile, nonsporulating, obligate, aerobic, Gram-positive, elongated pleomorphic rods.

Infection with these organisms most commonly produces pulmonary infection in the elderly, cervical lymphadenopathy in children, or disseminated disease in immunosuppressed patients. Infection of the skin, soft tissues, lymph nodes, bone, eye, and heart have been described. In 1959, Runyon proposed a working classification of these organisms based on rates of growth and response of the culture to light. A modified Runyon classification is presented in Table 12.1. The spectrum of disease caused by these organisms is presented in Table 12.2.

The mycobacteria responsible for most cutaneous disease include *Mycobacterium marinum, M. ulcerans, M. fortuitum, M. chelonae,* and *M. avium-intracellulare*. Cutaneous disease may be acquired by inoculation, either traumatically or iatrogenically; may be contiguous with underlying osteomyelitis or lymphadenitis; or may be secondary to disseminated disease. Numerous clinical lesions have been described, including pustules, hyperkeratotic plaques, suppurative and nonsuppurative

Table 12.1 Modified Runyon Classification

Groups	Clinically Significant Species
I. Photochromogens (yellow color on light exposure)	*M. kansasii* *M. marinum*
II. Scotochromogens (yellow color in the dark)	*M. scrofulaceum*
III. Nonphotochromogens (nonpigmented)	*M. avium* *M. intracellulare* *M. ulcerans* *M. haemophilum*
IV. Rapid growers (colony formation in 5 to 7 days)	*M. fortuitum* *M. chelonae*

Table 12.2 Spectrum of Disease with Nontuberculous Mycobacteria

Disease	Most Common Species
Chronic pulmonary disease adults	*M. avium* complex *M. kansasii* *M. fortuitum* complex
Lymphadenitis (children)	*M. scrofulaceum* *M. avium* complex

Skin and soft tissue
  Swimming pool granuloma
  Sporotrichoid
	
	M. marinum
	M. marinum
	M. kansasii

Abscess	*M. fortuitum* complex
Buruli ulcers	*M. ulcerans*
Skeletal	*M. kansasii*
Bone, tendon, joints	*M.. avium* complex
Postsurgical infection (mammoplasty)	*M. fortuitum* complex
Laparotomy, other type of surgery	*M. fortuitum* complex
Disseminated infection	*M. avium* complex *M. fortuitum* complex *M. kansasii*
Keratitis	*M. fortuitum* complex
Endocarditis	*M. fortuitum* complex
Lymphadenitis	*M. fortuitum* complex

nodules, sporotrichoid-pattern nodules, ulcers, and draining sinuses.

Pathogenic nontuberculous mycobacteria are not usually transmitted from person to person. These environmental saprophytes are found in soil, animal and human feces, human skin and sputum, lakes, rivers, swimming pools, aquariums, domestic water supplies, and vegetation. Entry is usually by direct inoculation, but may be by ingestion or inhalation. In most instances, it is not known what allows these microorganisms to become pathogenic.

Most infections of the skin are caused by *M. marinum* in immunocompetent patients. Localized skin involvement is also not uncommon in healthy persons infected with *M. chelonae*, *M. fortuitum*, *M. kansasii*, and *M. scrofulaceum* from surgery, puncture wounds, or accidental inoculation. Other nontuberculous mycobacterial cutaneous infections occur in immunocompromised persons, particularly transplant recipients on immunosuppressive drugs and patients with AIDS, often as part of disseminated disease involving predominantly the lungs, lymph nodes, joints, and bones.

In summary, although immunosuppression facilitates dissemination of the disease to the skin, and skin lesions can be a sign of disseminated disease, it should be kept in mind that primary cutaneous disease is not uncommon with many species of mycobacteria.

• PATHOGENESIS AND CLINICAL FEATURES •

Mycobacterium Marinum

M. marinum, a Runyon group I mycobacteria, causes cutaneous disease more frequently than any other nontuberculous mycobacteria. Primary cutaneous infection is acquired after trauma while in contact with either salt water or water from lakes, rivers, swimming pools, or aquariums (Fig. 12.1).

After an incubation period of 2 to 8 weeks, the primary lesion begins as a violaceous papule, or a scaly, verrucous, or ulcerated plaque most commonly on the hands, feet, elbows, or knees (Figs. 12.2–12.6). Occasionally, a sporotrichoid pattern of nodules, which may suppurate and drain, develops along the lymphatics of an extremity (Figure 12.7). Regional lymph nodes occasionally become enlarged but do not break down. Sometimes penetration to underlying structures (bursa and joints) occurs (Figure 12.8). Disseminated cutaneous disease has been reported in an HIV-positive patient with *M. marinum* cultured from blood, bone marrow, skin, and bronchial secretions (1).

Mycobacterium Fortuitum Complex

The *Mycobacterium fortuitum* complex includes the species *M. fortuitum* and *M. chelonae*. They are ubiquitous in the environment and have been isolated from water, milk, soil, dust, fish, dogs, frogs, cows, and the saliva of healthy humans. These organisms are classified by Runyon as type IV rapid growers, based on their rapid growth in culture. The incidence of infection by these two organisms is roughly equal, and they are second only to *M. marinum* for causing cutaneous infections in the United States.

Disease can be cutaneous, systemic, or both. Systemic involvement from these organisms includes pneumonia, osteomyelitis contiguous from soft tissue infection, lymphadenitis, bacteremia, mastoiditis, meningitis, keratitis, corneal ulceration, hepatitis, synovitis, and prosthetic valve endocarditis.

Cutaneous lesions may occur in three settings. Postoperative wound infections have been described after augmentation mammoplasty, median sternotomy, and percutaneous catheter place-

ment. One cluster of postoperative infections was traced to a contaminated gentian violet marking solution (2). Primary cutaneous infections have also been reported after injections of vaccines and insulin. Traumatic abrasions constitute the second setting for primary, localized cutaneous infections in immunocompetent patients. A third group are immunocompromised patients with disseminated disease involving the skin without an identifiable source of primary infection.

The incubation period for postoperative and postraumatic infections ranges from 3 weeks to 12 months, most commonly 4 to 6 weeks. Primary cutaneous disease usually presents as a localized area of cellulitis with multiple draining abscesses that are minimally tender (Figure 12.9). The drainage is usually thin and watery. Cutaneous manifestations of disseminated disease include multiple soft tissue abscesses without a history of skin trauma, primarily involving the extremities.

The natural history of these infections is that of chronicity and slow healing, even with treatment. Spontaneous resolution occurs in 10% to 20% of cutaneous infections in an average of 8 months.

Mycobacterium Avium-Intracellulare (MAI) Complex

Mycobacterium avium and *M. intracellulare* are closely related organisms found throughout the world. They have been isolated from many environmental sources, including soil, fresh water, sea water, dairy products, animal tissue, house dust, dry plants, and bedding. The usual portal of entry for human infection is the respiratory tract, and the most common form of disease in children is chronic pulmonary infection. Less frequently, the organism produces osteomyelitis or cervical lymphadenitis with sinus formation, clinically indistinguishable from scrofuloderma. Although disseminated disease may occur in immunocompetent patients, it occurs most frequently in hosts who are immunosuppressed from malignant disease or medications. Disseminated MAI infection usually results in diffuse involvement of the reticuloendothelial system with disease in lymph nodes, bone marrow, liver, and spleen.

Cutaneous involvement in MAI infection can occur under three circumstances. First, it may represent a primary infection following traumatic inoculation, but this is very rare. Second, cutaneous involvement may complicate cervical adenitis with the development of scrofuloderma-like draining sinuses. Third, skin infection may occur as a manifestation of disseminated disease, a situation becoming more prevalent in patients with AIDS.

The morphology of cutaneous infection with MAI includes ulcerations, pustular lesions, suppurative nodules, draining sinuses, soft tissue induration, and infiltrative erythematous plaques. Oral ulcers have also been reported.

Mycobacterium Kansasii

This organism has been found in tap water and in wild and domestic animals, but its natural reservoir is unknown. The disease is endemic in Texas, Louisiana, California, the Chicago area, and Japan.

The most common presentation by *Mycobacterium kansasii* is a pulmonary infection in elderly men with chronic underlying pulmonary disease, such as silicosis or emphysema. It frequently disseminates in those with impaired cellular immunity, affecting the skin, lymph nodes, and musculoskeletal system. Musculoskeletal involvement has included synovitis, arthritis, carpal tunnel syndrome, fasciitis, and osteomyelitis.

Patients with disseminated disease have fever, constitutional symptoms, pulmonary involvement, hepatosplenomegaly, leukopenia, or pancytopenia. Dissemination appears to be not uncommon in patients with hairy cell leukemia.

Primary skin infections caused by *M. kansasii* are rare—only 9 cases were reported in the literature as of August, 1991. Three of these were renal transplant patients who had received immunosuppressive chemotherapy. A fourth patient demonstrated marked impairment of cell-mediated immunity. Three of these four immunosuppressed patients also had extracutaneous foci of *M. kansasii* (3). The route of infection in these cases was usually through minor trauma, such as a puncture wound.

The clinical appearance of *M. kansasii* skin lesions varies widely. Crusted ulcers, verrucous nodules exhibiting a sporotrichoid pattern, granulomatous plaques, necrotic papulopustules, and cellulitis have been described.

Mycobacterium Scrofulaceum

This Runyon group II organism has been isolated from tap water, soil, and other environmental sources. The infection occurs mainly in children between 1 and 3 years of age. Scrofulodermatous skin lesions caused by *M. scrofulaceum* now far outnumber such lesions produced by *M. tuberculosis* in children.

The portal of entry is most commonly the oropharynx, resulting in a cervical lymphadenitis that quickly ruptures to form draining sinus tracts. The submandibular or maxillary nodes are usually involved, in contrast to the tonsilar and anterior cervical nodes involved in *M. tuberculosis*. These patients exhibit no constitutional symptoms, and the disease is benign and self-limited.

Less commonly, traumatic inoculation of an extremity can result in inguinal or epitrochlear lymphadenitis. Pulmonary infections also occur occasionally in elderly patients with underlying malignant disease, and their skin may be involved in disseminated disease.

Mycobacterium Haemophilum

Mycobacterium haemophilum infects the skin and underlying tissues because of its propensity for growth in a cooler environment. Cutaneous infection caused by *M. haemophilum* is rare, however, except in AIDS patients. When AIDS patients develop disseminated disease that reveals acid-fast organisms, *M. haemophilum* infection should be suspected, especially if the organism fails to grow on standard media (Löwenstein-Jensen or H-1011). Cutaneous nodules or ulcerations may also occur

in renal transplant patients. The infections may be localized or disseminated.

Mycobacterium Ulcerans

Mycobacterium ulcerans causes chronic cutaneous ulceration in Africa, Australia, and Papua-New Guinea. The portal of entry is usually a small puncture wound such as that caused by thorny plants. After an incubation period of about 3 months, a painless subcutaneous swelling develops. The swelling enlarges and eventually ulcerates, producing a deeply undermined ulcer through which necrotic fat is discharged. The disease is most commonly found on the extremities of young adults, although lesions may occur anywhere on the body. The lesion is painless and the patient feels well. The condition may persist for months and years and then heal spontaneously.

• DIAGNOSIS AND DIFFERENTIAL DIAGNOSIS •

Biopsy material from the margin of the cutaneous lesion should be submitted for both culture and histopathology with special stains for mycobacteria. The laboratory should be notified that nontuberculous mycobacteria are suspected because of the special culture requirements for these organisms with regard to incubation temperatures, media, and length of culture. Specimens should not be brought into contact with saline solutions, as this may result in false-negative results.

Mycobacterioses can be clinically, radiologically, and histologically indistinguishable from tuberculosis. The diagnosis of opportunistic mycobacterial disease is made bacteriologically; only culture procedures can unequivocally determine the species responsible. Histopathology and special stains can only make a presumptive diagnosis of nontuberculous mycobacterial infection.

The histopathologic picture in nontuberculous mycobacteriosis may include nonspecific acute and chronic inflammation, suppuration, abscess formation, or tuberculoid granulomas with or without caseation. The presence or absence of acid-fast bacilli is dependent on the tissue reaction. A suppurative lesion is more likely to harbor acid-fast organisms than a tuberculoid granuloma. Acid-fast bacilli may also be identified in the necrotic centers of granulomas. Sporotricoid nodules in the first few weeks show tuberculoid granulomas and a lack of acid-fast bacilli.

The histopathology of *M. ulcerans* is distinctive, showing extensive areas of subcutaneous necrosis characterized by ghost outlines of tissue structures. Fat cells are enlarged, without nuclei. Acid-fast organisms are found in the necrotic tissue but not in areas of granuloma formation.

The usual stain for mycobacteria is the Ziehl-Neelsen acid-fast stain. Slide preparations must be closely scanned with an oil immersion objective. The nontuberculous mycobacteria appears slightly larger than *M. tuberculosis* and may show transverse striations.

The species identification of nontuberculous mycobacteria from culture depends on growth rates, optimal temperature of growth, colony photoreactivity, biochemical properties, and growth inhibition tests; the role of colony morphology is limited. Freshly isolated strains may show smooth colonies whereas strains stored in the laboratory may show rough colonies. Cultures should be examined at 3 and 7 days and weekly thereafter for 6 to 8 weeks. Rapidly growing organisms, including *M. chelonae*, *M. fortuitum*, and many other saprophytic species, will commonly produce visible colonies in less than 1 week. However, *M. fortuitum* does not always grow rapidly, at times requiring up to 12 weeks before identification is possible. Other species grow in approximately 3 weeks.

The majority of *Mycobacterium* species can be grown at 35°–37°C. However, *M. ulcerans*, *M. haemophilum*, *M. marinum*, and some varieties of *M. chelonae* and *M. fortuitum* grow best at temperatures of 30°–32°C. All suspected specimens should be incubated at 35°–37°C and also at 32°C. Additionally, laboratories should be notified if *M. haemophilum* is suspected because this organism requires hemin or ferric ammonium citrate in the culture medium.

The extensive differential diagnosis of these infections includes tuberculosis, leprosy, syphilis, leishmaniasis, mycoses, verrucae, and bacterial infections. Noninfectious diseases, including sarcoidosis, panniculitis, vasculitis, and carcinomas of the skin should also be considered.

Sporotrichoid clinical presentations from mycobacterial disease may be caused by *M. marinum*, *M. kansasii*, *M. scrofulaceum*, and *M. chelonae*, in addition to *M. tuberculosis*. Sporotrichosis and other primary inoculation complex infections must be considered.

Differential diagnosis of enlarged and draining cervical lymph nodes includes cat-scratch disease, infectious mononucleosis, mumps, parotid disease, branchial cleft cysts, lymphoma, and metastatic tumors. Mycobacterial diseases producing a scrofulodermatous appearance may be caused by *M. scrofulaceum*, *M. intracellulare*, *M. kansasii*, and *M. fortuitum*, in addition to *M. tuberculosis*.

The differential diagnosis of *M. ulcerans* in the nodular stage includes foreign-body granuloma, panniculitis, vasculitis, epidermal cyst, or appendageal tumor. In the ulcerative stage, the differential diagnosis includes deep fungal infection, pyoderma gangrenosum, suppurative panniculitis, and squamous cell carcinoma.

• TREATMENT AND CLINICAL COURSE •

The choice of chemotherapeutic agents in nontuberculous mycobacterial infections should be guided by in vitro sensitivity results, but in vivo response does not always parallel these sensitivities. Some *Mycobacterium* species are poorly sensitive to chemotherapeutic agents; therefore, surgical management must be an important part of their treatment.

Minocycline or other tetracyclines are often considered the drugs of first choice for the treatment of *M. marinum* infections. Alternatives are the antituberculous drugs, including rifampin, and other antibiotics such as trimethoprim-sulfamethoxazole and clarithromycin. Surgical management may be needed in some instances.

When feasible, surgical treatment of *M. avium-intracellulare* infection is advisable because the organisms are poorly responsive to chemotherapeutic agents. If the extent of disease does not allow curative surgery, combination therapy with antituberculous drugs is suggested. Some authorities recommend combinations of clarithromycin, rifampin, ethambutol, and clofazimine as drugs of first choice. Alternative drugs include ciprofloxacin, amikacin, azithromycin, ethionamide, cycloserine, rifabutin, and imipenem.

Multi-drug regimens have been of value in the treatment of *M. kansasii* infections. Isoniazid and rifampin with or without ethambutol or streptomycin are considered first-line drugs; alternative drugs include ethionamide and cycloserine. Both localized skin disease and cervical lymphadenitis require surgical excision. The therapeutic outcome in nondisseminated disease is satisfactory, but the course of disseminated disease is often uncertain in spite of intensive therapy.

Mycobacterium fortuitum and *M. chelonae* infections usually require aggressive surgical therapy. Excision, debridement, or incision and drainage is usually combined with chemotherapeutic regimens that include combinations of amikacin, doxycycline, cefoxitin, rifampin, erythromycin, and sulfonamides. Conventional antituberculous drugs have no significant activity against these rapidly growing mycobacteria.

Mycobacterium scrofulaceum is not very sensitive to antituberculous drugs. The treatment of choice for cutaneous lymph node disease is surgical excision. For more widespread disease, combinations of antituberculous drugs are used until results from sensitivity tests are available.

REFERENCES

1. Fitzpatrick TB, et al, eds. Dermatology in general medicine. 4th ed. New York: McGraw-Hill, 1993:2671.
2. Safranek TJ, et al. *Mycobacterium chelonae* wound infections after plastic surgery employing contaminated gentian violet skin-marking solution. N Engl J Med 1987;317:197.
3. Hanke CW, Temofeew RK, Slama SL. *Mycobacterium kansasii* infection with multiple cutaneous lesions. J Am Acad Dermatol 1987;16(5):1122.

ANNOTATED BIBLIOGRAPHY

Balows A, et al, eds. Laboratory diagnosis of infectious diseases. New York: Springer-Verlag, 1988:382.
   An excellent chapter on laboratory techniques used to isolate and differentiate nontuberculous mycobacteria.
Blauvelt A, Kerdel F. Widespread primary cutaneous infection with *Mycobacterium fortuitum*. Int J Dermatol 1993;32:512.
   A case report and discussion of the histology and treatment of this infection.
Hanke CW, Temofeew RK, Slama SL. *Mycobacterium kansasii* infection with multiple cutaneous lesions. J Am Acad Dermatol 1987;16:1122.
   A discussion of the nine reported cases of cutaneous lesions due to *Mycobacterium kansasii* infection—physical examination, histopathology, culture, and treatment.
Moschella SL, Cropley TG. Diseases of the mononuclear phagocytic system. In: Moschella SL, Hurley HJ, eds. Dermatology. 3rd ed. Philadelphia: WB Saunders, 1992:1077.
   A comprehensive, well-referenced chapter on the cutaneous manifestations of nontuberculous mycobacteria.

Nedorost ST, Elewski B, Tomford JW, Camisco C. Rosacea-like lesions due to familial *Mycobacterium avium-intracellulare* infection. Int J Dermatol 1991;30:491.

   Provides a referenced list of reported cutaneous manifestations of culture-proven MAI infections.

Street ML, Umbert-Millet IJ, Roberts GD, Su WPD. Nontuberculous mycobacterial infections of the skin. J Am Acad Dermatol 1991;24:208.

   Addresses the clinical manifestations, histopathologic patterns, and culture requirements of 14 cases of nontuberculous mycobacteria infections of the skin, including *Mycobacterium marinum, M. chelonae, M. fortuitum, M. ulcerans, M. kansasii, and M. avium-intracellulare.*

Tappeiner G, Wolff K. Tuberculosis and other mycobacterial infections. In: Fitzpatrick TB, et al, eds. Dermatology in general medicine, 4th ed. New York:McGraw-Hill, 1993:2387.

   A comprehensive well-referenced chapter on the cutaneous manifestations of nontuberculous mycobacteria.

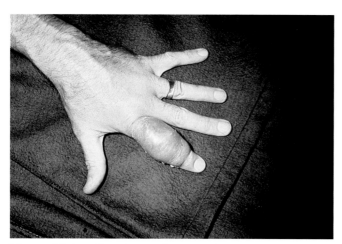

Figure 12.1. *Mycobacterium marinum* **infection**. Severe swelling of the index finger following puncture from a fish hook. The patient subsequently developed osteomyelitis. (Courtesy of Dr. Charles V. Sanders. From Williams CS, Riordan DC. J Bone Joint Surg (Am) 1993;55A(5):1042)

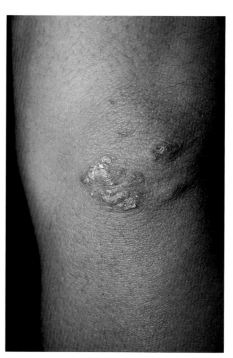

Figure 12.2. *Mycobacterium marinum* **infection**. Erythematous-to- violaceous plaque on the knee. (Courtesy of Dr. Lee T. Nesbitt, Jr.)

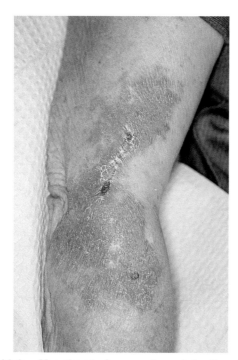

Figure 12.3. *Mycobacterium marinum* **infection**. Large, ill-defined erythematous plaques on the arm following trauma. (Courtesy of Dr. Lee T. Nesbitt, Jr.)

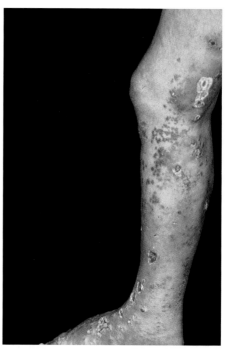

Figure 12.4. *Mycobacterium marinum* **infection**, disseminated. Ulcerative erythematous plaques of the leg and foot in a patient with Cushing's disease. (Courtesy of Dr. James Altick)

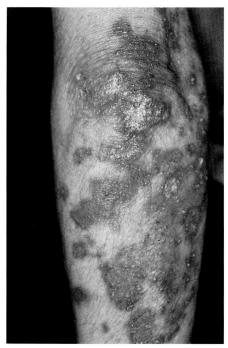

Figure 12.5. *Mycobacterium marinum* **infection**, disseminated. Erythematous plaques on the arm of the patient shown in Figure 12.4. (Courtesy of Dr. James Altick)

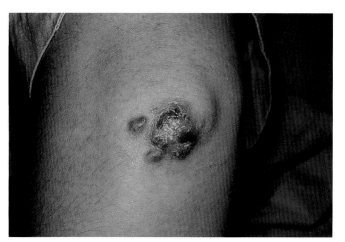

Figure 12.6. *Mycobacterium marinum* **infection**. Nodular plaques on the elbow. (Courtesy of Dr. Lee T. Nesbitt Jr.)

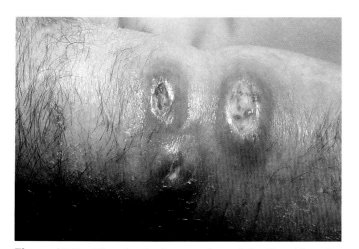

Figure 12.7. *Mycobacterium marinum* **infection**. Ulcerative nodules on the arm. (Courtesy of Dr. Charles V. Sanders)

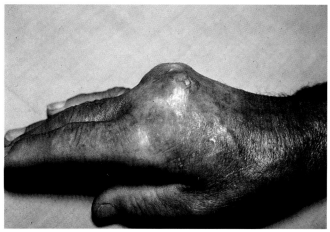

Figure 12.8. *Mycobacterium marinum* **infection**. Severe arthritis and tenosynovitis. (Courtesy of Dr. Lee T. Nesbitt, Jr.)

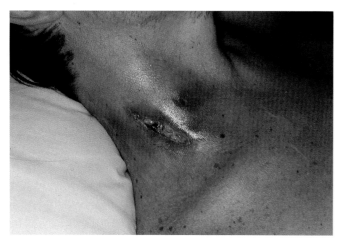

Figure 12.9. *Mycobacterium fortuitum* **infection**. Ulceration and surrounding cellulitis of the neck. (Courtesy of Dr. Charles V. Sanders)

CHAPTER **13**

Leprosy

BRUCE H. CLEMENTS

Skin Signs of *Mycobacterium Leprae* Infection

Leprosy, or Hansen's disease, is a chronic infectious communicable disease affecting primarily the cooler areas of the body, especially the skin, superficial peripheral nerves, eyes, testes, nose, and larynx. It is a worldwide public health problem with 81 countries regarded as endemic according to statistics released after a meeting of the World Health Organization (WHO) Leprosy Working Group in 1993. Twenty-five countries are badly affected—with India, Indonesia, and Myanmar (formerly Burma) accounting for 70% of all cases. The estimated number of cases requiring treatment in 1993 is 3.1 million, with multidrug therapy covering about half of these. More than 600,000 new cases are diagnosed every year.

According to the Ridley-Joplin classification of leprosy, the type of leprosy that develops depends on the body's ability to generate a cell-mediated immune response to invasion by the relatively avirulent *Mycobacterium leprae*. Skin manifestations of the disease are protean, ranging from a single hypopigmented lesion to multiple skin eruptions with systemic symptoms.

• PATHOGENESIS •

Leprosy is probably highly infectious but with low pathogenicity. While it is not hereditary, about 10% of the population appears susceptible to the disease, perhaps genetically. These persons are postulated to have a defect in their cell-mediated immune system specific for *M. leprae* that may persist for life. The incubation period averages 3 to 5 years, although it ranges from several months to over 20 years. All races are susceptible, and men are twice as likely as women to contract the more severe form of the disease.

The earliest form of the disease detectable after exposure to *M. leprae* is indeterminate leprosy (I). This condition may self-heal or progress to one of the more severe forms of the disease, depending on the person's immune response. For those with a relatively intact immunity, a localized form called tuberculoid disease (TT) develops. For those with a diminished or absent immune response, a widespread, generalized form called lepromatous leprosy (LL) emerges. Between these two extremes is the broader portion of the leprosy spectrum called borderline leprosy, comprising borderline tuberculoid (BT), basic borderline (BB), and borderline lepromatous (BL) disease.

The exact mode of transmission is not known, but the respiratory transmission theory is presently favored. Patients with borderline and lepromatous leprosy, the more severe forms of the disease, spread bacteria from their noses and upper respiratory tracts while coughing and sneezing. If a susceptible person inhales these *M. leprae*, the bacteria can be disseminated by the bloodstream to various parts of the body. Other transmission possibilities are skin-to-skin contact, insect vectors, and infected animals, especially the nine-banded armadillo. *M. leprae* has not been grown in an artificial medium. Shepard, in 1960, grew *M. leprae* in the footpads of mice, leading to methods of determining drug resistance to the organism.

At both extremes of the spectrum, TT and LL, the disease is relatively stable, but the borderline portion is characterized by instability. With treatment, the tendency of the condition is to shift toward the less severe tuberculoid end of the spectrum with an enhanced immune response; without treatment, the shift is toward the lepromatous end of the spectrum.

These shifts may be accompanied by acute episodes, known as reactions, that produce changes in the appearance of old lesions and sometimes the development of new lesions. Reactions that occur before treatment when the disease is moving toward the lepromatous end of the spectrum are known as downgrading reactions. Those that accompany effective treatment occur in about half the patients and are known by leprologists as reversal or Type 1 reactions, which have a cell-mediated immunologic mechanism. Another type of reaction that can occur before and after treatment, but only toward the lepromatous end of the spectrum, is erythema nodosum leprosum or Type 2 reaction. This reaction is characterized by the deposition of immune complexes around blood vessels with vasculitis, and occurs when there are large numbers of mycobacterial antigens and antibodies. It is similar to an Arthus-type reaction, and is characterized by erythema nodosum leprosum manifested by the sudden onset of painful red nodules associated with chills and fever (Figs. 13.1–13.3).

• CLINICAL FEATURES •

INDETERMINATE LEPROSY (I)

The earliest form of the disease characteristically presents as a hypopigmented macular lesion on the face, extremities, or buttocks (Fig. 13.4). It is symptomless and may be single or multiple. Skin sensation in the lesion may be slightly diminished but peripheral nerves are normal. Most of the lesions appear very innocuous, are self-healing, and remain undetected unless they are found during population surveys or contact examinations. The disease can be confirmed only by a biopsy of the suspected skin lesion.

TUBERCULOID LEPROSY (TT)

Tuberculoid leprosy usually presents as a fairly large, single, anesthetic lesion with variable loss of pigmentation, sweating, and tactile sensitivity inside the lesion (Fig. 13.5). Lesions are macular or plaque-like and may occasionally be multiple. The longer the lesion persists before treatment, the greater the area of skin involvement. The skin around the lesion may show some reaction with involvement of cutaneous or peripheral nerves in the area, resulting in tenderness and enlargement.

The sites of predilection for nerve involvement in all kinds of leprosy, except indeterminate, are the ulnar nerve proximal to the elbow (Fig. 13.6), the median and radial cutaneous nerves at the wrist, the posterior tibial nerve at the ankle, the peroneal nerve on the lateral aspect of the knee, the facial nerve, and the greater auricular nerve of the neck. Any superficial nerve in the vicinity of a lesion may be affected, however.

BORDERLINE LEPROSY

Most of the lesions of leprosy fall into the broad, unstable, intermediate zone of the spectrum called borderline. Reactive episodes before and after treatment occur often in this form of the disease, and widespread and severe neuropathy can occur.

In borderline tuberculoid (BT) disease, lesions tend to be larger, often with diminished hair growth and sensation (Figs. 13.7–13.9). As the disease progresses across the spectrum toward lepromatous, the lesions become more numerous, with increasing sensory loss in the lepromatous pattern (Fig. 13.10). In basic borderline (BB) disease, the lesions are smaller with punched-out centers, and *M. leprae* may be found on biopsy or in skin scrapings. In borderline lepromatous disease (BL), the lesions tend to be extensive, fairly symmetrical, and smaller. Lesions may also have the classic punched-out center, and a few nodules may be present (Figs. 13.11–13.13). Bacilli are usually numerous in the lesions.

LEPROMATOUS LEPROSY (LL)

Papules and nodules may be symmetrically distributed on the face, buttocks, and limbs (Figs. 13.14–13.20). Vague erythematous macular lesions may coalesce into plaque-like lesions (Fig. 13.21). Another form with diffuse nonnodular infiltrative disease that lacks discernible plaques or nodules is accompanied by loss of eyebrows and eyelashes (Fig. 13.22), distal extremity sensory loss, and numerous *M. leprae* in the skin, associated with loss of body hair and loss of sweating.

Years after onset, these patients are prone to severe reactive episodes with sudden and widespread tissue breakdown, called the Lucio phenomenon (Fig. 13.23). Untreated, the course of lepromatous leprosy is slowly progressive with involvement of nearly the entire skin. Involvement of the upper respiratory tract may eventually cause septal perforation with nasal collapse (Fig. 13.24). The skin, especially of the face, becomes corrugated and shiny with the so-called leonine facies. Granulomatous tissue may infiltrate the nose, ears, soft and hard palate, uvula, and larynx. Gradually, the peripheral nerves are infiltrated and destroyed by invasion of *M. leprae*, with resulting sensory and motor deficits followed by neurotrophic ulcerations of the hands and feet.

OTHER MANIFESTATIONS

Miscellaneous manifestations usually occurring toward the lepromatous end of the spectrum are ocular damage, bone changes, and involvement of the testes. Ocular damage, however, can occur across the entire spectrum, with damage to the zygomatic branch of cranial nerve VII, causing paralysis of the orbicularis oculi muscle and lagophthalmos. Damage to the ophthalmic branch of cranial nerve V can cause sensory loss to the cornea, resulting in superficial punctate keratitis, which can lead to pannus formation and a sclerosing keratitis if untreated. Reactive episodes in the eye lead to acute and chronic iridocyclitis, followed by iris atrophy and blindness.

Bone changes are essentially confined to the skull and the small bones of the hands and feet, which may appear cystic on X-ray due to bacillary deposits in the phalanges. Repeated episodes of trauma and infection in the insensitive extremity lead to bone absorption with concentric bone atrophy. In the skull, atrophy of the anterior nasal spine contributes to nasal collapse and atrophy of the maxillary alveolar process with loss of both upper incisors.

The testes may be destroyed by a granulomatous process in lepromatous leprosy and also by repeated episodes of Type 2 lepra reaction, causing sterility and gynecomastia.

• DIAGNOSIS AND DIFFERENTIAL DIAGNOSIS •

Leprosy should be suspected in any patient with skin lesions and signs of peripheral neuropathy. Clinicians should maintain a high degree of suspicion of leprosy in such patients, particularly if the patients live in or immigrate from an endemic area. Diagnosis can be confirmed by biopsy and/or the demonstration of acid-fast organisms in skin scrapings from selected lesions. Any biopsy specimen should be stained by hematoxylin and eosin and Fite-Faraco procedure for acid-fast organisms. The lepromin skin test is useful in classifying the disease and establishing prognosis, but it rarely helps in making the diagnosis.

Skin scrapings are taken from skin lesions or from cooler

Table 13.1   Bacterial Index in Relation to Bacilli

Bacterial Index	Number of Bacilli in Oil Immersion Field (OIF)
0	0 bacilli per 100 OIF
1+	1-10 bacilli per 100 OIF
2+	1-10 bacilli per 10 OIF
3+	1-10 bacilli per 1 OIF
4+	10-100 bacilli per 1 OIF
5+	100-1000 bacilli per 1 OIF
6+	Over 1000 bacilli per 1 OIF

areas of the body and stained with an acid-fast stain such as Fite-Faraco. The number of bacilli present in scrapings or biopsy slides is determined and reported as the bacterial index (BI) (Table 13.1). The BI on skin scrapings and biopsy will usually be 0 to 1+ in indeterminate and tuberculoid, 0 to 4+ in borderline, and 3+ to 6+ in lepromatous patients. Also determined is the morphological index (MI), which is the percentage of solid-staining and presumably viable organisms. The MI in an untreated borderline or lepromatous case is 1% to 5%, which should fall to zero within 4 months of effective therapy.

Other evidence of the presence of leprosy may be found by careful neurological examination, which should include palpation of the peripheral nerves, a detailed sensory examination, and testing of motor strength in the muscles of the hands, feet, and face. In cases that are difficult to diagnose, a small twig of an enlarged, superficial nerve may be removed for histological examination.

The differential diagnosis in skin lesions is broad. Raised lesions can be confused with lupus vulgaris, granuloma annulare, psoriasis, sarcoidosis, and treponemal lesions. The macular lesions of indeterminate or tuberculoid leprosy can be confused with birthmarks, contact dermatitis, vitiligo, tinea versicolor, seborrheic dermatitis, and postinflammatory hypochromia. The nodular lesions of lepromatous leprosy can be confused with acne vulgaris, treponematosis, atypical mycobacterial infections, leishmaniasis, leukemia cutis, histoplasmosis, neurofibromatosis, and multiple lipoma. By careful history and physical examination, the condition can usually be diagnosed correctly.

The use of smears and cultures to rule out other acid-fast and fungal diseases can also be helpful. Disease toward the tuberculoid end of the spectrum, where acid-fast bacilli are sparse, is the most difficult type of leprosy to diagnose by laboratory tests. As the disease progresses across the spectrum to lepromatous, acid-fast bacilli become easier to find. The culture of these organisms will show no growth despite their plentiful number.

Damage to the peripheral nerves causing motor and sensory impairment can also occur in diabetic neuropathy, syringomyelia, and polyneuropathies, caused by infection or toxic substances. Sometimes, an extremely rare syndrome, such as congenital indif-ference to pain or familial hypertrophic peripheral neuropathy, should be considered in the differential diagnosis.

• TREATMENT AND CLINICAL COURSE •

The sulfones have been the treatment of choice for leprosy since their introduction in the 1940s as single-drug therapy. Due to the rising incidence of sulfone-resistant disease since the early 1970s, multidrug therapy (MDT) has been the standard therapy for leprosy at the Gillis W. Long Hansen's Disease Center at Carville, LA. In 1982, a World Health Organization Study Group recommended multidrug therapy on a short-term basis for all types of leprosy. In 1990, investigational short-term therapy was introduced in the United States.

The standard therapy in the United States for paucibacillary cases (those with BI of 0 at all sites on skin scrapings, which usually includes all I, TT, and BT cases) is dapsone 100 mg daily and rifampin 600 mg daily for 6 months, followed by dapsone monotherapy for 3 years in I, and 5 years in TT and BT. Multibacillary cases (those with a BI of 1+ or more at any site on skin scrapings, which would include all BB, BL, and LL cases) infected with sulfone-sensitive bacilli are treated with dapsone 100 mg daily and rifampin 600 mg daily for 3 years, followed by dapsone monotherapy for 10 years in BB, and for life in BL and LL. Clofazimine is given at 50 mg daily for 3 years if there is any uncertainty as to whether the bacilli are sulfone-sensitive.

The short-term therapy approaches that are investigational in the United States consist of two regimens for paucibacillary cases: PB-1, which consists of dapsone 100 mg daily and rifampin 600 mg daily for 12 months, and PB-2, which consists of dapsone 100 mg daily and rifampin 600 mg monthly for 12 months. Multibacillary disease has three different regimens: MB-1, which is dapsone 100 mg daily and rifampin 600 mg daily for 2 years with all treatment stopped if a mouse footpad study is successful; MB-2, which is dapsone 100 mg daily, rifampin 600 mg daily, and clofazimine 50 mg daily for 2 years, with all therapy stopped thereafter; and MB-3, which is dapsone 100 mg daily, rifampin 600 mg monthly directly observed, and clofazimine 50 mg daily with 300 mg monthly directly observed for 2 years, with therapy then discontinued. Protocols for using these investigational treatments (1) can be obtained by contacting the Clinical Branch at the Gillis W. Long Hansen's Disease Center.

The WHO regimens for paucibacillary include dapsone 100 mg daily and rifampin 600 mg monthly, directly observed, for 6 months. The multibacillary regimen is dapsone 100 mg daily plus clofazimine 50 mg daily and 300 mg monthly directly observed, plus rifampin 600 mg monthly directly observed for 2 years, preferably until the skin smear is negative. The 1992 Consensus Development Statement on the Chemotherapy of Leprosy based on 7 years of follow-up data pronounced these regimens effective, with low relapse rates of 0.12% per year for paucibacillary and 0.22% for multibacillary cases (2). Even shorter drug regimens have been evaluated under the auspices of the WHO since February, 1992, using rifampin 600 mg daily and ofloxacin 400 mg daily for 1 month (3).

REFERENCES

1. Yoder LJ. Leprosy (Hansen's Disease). In: Rokel RE, ed. Conn's current therapy. 45th ed. Philadelphia:WB Saunders, 1993:94–99.
2. Jacobson RR, et al. Consensus development statement on the chemotherapy of leprosy. Int J Lepr 1992;60(Spec Sect 4):644.
3. Anonymous. New leprosy treatment. Trop Dis Res News 1992;38:1.

ANNOTATED BIBLIOGRAPHY

Becx-Bluemink M, Berhe D. Occurrence of reactions, their diagnosis and management in leprosy patients treated with multidrug therapy: Experience in the Leprosy Control Program of All Africa Leprosy and Rehabilitation Training Center (ALERT) in Ethiopia. Int J Lepr 1992;60:173.

Type 1 and Type 2 reactions cause most of the disability and deformities in leprosy. This article addresses the diagnosis and management of these reactions.

Bryceson A, Pfaltzgraff RE. Leprosy. 3rd ed. Edinburgh: Churchill Livingstone, 1990.

A concise handbook of leprosy covering all aspects of the disease under field conditions as part of the *Medicine in the Tropics* series.

Hastings RC. Leprosy. New York: Churchill Livingstone, 1985.

A comprehensive textbook of leprosy written by various experts in their fields of expertise in the disease.

Kaur S, Sharma VK, Basak P, Kaur I. Paucibacillary multidrug therapy in leprosy: 7½ years experience. Indian J Lepr 1992;64:153.

Long-term follow-up of 323 paucibacillary (PB) leprosy patients treated with the WHO-recommended multidrug therapy (MDT), including incidence of reversal reactions.

Noordeen SK. A look at world leprosy. Lepr Rev 1991;62:721.

Comprehensive review of world leprosy, including estimate of registered cases, progress in implementation of multidrug treatment (MDT), problems relating to MDT therapy, disability prevention, rehabilitation, and future prospects of MDT.

Ridley DS, Joplin WHA. Classification of leprosy according to immunity–a five group system. Int J Lepr 1966;34:255.

A five-group classification of leprosy in which the group represents five grades of resistance by the patient to the infection.

Rose P, Waters MFR. Reversal reactions in leprosy and their management. Lepr Rev 1991;62:113.

Review of Type 1 reactions along with recommendation for treatment to prevent the development of neuropathy and deformities.

Shepard CC. The experimental disease that follows the injection of human leprosy bacilli into footpads of mice. J Expr Med 1960;112:445.

Description of the first culture and sensitivity test for human leprosy bacilli as grown in the footpads of mice.

World Health Organization Study Group. Chemotherapy of leprosy control programmes. WHO Tech Rep Serv 675. Geneva: World Health Organization, 1982.

Rationale for the multiple drug treatment of leprosy with recommendations for using dual- and triple-drug therapy.

Yoder LJ. Leprosy (Hansen's Disease). In: Rakel RE, ed. Conn's current therapy. 45th ed. Philadelphia: WB Saunders, 1993.

Review of current therapeutics and dosages as well as treatment of the various reactions in leprosy.

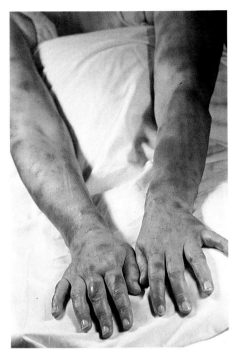

Figure 13.1. Erythema nodosum leprosum. Leprologist Type 2 reaction (immunologist Type 3), showing edema of the fingers. (Courtesy of Dr. Lee T. Nesbitt, Jr.)

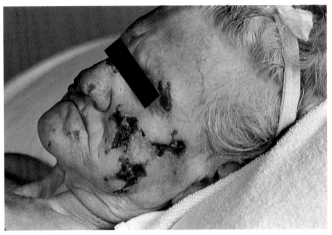

Figure 13.2. Erythema nodosum leprosum. Leprologist Type 2 reaction (immunologist Type 3), showing severe ulcerative lesion due to far advanced lepromatous leprosy. (Courtesy of Dr. Lee T. Nesbitt,Jr.)

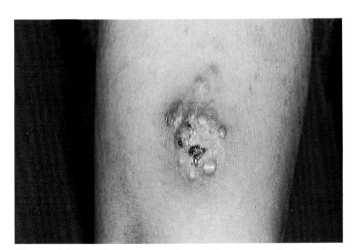

Figure 13.3. Erythema nodosum leprosum. Erythematous nodule with overlying pustules.

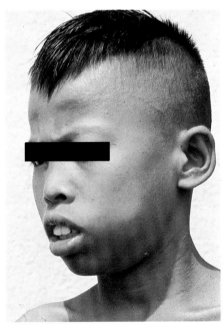

Figure 13.4. Indeterminate leprosy. Slightly hypopigmented patch on right cheek. (From Guinto RS, et al. An atlas of leprosey. Rev. ed. Tokyo: Sasakawa Memorial Health Foundation, 1984:4.)

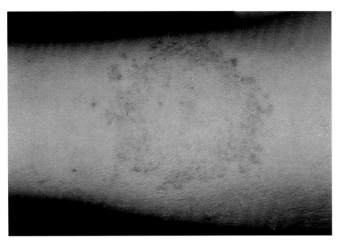

Figure 13.5.   Tuberculoid disease. A fairly typical, anesthetic, hyperpigmented lesion with raised erythematous borders. (Courtesy of Dr. Lee T. Nesbitt, Jr.)

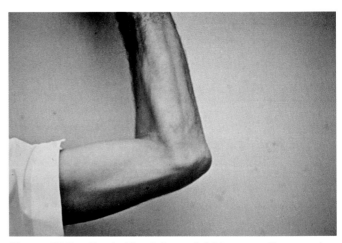

Figure 13.6.   Borderline-tuberculoid leprosy. Close-up of an enlarged ulnar nerve.

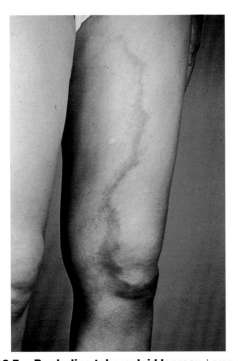

Figure 13.7.   Borderline-tuberculoid leprosy. Large, irregularly shaped anesthetic lesion. (Courtesy of Dr. Lee T. Nesbitt, Jr.)

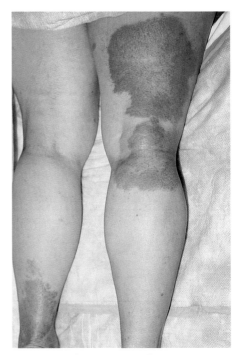

Figure 13.8.   Borderline-tuberculoid leprosy. Large, red, scaly, erythematous anesthetic plaques.

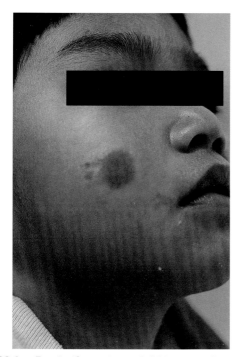

Figure 13.9. Borderline-tuberculoid leprosy. Southeast Asian child with anesthetic erythematous lesion of face and surrounding hypopigmentation. Lesions were also present on his trunk and extremities.

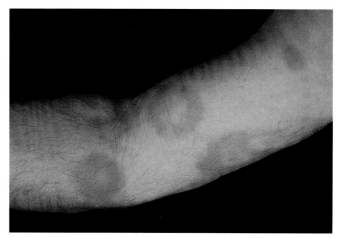

Figure 13.10. Borderline-to-borderline-lepromatous leprosy. Besides these lesions on her arm, this 47-year-old had anesthetic lesions on her other arm, legs, and face.

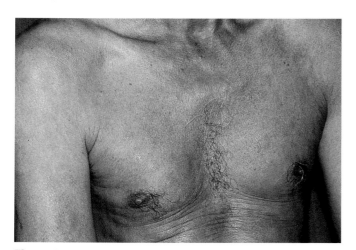

Figure 13.11. Borderline-lepromatous leprosy. Erythematous maculopapular and nodular lesions. Skin smears showed a BI of 3+ to 4+. (Courtesy of Dr. Lee T. Nesbitt, Jr.)

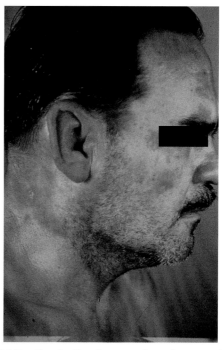

Figure 13.12. Borderline-lepromatous leprosy. Leprologist Type 1 (or immunologist Type 4) reaction, with edema of ear and erythematous skin lesions. (Courtesy of Dr. Lee T. Nesbitt, Jr.)

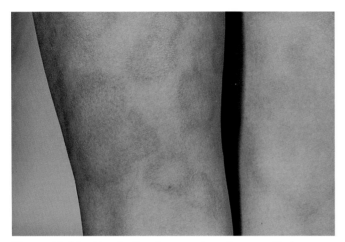

Figure 13.13.   Borderline-lepromatous leprosy. Erythematous lesions, some anesthetic, with central clearing and skin smears of 3+ and 4+.

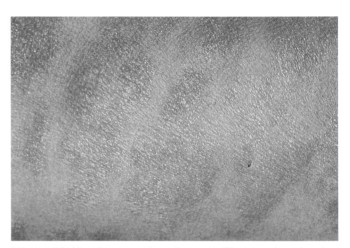

Figure 13.14.   Lepromatous leprosy. Close-up view of erythematous nodules. (Courtesy of Dr. Lee T. Nesbitt, Jr.)

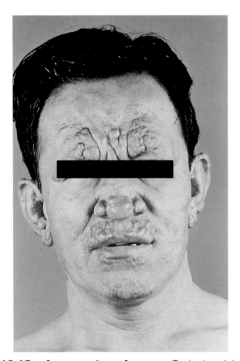

Figure 13.15.   Lepromatous leprosy. Typical nodular lesions, which will clear completely with antileprotic medication. (Courtesy of Dr. Lee T. Nesbitt, Jr.)

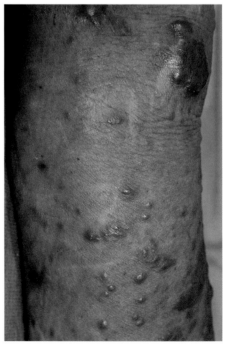

Figure 13.16.   Lepromatous leprosy. Active disease in a 52-year-old Texas female with skin smears showing a BI of 5+.

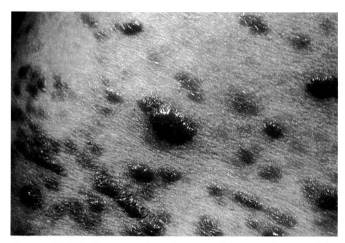

Figure 13.17. Lepromatous leprosy. Sulfone-resistant, nodular form. Skin smears showed a BI of 4+ to 6+ with an MI of 2% to 3%.

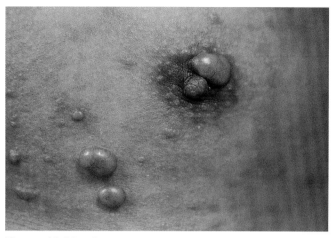

Figure 13.18. Lepromatous leprosy. Histoid-type nodules of sulfone-resistant disease on the chest of a 23-year-old Mexican-American male.

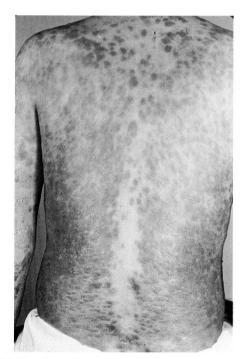

Figure 13.19. Lepromatous leprosy. Widespread lesions showing relative sparing of the warmer mid-line area. (Courtesy Dr. Lee T. Nesbitt, Jr.)

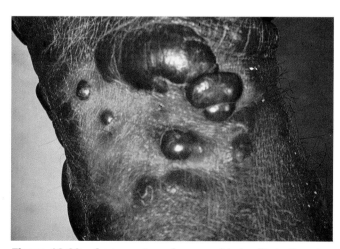

Figure 13.20. Lepromatous leprosy. A lesion filled with watery fluid, which is another manifestation of this form.

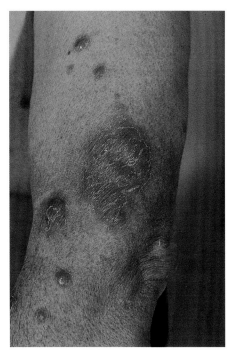

Figure 13.21.   Lepromatous leprosy. Nodules and plaque-like lesions in a 63-year-old patient. All skin smears showed a BI of 3+.

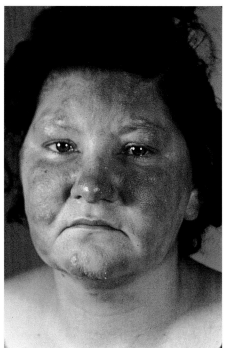

Figure 13.22.   Lateral madarosis. Loss of eyebrows, which is common in borderline-lepromatous and polar lepromatous leprosy. (Courtesy of Dr. Lee T. Nesbitt, Jr.)

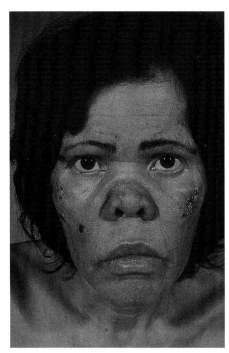

Figure 13.23.   Lucio's phenomenon. An untreated patient with lepromatous leprosy, who subsequently died of Gram-negative septicemia.

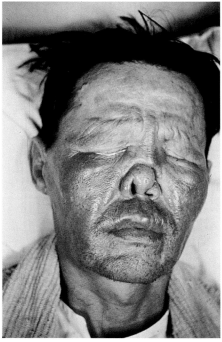

Figure 13.24.   Lepromatous leprosy. Madarosis, collapsed nose, and blindness due to far advanced, untreated lepromatous leprosy.

CHAPTER 14

Superficial Fungal Infections

ANDREW RUDOLPH and DEBRA CHESTER KALTER

Fungal infection of the skin is a common human condition, ranging from subclinical involvement to serious morbidity. In the United States, 10% of the population has cutaneous fungal infection at any given time, and at least 40% may have it at some time during life. Mycotic skin infestation can be divided into three groups: superficial mycoses, dermatophytosis, and candidiasis.

The superficial mycoses involve only the stratum corneum or the outer hair shaft, and include tinea versicolor, tinea nigra palmaris, white piedra, and black piedra. Host response is negligible because these infections are superficial.

Cutaneous infection by dermatophytes does induce a greater clinical response from the host. The intensity of the response varies, depending primarily on the host's ability to mount an immunologic reaction and, to a lesser extent, on the type of infecting organism. Dermatophytosis is usually subdivided according to the anatomic area affected, which, in turn, determines the clinical manifestation. Hair, skin, and nails are all subject to parasitization. Geographical distribution of certain fungal species also determines distinctive patterns in dermatophytosis.

Candidiasis includes a spectrum of clinical diseases associated with infection by the yeast-like fungus *Candida*. Mucous membrane involvement is common, in addition to skin and nail infection. Serious systemic disease can occur in predisposed patients, leading to great morbidity and even death.

Other fungi, considered nonpathogenic or saprophytic, can produce disease in certain unusual situations fortuitous to their growth.

• PATHOGENESIS •

In general, all superficial fungal infections are more likely to develop in conjunction with predisposing factors. The source of infection may be from the soil, animals, infected humans, or infected fomites. Suitable contact with the infecting agent is, of course, essential in initiating disease. Not all exposed persons will develop infection in the same environmental situation. Host resistance is probably the most important single factor in determining the extent of disease.

Acute inflammatory reactions tend to be associated with a limited area of involvement, the development of an immunologic response, and, at times, spontaneous cure. Minimal inflammation is associated with chronic, extensive disease, and failure to develop delayed-type hypersensitivity. Interference with normal immunologic capabilities leads to an increased susceptibility to fungal infection, as occurs in endocrinopathies, use of corticosteroids, chemotherapeutic or immunosuppressive agents, inborn immune defects, pregnancy, debilitating systemic disease, and malnutrition. Environmental conditions of high heat, humidity, maceration, occlusive garb, and poor hygiene are also influential. Often, proper therapy is ineffective until the environmental or predisposing factor is corrected.

Brief clinical descriptions of more common superficial fungal infections are presented below, followed by a therapeutic overview.

• CLINICAL FEATURES •

The Superficial Mycoses

TINEA VERSICOLOR

A common, chronic fungal infection, tinea versicolor is caused by the lipidophilic *Pityrosporum orbiculare* (*Malassezia furfur*). Young adults of both sexes are prone to infection worldwide, with episodic worsening in the hot months. Genetic predisposition and hyperhidrosis also play a role.

Slightly scaly, round-to-oval macules may be scattered individually or coalesce on the upper portion of the trunk (Figs. 14.1, 14.2), shoulders, and neck, occasionally extending to the groin area, thighs, arms, or face. Lesions may be hypopigmented or hyperpigmented, and vary from white to fawn, red, or brown. Suntanning of the surrounding skin makes the macules more obvious, as does illumination with a Wood's light. The condition is asymptomatic or variably pruritic. Occasionally, perifollicular papules or pustules develop and may become inflamed.

Scratching the macular lesions emphasizes their scaly nature. Although response to therapy is good, recurrence is extremely common. Pigmentary changes take months to correct after treatment. Differential diagnosis includes vitiligo, chloasma, seborrheic dermatitis, dermatophytosis, pityriasis rosea, secondary syphilis, erythrasma, and pinta.

TINEA NIGRA PALMARIS

This asymptomatic, hyperpigmented macule is infrequently reported. Infection with *Exophiala werneckii* leads to a chronic, slowly enlarging, single, brown-to-black macule with sharply defined but irregular borders. The palmar aspect of the hand is the most common locale (Fig. 14.3), but others include the plantar surface of the foot, the trunk, or the neck. It must be distinguished from malignant melanoma, junctional nevus, stains, syphilis, talon noir, and Addison's disease.

WHITE PIEDRA

Infection with the yeast-like *Trichosporon beigelii* may be asymptomatic or may lead to the accumulation of multiple, white-to-brown firm nodules, up to 0.5 mm in diameter, along the shaft of any of the terminal hairs of the body. Affected hairs break more easily and feel gritty. Mild, persistent pruritus or involvement of the surrounding skin may lead the patient to seek medical attention. Infection is more commonly encountered than previously thought. The differential diagnosis includes trichomycosis axillaris, pediculosis, monilethrix, trichorrhexis nodosa, hair casts, and artifacts.

BLACK PIEDRA

Black piedra also leads to nodule formation on terminal hair shafts, but is due to the ascomycete *Piedraia hortae*. The nodules are black, harder, more discrete, and more adherent than those of white piedra. Normal hair intervenes between nodules and does not appear to be significantly weakened. Infestation is endemic to tropical areas of Central and South America, Africa, and Malaysia, where some consider these lesions a mark of beauty. The differential diagnosis is that described for white piedra.

Dermatophytosis

TINEA CAPITIS

The scalp, eyebrows, and eyelashes are subject to infection by *Microsporum* and *Trichophyton* species. Young school-aged children are most commonly affected. In adults, infection in women predominates. Infections by *Microsporum* may clear spontaneously at puberty, whereas infections by *Trichophyton* do not. The agents that cause tinea capitis may also cause tinea corporis in the same person or in family members in close contact with affected children. *T. tonsurans* is the most common cause in the United States, followed by *M. canis*. The preponderant organism varies according to geographic location worldwide.

The terminology used to describe and subdivide tinea capitis is confusing. Ectothrix infection implies the development of arthroconidia around the hair shaft that may destroy the cuticle.

"Gray-patch" tinea is of this type, presenting with one large noninflammatory patch and several smaller ones with grayish scale and broken stubble of lusterless hair. Pruritus is a common complaint. It is highly contagious and may lead to urban epidemics. Ectothrix tinea may fluoresce yellow-green with Wood's lamp examination. Fluorescence may be lost during acute inflammation. Ectothrix agents include *M. audouinii*, *M. canis*, *M. ferrugineun*, *M. gypseum*, *T. verrucosum*, and *T. mentagrophytes*.

Endothrix infection causes "black-dot" tinea, as the arthroconidia form within the hair shaft, leading to hair breakage at the scalp surface (Fig. 14.4). It tends to be more severe, chronic, and resistant to therapy than is ectothrix infection. Multiple small, nonfluorescent areas, involving only a few hairs, may be scattered throughout the scalp. Endothrix infection may be due to *T. tonsurans*, *T. schoenleinii*, *T. violaceum*, *T. soudanense*, *T. gourvilii*, and *T. yaoundei*. These last three organisms are restricted to Africa.

Tinea capitis is also described as inflammatory or noninflammatory. In general, zoophilic and geophilic fungi produce more inflammatory lesions that tend to have a rapid course and may involute spontaneously. *M. canis* and *M. gypseum* are typical; *T. mentagrophytes*, *T. tonsurans*, *T. verrucosum*, and *T. rubrum* may lead to an inflammatory tinea (Fig. 14.5). Clinically, a painful, elevated, boggy, erythematous mass, or kerion, develops (Fig. 14.6). Suppurative folliculitis may ensue, followed by patchy, scarring alopecia (Fig. 14.7).

Favus is a rare type of inflammatory tinea capitis, usually due to *T. schoenleinii* but occasionally secondary to *M. gypseum* or *T. violaceum*. It is endemic to certain geographical areas, and may affect several family members. Infection begins with yellow, follicular crusts penetrated by hairs. These enlarge to form cup-shaped crusts, or scutula, that overlie oozing, erythematous ulcers. The surrounding scalp is scaly and erythematous and exudes a "mousy" odor. Involved hairs are lusterless, turn gray, and are shed to produce scarring alopecia and central atrophy. Spontaneous involution does not occur and the entire scalp may become involved. The neck and shoulders may be infected by contiguous spread, clinically resembling scutula or typical tinea corporis. Nail infection may also develop. Fluorescence with Wood's lamp may be dull green or bluish-white.

The differential diagnosis of tinea capitis should include seborrheic dermatitis, psoriasis, trichotillomania, alopecia areata, pityriasis amiantacea, impetigo, pyoderma, folliculitis decalvans, pseudopelade, lupus erythematosus, and lichen planopilaris.

TINEA BARBAE

Dermatophyte infection of the beard area has most frequently been caused by *T. mentagrophytes* and *T. verrucosum*, although other species have been implicated. Infection is usually acquired from close contact with animals, especially in rural areas. A mild superficial type with central scaling and vesiculopustular borders resembles lesions seen in tinea corporis. A more severe, deep pustular folliculitis can develop with progression to nodular, kerion-like plaques that are erythematous and boggy (Fig. 14.8). Much of the beard area can become involved with purplish verrucose induration and eventuate into scarring alopecia. Fever, malaise, and regional lymphadenopathy may be associated. Spontaneous resolution can occur in the inflammatory type. Sycosis barbae, cystic acne, contact dermatitis, acneiform drug eruptions, actinomycosis, and secondary syphilis should be excluded.

TINEA FACIEI

Facial involvement by dermatophytes, other than in the beard area, is basically localized tinea corporis. Concurrent tinea capitis or corporis may be present. *T. mentagrophytes, T. rubrum,* and *M. canis* are common causative agents. Lesions may be annular, circinate, or plaque-like, with erythema and fine scale (Figs. 14.9, 14.10). The appearance is often misleading, especially if modified by topical steroid use so that scale is minimal and tinea is not suspected. Patients complain of itching, burning, and exacerbation with sun exposure, which further encourages misdiagnosis. The differential diagnosis of such facial lesions includes polymorphic light eruption, lupus erythematosus, eczema, actinic keratosis, psoriasis, impetigo, rosacea, and benign lymphocytic infiltrate of the skin.

TINEA CORPORIS

Ringworm may involve any part of the body in any part of the world. Exposed skin areas are those most affected. *T. rubrum* is the most common cause, followed by *T. mentagrophytes,* and whichever species that predominates in producing tinea capitis in that geographic region. *Epidermophyton floccosum,* although more common in crural locations, can occasionally spread to adjacent body parts and rarely induce verrucous nodules. Typical lesions can be dry and scaly, or vesicular and exudative, or both. Annular or serpiginous configurations with erythematous, slightly elevated or vesicular active borders are produced by central clearing of infection and centrifugal spread (Figs. 14.11, 14.12). Scaling is a hallmark. Papular lesions may coalesce to form solid plaques or appear psoriasiform. In certain geographic areas, *T. concentricum* produces a distinctive pattern of concentric, gyrate rings.

Follicular involvement may serve as a reservoir for recurrent or relapsing infection. Granulomas and suppurative folliculitis can sometimes develop, especially on the wrists and forearms of livestock workers (Fig. 14.13). Immunosuppressed patients may also develop these dark red nodules, pustules, and plaques. This kerion of the skin is known as Majocchi's granuloma, or tinea profunda and may be aggravated by steroid use. Pruritus and irritation with warm weather is typical of dermatophytosis. Although tinea corporis is less inclined to chronicity than is tinea pedis or cruris, *T. rubrum* infection is especially difficult to eradicate.

The differential diagnosis should include psoriasis, eczema, pityriasis rosea, secondary syphilis, annular erythemas, seborrheic dermatitis, contact dermatitis, tinea versicolor, candidiasis, and lichen planus.

TINEA CRURIS

Dermatophyte infection of the groin and gluteal regions tends to be bilateral, although not necessarily symmetric. *T. rubrum, T. mentagrophytes,* and *E. floccosum* are most often at fault. Coexistent tinea pedis is frequent, and males are most commonly affected. Epidemics can occur in close quarters, especially from *E. floccosum.* Typical lesions of *E. floccosum* are well-marginated, reddish-brown, dry, scaly areas bordered by tiny vesicopustules. *T. rubrum* is more chronic, may be unilateral, and may spread widely to form thick, scaly, dull red plaques. Pruritus and irritation may be intense. In contrast to candidal intertrigo, the penis and scrotum tend to be spared (Fig. 14.14). Erythrasma, intertrigo, seborrheic dermatitis, psoriasis, contact dermatitis, and lichen planus should be excluded.

TINEA PEDIS

"Athlete's foot" is a universal affliction with several clinical manifestations. The most common causative organisms are *T. rubrum, T. mentagrophytes,* and *E. floccosum.* The moccasin or hyperkeratotic type is the most common clinical presentation. Skin that is pink to dull-red is covered by branny, whitish scales involving the soles and extending up the sides of both feet to resemble moccasins. This chronic infection is extremely resistant to therapy and relapse is almost inevitable, especially in the presence of coexistent onychomycoses.

A vesicular or vesiculopustular type is also common, appearing between the toes or on the instep. Tense vesicles on erythematous bases rupture, leak serous exudate, and may progress to maceration and fissures. Interdigital infection similarly leads to tender erythema, maceration, and fissuring, especially between the 3rd, 4th, and 5th toes (Fig. 14.15). Foul smelling keratotic debris accumulates and promotes the moist environment. Secondary bacterial infection can intervene and progress to cellulitis and lymphangitis. Candidiasis, erythrasma, pyoderma, dyshidrosis, contact dermatitis, psoriasis, secondary syphilis, arsenical keratosis, and other keratodermas must be excluded.

Dermatophytid, or "id," reactions are not infrequently associated with tinea pedis, but may also occur with any fungal infection. Pruritic or painful vesicles develop along the sides of the fingers and the palms. More rarely, a widespread folliculopapular eruption may develop. These noninfective cutaneous eruptions represent a systemic allergic response to fungal antigens; adequate treatment of the primary infection is necessary for clearing.

TINEA MANUM

Fungal infection of the hand is usually unilateral and associated with tinea pedis (two feet-one hand syndrome); therefore, it can be assumed that the organisms are usually the same (Fig. 14.16). Like tinea pedis, infection may produce diffuse hyperkeratosis, scaling, fissuring, or vesicles. Palmar and interdigital surfaces are more commonly involved, but the dorsum may be involved as well. Although the differential diagnosis is similar to that of tinea pedis, it is important to distinguish it from an id reaction.

TINEA UNGUIUM (ONYCHOMYCOSIS)

Nail invasion by fungus usually begins subungually at the distal or lateral margin and progresses proximally. Once entrenched, it is very difficult to eradicate. *T. mentagrophytes, T. rubrum,* and *E. floccosum* are again the usual agents. The nail becomes gradually opaque, discolored, thickened, and brittle (Fig. 14.17). Subungual debris accumulates under the dystrophic nail and onycholysis loosens the nail plate further. A more benign nail disease is represented by white superficial onychomycosis restricted to circumscribed patches or pits on the surface of the toenail. *T. mentagrophytes, Cephalosporium* species, *Aspergillus* species, and *Fusarium* species have been held responsible. Proximal subungual infection beginning at the proximal nail fold is an uncommon variant. *Candida* and other nondermatophyte fungi can produce nail infection, especially in the presence of preexisting nail pathology. Bacterial and noninfectious causes of onychodystrophy must be considered.

Candidiasis

Candida albicans is a normal commensal organism on mucous membranes, skin, and the gastrointestinal tract. Its proliferation is held in check by host factors and by the normal bacterial flora of the body. Predisposing factors, as mentioned in the discussion of pathogenesis above, play a major role in disease initiation and maintenance. Use of antibiotics, corticosteroids, or oral contraceptives in otherwise normal hosts may be sufficient to allow candidiasis to occur, especially vulvovaginitis.

Thrush is common in infants and prone hosts (Fig. 14.18). Soft white plaques are loosely attached on oral mucous membranes and can be scraped off to reveal bright red, superficial erosions. Infection may extend into the esophagus; associated pain may interfere with oral intake. Perleche refers to candidal angular cheilitis. Moist, fissured, erythematous plaques develop in any warm, macerated area, such as the axilla, groin, gluteal cleft, and inframammary, or infrapanniculus regions. The skin is tender and irritated; erythematous, moist expanses are surrounded with well-defined borders and satellite papules and pustules (Figs. 14.19, 14.20).

Thrush in AIDS patients is discussed in Chapter 21.

Candidal paronychia produces tenderness, erythema, and swelling of the nail folds, without purulence (Fig. 14.21). The nail may become discolored or ridged, or undergo onycholysis in the absence of subungual debris. Vulvovaginitis usually involves vulvar intertrigo in association with a thick, white, curd-like vaginal discharge. Pruritus and irritation may be intense. Secondary infection with Gram-negative bacilli is not uncommon in cutaneous candidiasis.

Chronic mucocutaneous candidiasis is usually a lifelong, granulomatous candidal infection, associated with various defects in host immunologic reaction. The patients are anergic to skin testing with candidal antigen. Severe, hypertrophic mucous membrane, skin, and nail changes occur but without systemic dissemination (Figs. 14.22, 14.23).

• DIAGNOSIS AND DIFFERENTIAL DIAGNOSIS •

Scraping of suspicious lesions and examination with warmed potassium hydroxide at low-power magnification is usually sufficient to diagnose most superficial fungal infections. Removal and examination of the vesicle roof may reveal characteristic hyphae in vesicular eruptions. Extreme inflammation, debris, or medicaments may interfere with positive findings. Multiple examinations may be necessary. Fungal culture on various media will often confirm a diagnosis and allow for specific identification. Biopsy and special stains may be helpful in isolated cases. Dermatophyte and yeast forms can be distinguished microscopically, but rarely can species be determined.

Differential diagnoses have been listed in previous sections according to infection.

• TREATMENT AND CLINICAL COURSE •

Topical antifungal therapy is very effective in treating tinea versicolor, localized tinea corporis, mild tinea cruris and pedis, and mild-to-moderate candidiasis. Tinea versicolor also responds to a variety of keratolytic and selenium-containing topicals. Maintenance therapy is frequently necessary to retain a remission. Oral therapy with griseofulvin is excellent in treating more serious dermatophytic infections, but may need to be prolonged.

Adequate therapy in onychomycosis often exceeds a year in duration, and reinfection is the rule. Nail avulsion, by surgery or keratolysis, is thought to be adjunctive in response time only. Topical therapy in addition to oral medication offers little statistical advantage, but may be introduced at the end of the systemic regimen to maintain the "cure."

Griseofulvin is ineffective against yeast forms. The imidazoles and nystatin in cream, lotion, tablet, troche, and powder preparations help control candidal infections. Topical amphotericin B, gentian violet, and Castellani's paint may also be useful. Drying soaks decreases inflammation and weeping in macerated lesions.

Ketoconazole may be appropriate in serious, persistent fungal infections that are unresponsive to other therapy. It has been extremely useful in chronic mucocutaneous candidiasis, but may need to be maintained indefinitely. Ketoconazole has also been useful in significant dermatophytic infections and in single-dose intermittent therapy for tinea versicolor. One should watch for the occurrence of hepatotoxicity as a rare side effect of Ketoconazole therapy.

ANNOTATED BIBLIOGRAPHY

Ahmed AR. Immunology of human dermatophyte infections. Arch Dermatol 1982;118:521.
    The host-parasite interaction is investigated.
Arndt KA. Manual of dermatologic therapeutics. 4th ed. Boston: Little Brown, 1989.
    An overview of antifungal therapy.
Bronson D, Desai D, Barsky S, Foley S. An epidemic of infection with *Trichophyton tonsurans* revealed in a 20-year survey of fungal infections in Chicago. J Am Acad Dermatol 1983;8:322.
    The connection between tinea capitis and tinea corporis highlighted in a population study.

Jorizzo J. Chronic mucocutaneous candidiasis. Arch Dermatol 1982;118:963.

A discussion of chronic mucocutaneous candidiasis with an emphasis on immunologic aspects.

Laude TA, Shah B, Lynfield Y. Tinea capitis in Brooklyn. Am J Dis Child 1982;136:1047.

Analysis of 96 cases of tinea capitis revealed *Trichophyton tonsurans* in 89%, an inflammatory pattern in 40%, and a cure with griseofulvin after 4.7 weeks.

Rippon JW. Medical Mycology. 2nd ed. Philadelphia: WB Saunders, 1982.

In-depth review of pathogenic fungal infections.

Smith EB, ed. Symposium on superficial fungal infections. Dermatol Clin 1984:2(1).

A collection of 15 articles pertaining to various aspects of superficial fungal infections.

Zaias N. Onychomycosis. Arch Dermatol 1972;105:263.

Summary of various etiologies and pathogenesis in onychomycosis.

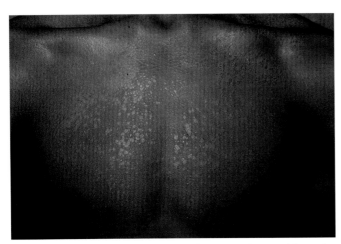

Figure 14.1.   Tinea versicolor. Slightly scaly, round hypopigmented macules coalesce over the chest. (Courtesy of Dr. Lee T. Nesbitt, Jr.)

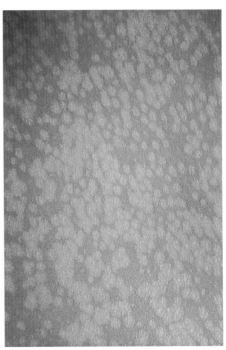

Figure 14.2.   Tinea versicolor. Close-up view of hypopigmented macules on the back. Scratching the lesions will emphasize their borders.

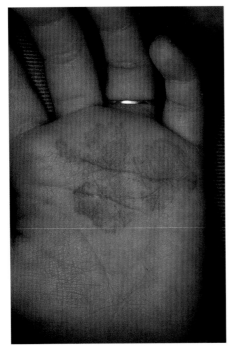

Figure 14.3.   Tinea nigra palmaris. The palm and sides of fingers are common locations for this slowly growing, asymptomatic superficial fungal infection. (Courtesy of Dr. Lee T. Nesbitt, Jr.)

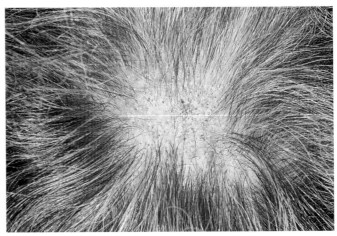

Figure 14.4.   Tinea capitis. Black dot type. This noninflammatory endothrix infection by *Trichophyton tonsurans* causes breakage of affected hair shafts at the scalp.

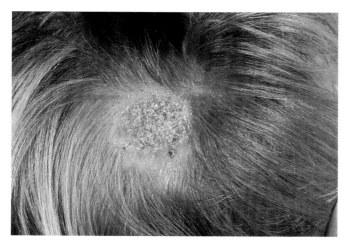

Figure 14.5. **Tinea capitis.** Slightly more inflammation is seen with this lesion. (Courtesy of Dr. Lee T. Nesbitt, Jr.)

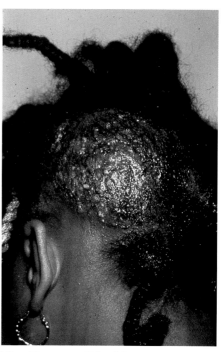

Figure 14.6. **Tinea capitis.** *Microsporum canis* infection can result in a painful, boggy, inflammatory mass called a kerion.

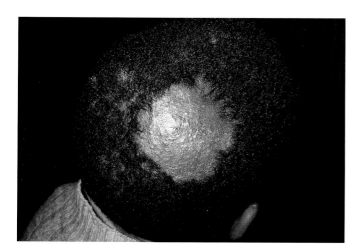

Figure 14.7. **Tinea capitis.** Subsequent scarring. (Courtesy of Dr. Lee T. Nesbitt, Jr.)

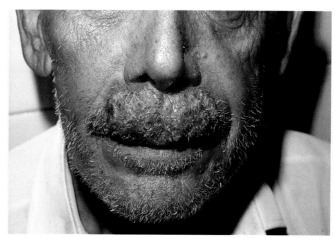

Figure 14.8. **Tinea barbae.** Nodular erythematous swelling of the beard around the upper lip. (Courtesy of Dr. Charles V. Sanders)

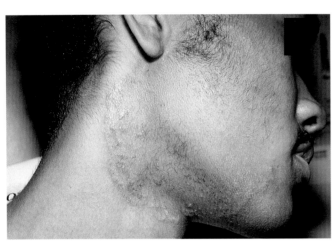

Figure 14.9.   Tinea faciei. Large annular lesion of the right face and neck with raised border. (Courtesy of Dr. Charles V. Sanders)

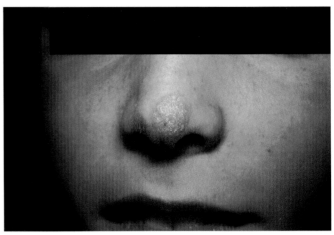

Figure 14.10.   Tinea faciei. Erythematous scaly patch on the nose of a child. (Courtesy of Dr. Lee T. Nesbitt, Jr.)

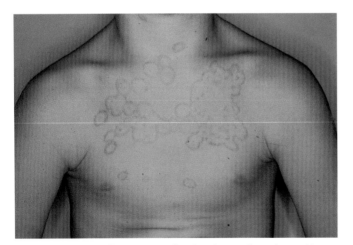

Figure 14.11.   Tinea corporis. Annular configurations with erythematous, active borders are produced by central clearing of infection and centrifugal spread.

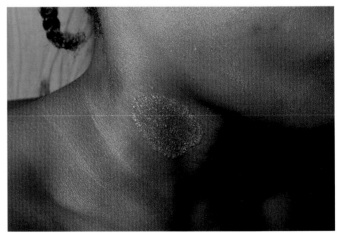

Figure 14.12.   Tinea corporis. Annular patch on the neck with sharp border. (Courtesy of Dr. Lee T. Nesbitt, Jr.)

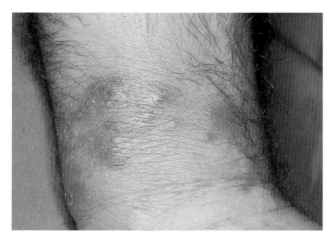

Figure 14.13.   Tinea profunda (Majocchi's granuloma). Dark red nodules, pustules, and plaques may form under watchbands and other areas of occlusion or in immunocompromised patients.

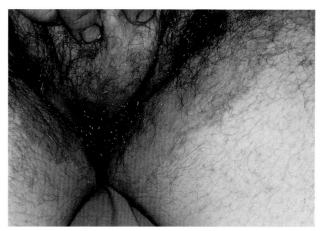

Figure 14.14.   Tinea cruris. Well-marginated, erythematous, and irritating patches involve the groin bilaterally, but tend to spare the scrotum and penis.

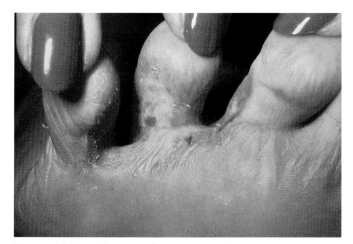

Figure 14.15.   Tinea pedis. Interdigital infection with *Trichophyton mentagrophytes* leads to painful maceration, fissuring, and, often, secondary bacterial infection.

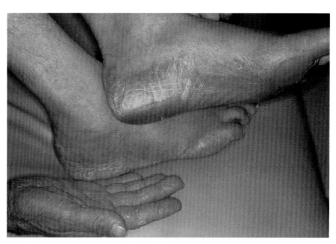

Figure 14.16.   Two feet-one hand syndrome. Diffuse hyperkeratosis and scaling affect the palmar aspect of only one hand and the plantar aspect of both feet.

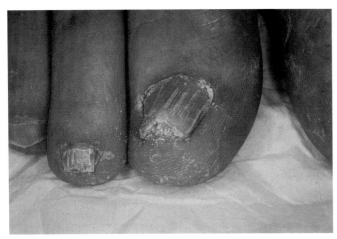

Figure 14.17.   Tinea unguium. Subungual debris and discoloration of the nail.

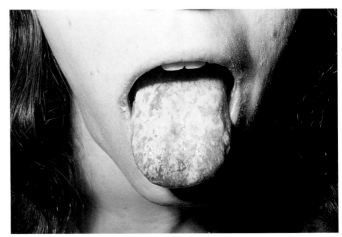

Figure 14.18.   Candidiasis. Chronic mucocutaneous candidiasis leads to exudative infection of the mucous membranes known as thrush. (Courtesy of Dr. Lee T. Nesbitt, Jr.)

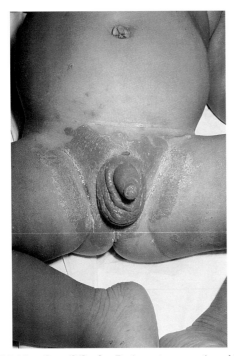

Figure 14.19.   Candidiasis. Erythematous eruption of the diaper area. (Courtesy of Dr. Lee T. Nesbitt, Jr.)

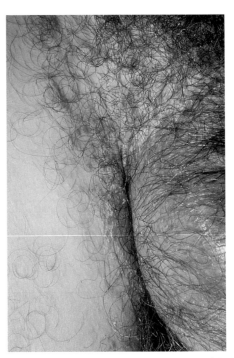

Figure 14.20.   Candidal intertrigo. Involvement of the inner thigh and scrotum showing satellite lesions. (Courtesy of the American Academy of Dermatology)

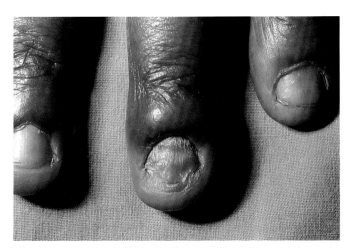

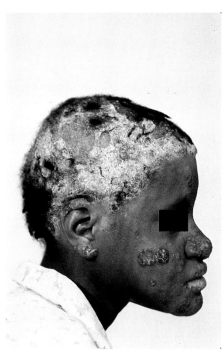

Figure 14.21. Candidiasis. Paronychial swelling and dystrophy of nail. (Courtesy of Dr. Lee T. Nesbitt, Jr.)

Figure 14.22. Candidiasis. Chronic mucocutaneous candidiasis in an immunodeficient patient. Thick, hyperkeratotic plaques of the scalp and face.

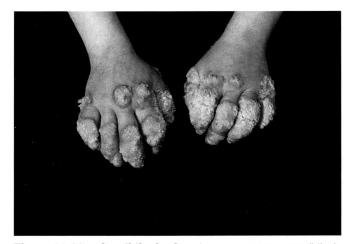

Figure 14.23. Candidiasis. Chronic mucocutaneous candidiasis with severe verrucoid plaques of fingers and dorsal hands. (Courtesy of Dr. Charles V. Sanders)

CHAPTER **15**

Systemic Fungal Infections

ALAN M. STAMM and WILLIAM E. DISMUKES

Each of the systemic mycoses may cause cutaneous disease. The majority of these mycoses are acquired by inhalation of organisms with patients developing skin lesions as part of subsequent disseminated disease. Some of these diseases are initiated by direct inoculation of organisms, with patients having progressive but localized skin and soft tissue disease. Cutaneous lesions in both situations are often prominently manifested and represent a major area for examination and evaluation in the diagnosis of these deep fungal infections.

Blastomycosis

• PATHOGENESIS •

Blastomycosis is endemic in the southeastern United States and Africa. The disease most commonly affects middle-aged men with extensive rural or feral outdoor activities. Inhalation of spores of *Blastomyces dermatitidis* elicits an inflammatory response with the eventual formation of granulomas in the lung. The primary pulmonary infection may be asymptomatic, acute and influenza-like, or chronic and progressive. The infection may spread via the lymphatics to the bloodstream with consequent hematogenous dissemination and secondary skin involvement. Rarely, infection is acquired by direct cutaneous inoculation, mostly in laboratory workers.

• CLINICAL FEATURES •

The majority of patients who develop disseminated blastomycosis have cutaneous lesions. Although any area of the body may be involved, lesions are often prominently displayed on the distal exanthem or face (Figs. 15.1–15.5). Most commonly, one to many papulonodules evolve over weeks or months into verrucous lesions characterized by induration and crusting, with possible areas of healing marked by pigmentary changes and scarring. Alternatively, one to many pustules may appear and rapidly progress into superficial ulcers (Fig. 15.6). These disseminated lesions are generally painless and not associated with lymphangitis or lymphadenopathy. Mucous membranes are uncommonly involved.

Direct cutaneous inoculation of *B. dermatitidis* results in a chancriform lesion—a painless papule or pustule that evolves over weeks into an ulcer. Ascending, nodular lymphangitis and regional lymphadenitis develop, but there have been no reports of hematogenous dissemination from one of these primary skin lesions. Erythema nodosum may occur in association with either direct inoculation or disseminated cutaneous blastomycosis.

• DIAGNOSIS AND DIFFERENTIAL DIAGNOSIS •

A potassium hydroxide (KOH) wet preparation made from pus or tissue scrapings demonstrates the yeast in most cases. Histologic examination of tissue obtained by skin biopsy after staining with periodic acid-Schiff (PAS) or Gomori's methenamine silver (GMS) usually reveals the 8–15-μm, thick-walled, broad-based budding yeasts. Pseudoepitheliomatous hyperplasia and microabscess formation in the epidermis are also noted. Demonstration of *B. dermatitidis* in a culture of pus or tissue on Sabouraud's dextrose agar is definitive.

Cutaneous lesions of disseminated or direct inoculation blastomycosis must be differentiated from other mycoses, bacterial pyoderma, tuberculosis, syphilis, bromoderma, pyoderma gangrenosum, and squamous cell carcinoma.

• TREATMENT AND CLINICAL COURSE •

Patients with non-life-threatening disease are treated with an oral azole drug, such as ketoconazole or itraconazole. Those with more serious or widely disseminated disease require amphotericin B. Lesions heal over weeks to months, often with pigmentary changes and scarring.

Chromoblastomycosis

• PATHOGENESIS •

Chromoblastomycosis, also called chromomycosis, occurs most commonly in the tropical and subtropical regions of America, Africa, and Australia. Most victims are adult male farm workers who go barefoot. The etiologic agents are dematiaceous (dark-walled) fungi, such as *Fonsecaea pedrosoi, Rhinocladiella aquaspersa, Cladosporium carrionii, Phialophora verrucosa,* and *Fonsecaea compacta,* present in soil and on vegetation. Infection is acquired by direct inoculation.

Phaeohyphomycosis is the diagnosis used for subcutaneous infections caused by numerous species of dematiaceous fungi that produce hyphae and/or yeast forms in tissue.

• CLINICAL FEATURES •

The typical primary lesion is a small scaly papule on the foot or lower leg. Over months to years the papule enlarges into a fibrous nodule, the surface of which may be smooth, scaly, verrucous, crusted, or ulcerated (Fig. 15.7). Lesions may also evolve into large plaques with scaly, warty, or crusted surfaces, or into tumor-like masses (Figs. 15.8–15.10).

Lesions are not usually painful unless secondary infection occurs. Purulent material may be expressed by squeezing a nodule. Scratching may inoculate adjacent areas of the skin; satellite lesions may appear and subsequently coalesce. As a result, the disease tends to extend peripherally. Bacterial superinfections may cause lymphangitis, regional lymphadenopathy, and eventual lymphatic fibrosis with elephantiasis. Chromoblastomycosis frequently is present for decades without causing constitutional illness or bony invasion, and hematogenous dissemination is rare.

• DIAGNOSIS AND DIFFERENTIAL DIAGNOSIS •

The diagnosis of chromoblastomycosis is suggested by clinical findings and supported by detection of sclerotic bodies in KOH wet preparations of purulent exudate. Cultures on Sabouraud's dextrose agar are usually positive after 2 to 3 weeks. Histologically, this mycosis is characterized by hyperkeratotic pseudoepitheliomatous hyperplasia, epidermal microabscess formation, granulomatous dermal reaction with giant cells, and the presence of sclerotic bodies (round, thick-walled, brown, 8–12-μm, vegetative fungal cells).

The differential diagnosis includes blastomycosis, mycetoma, sporotrichosis, tuberculosis, tertiary syphilis, yaws, and leishmaniasis.

• TREATMENT AND CLINICAL COURSE •

Limited early lesions are best managed by surgical excision. For extensive lesions, either flucytosine plus amphotericin B or itraconazole is recommended. Intermediate cases may be treated with surgical resection, plus itraconazole. Incomplete responses to therapy and relapses are common.

Coccidioidomycosis

• PATHOGENESIS •

Coccidioidomycosis is endemic in the Lower Sonoran Life Zone of the southwestern United States and in Central and South America. The dimorphic fungus, *Coccidioides immitis,* exists in soil as a mold. Mechanical disruption of the soil results in dispersal of arthrospores, which cause primary pulmonary infection when inhaled.

About 60% of infections are asymptomatic or experienced as commonplace upper respiratory infections, while 35% are manifest as self-limited lower respiratory infections. About 5% of infected individuals develop chronic, progressive, sometimes cavitary pulmonary disease, and fewer than 1% develop extrapulmonary, disseminated disease due to hematogenous spread. Those at increased risk for dissemination include African Americans, Filipinos, American Indians, Mexicans, and pregnant women. The skin is involved in most cases; lesions generally appear within several months of primary infection. Rarely, primary cutaneous disease occurs following inoculation and an incubation period of 1 to 3 weeks.

• CLINICAL FEATURES •

Acute, self-limited, pulmonary coccidioidomycosis may be associated with three different eruptions, none of which are indicative of dissemination. Toxic erythema is a fine, diffuse, maculopapular erythema of the trunk and extremities that occurs early and fades after a few days. Erythema multiforme may occur at approximately the 3rd to 7th week as annular erythematous target-like lesions, primarily on the extremities, with lesions lasting 2 to 3 weeks. Erythema nodosum may occur as painful, erythematous, symmetrically distributed nodules on the legs, thighs, or forearms late in the pneumonic process and last for several weeks. Erythema multiforme and erythema nodosum are hypersensitivity reactions and may present in conjunction with fever, arthralgias, and other systemic symptoms.

The cutaneous manifestations of disseminated coccidioidomycosis are many and varied. They include verrucous lesions that frequently occur on the face, a diffuse pustular eruption, and subcutaneous abscesses (Figs. 15.11–15.12). These abscesses present as cool, painless, fluctuant nodules most commonly on the back, hip, or flank, which may ulcerate and drain purulent or blood-tinged material. Other draining lesions may represent sinus tracts from bone, joint, or visceral foci.

The rare condition of primary inoculation coccidioidomycosis appears as a chancriform lesion: a painless, nontender induration with central ulceration. Lymphangitis and regional lymphadenopathy ensue, but constitutional symptoms are lacking. The process usually heals spontaneously within 3 months, although hematogenous dissemination is possible.

• DIAGNOSIS AND DIFFERENTIAL DIAGNOSIS •

Histologically, the disease is characterized by granulomas and spherules, the tissue form of *C. immitis.* These 30–60-μm spheres can be shown in hematoxylin-eosin and GMS-stained tissue sections to contain numerous endospores 2 to 5 μm. They are present within the areas of granulomatous inflammation.

The diagnosis also can be made by demonstrating the characteristic spherules of *C. immitis* in KOH wet preparations of pus. Growth of cultures on Sabouraud's dextrose agar is usually apparent in 3 to 4 days, and patients with disseminated disease usually have detectable serum precipitin and complement-fixing antibodies. The differential diagnosis of secondary cutaneous coccidioidomycosis includes other mycoses, actinomycosis, syphilis, and tuberculosis. Primary cutaneous disease also can be confused with nocardiosis, yaws, and cutaneous leishmaniasis.

• TREATMENT AND CLINICAL COURSE •

The hypersensitivity eruptions accompanying primary pulmonary infection require only supportive therapy. Likewise, primary cutaneous disease generally resolves spontaneously. Cutaneous disease associated with hematogenous dissemination mandates systemic antifungal chemotherapy with amphotericin B or an azole compound. Lesions heal in weeks to months with scarring.

Cryptococcosis

• PATHOGENESIS •

Cryptococcosis is a deep mycosis caused by *Cryptococcus neoformans*. This microorganism exists as a yeast in tissue at 37°C and in culture at 20°C. In nature, it has been recovered from soils around the world, particularly those enriched by pigeon droppings or by detritus from eucalyptus trees.

Infection is acquired by inhalation, but most individuals remain asymptomatic, and there have been no airborne outbreaks of disease. While pneumonia does occur, the most common clinical presentation is as meningoencephalitis due to hematogenous dissemination. Among patients with disseminated disease, 30% are normal hosts and 70% are immunocompromised, often by chronic systemic glucocorticosteroid therapy. *Cryptococcus neoformans* is the most common cause of meningitis in patients with AIDS.

• CLINICAL FEATURES •

The skin is involved in 10% to 15% of cases (and in 20% to 30% of AIDS patients infected with cryptococcosis). Historically, the most commonly recognized skin lesions have been painless erythematous papules, pustules, or subcutaneous nodules on the face or scalp. These may enlarge, ulcerate, or drain purulent material, and they may be confused with lesions due to other mycoses. Maculopapular skin lesions resembling molluscum contagiosum are often observed in patients with AIDS.

More recently, cellulitis has become increasingly appreciated as a cutaneous manifestation of disseminated cryptococcosis, particularly in immunosuppressed patients. An erythematous, warm, tender area on an extremity may subsequently undergo vesiculation, hemorrhage, ulceration, or development of an eschar (Fig. 15.13). This process must be differentiated from bacterial cellulitis due to staphylococci, streptococci, or vibrios.

• DIAGNOSIS AND DIFFERENTIAL DIAGNOSIS •

A diagnosis of cryptococcosis may be established via microscopic examination and culture of pus or biopsy specimens. Purulent material can be mixed with India ink or smeared and stained using the Gram, Wright, or Papanicolaou techniques (Fig. 15.14). The yeasts are 4 to 20 μm in diameter and have a double-refractile cell wall and cytoplasmic inclusions. The entire cell is surrounded by a thick capsule, and reproduction is by budding. Histologic sections may reveal very little inflammation or, less commonly, a granulomatous reaction pattern. Yeasts are usually present in abundance in the dermis and/or subcutis. The cell wall is stained red with PAS or black with GMS; the capsule is red when stained with mucicarmine. With culture on Sabouraud's dextrose agar, colonies appear after 5 to 7 days. The cerebrospinal fluid (CSF) latex agglutination test for cryptococcal polysaccharide capsular antigen is positive in almost all patients. The same test in serum is more sensitive in those with AIDS.

As mentioned before, the differential diagnosis of cryptococcosis includes other mycoses, molluscum contagiosum, and bacterial cellulitis.

• TREATMENT AND CLINICAL COURSE •

The evaluation of individuals with cutaneous cryptococcosis must include sampling of cerebrospinal fluid to rule out concomitant meningoencephalitis. Patients with life-threatening or central nervous system disease are treated initially with amphotericin B plus flucytosine; others may be treated with fluconazole. About 15% to 20% of patients with serious disease fail to respond to therapy, and a similar percent relapse after seemingly successful treatment. AIDS patients must be kept on maintenance fluconazole or itraconazole indefinitely.

Histoplasmosis

• PATHOGENESIS •

Although the greatest incidence of disease caused by *Histoplasma capsulatum* is in the central United States, histoplasmosis also occurs in temperate zones around the world. The fungus, *H. capsulatum*, resides in soil with infection being acquired via inhalation of spores. The vast majority of human infections are asymptomatic and without clinical consequence. Acute pulmonary histoplasmosis, which may follow primary infection or a reinfection with a heavy inoculum, is characterized by fever, chills, headache, dry cough, and pleuritic chest pain, lasting for several days to 3 weeks. Lymphohematogenous disseminated disease occurs in less than 1% of those infected; infants, immunocompromised hosts, and the elderly are at increased risk.

• CLINICAL FEATURES •

Acute symptomatic pulmonary histoplasmosis is associated with erythema multiforme and/or erythema nodosum in up to

4% of cases. When they occur, erythema multiforme-like lesions usually appear at the end of the first week of illness as annular, target-like maculopapules on the hands, feet, extremities, and lips and persist for 2 to 3 weeks. The central areas may become vesicular and hemorrhagic. Erythema nodosum most commonly appears at the end of the 2nd week as tender, warm, red-brown nodules overlying the anterior tibial areas. Both eruptions are attributed to hypersensitivity and may have arthralgias and fever as associated symptoms.

Oropharyngeal ulcers, the most common mucocutaneous manifestation of disseminated histoplasmosis, occur in the majority of adults with chronic, mild disease but infrequently in infants with acute, widespread involvement. The ulcerated lesion, initially a plaque or nodule, is painful and has thick, rolled edges (Figs. 15.15, 15.16). Ulcers are frequently located on the tongue, buccal mucosa, larynx, lip, and/or gingiva. In children, the ulcers are usually small and shallow.

The skin is involved in only 5% of adults with disseminated histoplasmosis but is not uncommonly involved in immuno-compromised hosts, such as patients with AIDS. Painless papules or nodules evolve into pustules and ulcers with heaped-up margins and purulent discharge (Fig. 15.17). These lesions typically arise around body orifices, but may occur anywhere in patients with AIDS.

Primary cutaneous histoplasmosis follows local inoculation and runs a different course than the skin lesions of disseminated histoplasmosis. A painless nodule or ulcer occurs at the site of inoculation with subsequent lymphangitis and regional lymphadenopathy, healing spontaneously within several months.

• DIAGNOSIS AND DIFFERENTIAL DIAGNOSIS •

The diagnosis of acute pulmonary histoplasmosis is confirmed by serologic testing. The complement fixation titer should be equal to or greater than 1:32 or demonstrate a 4-fold rise on serial testing. The diagnosis of disseminated disease requires biopsy and culture. Histologically, the lesions are characterized by heavily parasitized macrophages and varying degrees of granulomatous reaction. In GMS-stained tissue sections, budding, 2–4-μm yeasts may be demonstrated in macrophages in the inflammatory reaction. The mold phase of *H. capsulatum* can be identified after isolation on Sabouraud's dextrose agar.

Oropharyngeal ulcers must be differentiated clinically from aphthous ulcers and carcinoma. Cutaneous lesions of histoplasmosis may be mistaken for those associated with other mycoses, actinomycosis, or nocardiosis.

• TREATMENT AND CLINICAL COURSE •

Patients with acute pulmonary or primary cutaneous disease generally recover spontaneously. Infants and immunocompromised adults with disseminated disease are treated with amphotericin B, whereas adults with chronic, non-life-threatening forms of histoplasmosis are effectively treated with an oral azole drug, such as ketoconazole or itraconazole. Mucosal and skin lesions heal within weeks or months.

Mycetoma

• PATHOGENESIS •

Mycetoma (maduromycosis) occurs primarily in the tropical regions of Central and South America, Africa, and Asia. The typical patient is a young or middle-aged male farmer who goes barefoot. The syndrome is caused by microorganisms living in the soil or on plants. The etiologic agents to be discussed in this section are true fungi (eumycetoma), although various actinomycetes (actinomycetoma) may also produce this disorder and are discussed in Chapter 5. In the United States, *Pseudallescheria boydii* is the most common cause of eumycetoma, whereas *Madurella mycetomatis* is the most frequently isolated pathogen worldwide.

Trauma of the involved area (foot, hand, buttock) with inoculation of organisms is usually the initiating event. The disease is slowly progressive, infrequently associated with constitutional symptoms, and rarely complicated by hematogenous dissemination.

Mycetoma can also be caused by various actinomycetes. For a discussion on actinomycetoma, see Chapter 5.

• CLINICAL FEATURES •

Eumycetoma may begin as a small papule or nodule, an indurated area, or an abscess with a sinus tract. The disease process spreads by contiguity along fascial planes and destroys subcutaneous tissue as well as deeper structures. As a result, there is ankylosis of the involved joint, with the involved extremity becoming progressively more indurated, deformed, and nonfunctional (Fig. 15.18). There is discoloration of the skin and scarring, but generally no pain or tenderness. Multiple deep abscesses drain serosanguinous-purulent material containing grains or granules. These grains, representing colonies of the offending microorganism, are about 1 mm in diameter and are white, yellow, or black, depending on the causative organism. After 10 to 15 years, the limb often appears globose or club-shaped. Bacterial superinfection may cause fever, pain, and regional lymphadenopathy.

• DIAGNOSIS AND DIFFERENTIAL DIAGNOSIS •

The diagnosis of eumycetoma is suggested by clinical findings and supported by detection and microscopic examination of grains. Black grains are seen only in eumycetoma and red grains only in actinomycetoma. White-to-yellow grains are the most common and may indicate either. Potassium hydroxide wet preparations of organisms reveal 2–5-μm septate hyphae in eumycetoma. Confirmation of the diagnosis is obtained by culture on Sabouraud's dextrose agar with appropriate lactophenol cotton blue-stained smears of colony growth. Histologically, the disease is characterized by necrosis, granulomatous inflammation with multinucleated giant cells, and fibrosis (Fig. 15.19).

The differential diagnosis of eumycetoma includes actinomycetoma, actinomycosis, and botryomycosis, all of which are also associated with grains in purulent drainage from skin lesions.

In actinomycetoma, the grains may be white, yellow, pink, red, or brown, depending on the species of actinomycete. Gram's stain of the exudate reveals filamentous, branching, Gram-positive bacteria. The various actinomycetes can be isolated on an enriched medium, such as brain heart infusion (BHI) agar in an aerobic environment. In actinomycosis, the grains are white or yellow "sulfur granules." *Actinomyces israelii* can be cultured on BHI agar under anaerobic conditions. In botryomycosis, the grains are also white or yellow, but Gram's stain demonstrates either Gram-positive cocci or Gram-negative bacilli, and aerobic cultures yield *Staphylococcus aureus* or *Pseudomonas aeruginosa*. Other diseases that should be included in the differential diagnosis of eumycetoma are tuberculosis, syphilis, and yaws.

• TREATMENT AND CLINICAL COURSE •

The treatment of eumycetoma is generally unsatisfactory. Disease caused by *Pseudallescheria boydii* may respond to miconazole or ketoconazole and surgery, including debridement, drainage of abscesses, exploration of sinus tracts, and removal of infected bone. Amputation with a wide margin is frequently necessary.

Paracoccidioidomycosis

• PATHOGENESIS •

Paracoccidioidomycosis, which is endemic in tropical and subtropical forested areas of Central and South America, is a disease predominantly of 30- to 50-year-old male farmers and ranchers. *Paracoccidioides brasiliensis* is a dimorphic fungus; mycelia in the soil produce arthroconidia and microconidia. Infection is almost always acquired by inhalation of conidia.

The primary pulmonary infection is rarely symptomatic, but often followed by spread to the reticuloendothelial system. In children, after a brief latent period, acute disseminated disease marked by fever, weight loss, malaise, hepatosplenomegaly, and lymphadenopathy may appear. In adults, after a latency of many years, chronic paracoccidioidomycosis may develop. Two-thirds of cases have hematogenously disseminated disease, usually in association with pneumonia.

• CLINICAL FEATURES •

Acute disseminated paracoccidioidomycosis in children may be associated with an acneiform eruption or subcutaneous abscesses; mucosal involvement is rare. In contrast, half of adults with chronic disseminated disease seek medical attention because of mucocutaneous involvement. The lesions are usually ulcerative with granulomatous, mulberry-like surfaces and occur most frequently on lips, gums, palate, and tongue (Figs. 15.20, 15.21). Gingivitis may result in loss of teeth. Lesions are painful, enlarge slowly, and spread to adjoining skin, producing crusted ulcers. Lymphadenitis is seen in association with mucocutaneous disease. Other manifestations of chronic dissemination include conjunctivitis and ulcerative or granulomatous lesions of the perianal mucosa and genitalia. Cutaneous inocu-

lation of *P. brasiliensis* is rare, but may result in a chancre with ascending lymphangitis and regional lymphadenopathy.

• DIAGNOSIS AND DIFFERENTIAL DIAGNOSIS •

The diagnosis of paracoccidioidomycosis is usually made by recognition of the yeast in KOH preparations of exudate. Large double-walled cells 10–40-μm in diameter surrounded by multiple 1–5-μm buds may be seen; this "pilot wheel" configuration is pathognomonic of *P. brasiliensis*. Histologic study of biopsy material reveals granulomas, multinucleated giant cells, necrosis, and fibrosis; GMS staining will accentuate the budding yeast. Cultures on Sabouraud's dextrose or Mycosel agar incubated at 25°C yield mycelial growth in 3 to 4 weeks; however, identification of the fungus requires transfer to Kelly agar and incubation at 37°C for another week or more to produce characteristic yeast forms. Serologic testing is also useful. The immunodiffusion test is sensitive and specific for active disease, and the complement-fixation titer can be followed to evaluate the response to therapy.

The differential diagnosis of mucocutaneous paracoccidioidomycosis includes other mycoses, tuberculosis, and malignancies. Coexistent tuberculosis is not uncommon.

• TREATMENT AND CLINICAL COURSE •

Itraconazole and ketoconazole have become the drugs of choice. Sulfonamides are preferable in under-developed areas based on cost. Although mucocutaneous lesions improve in weeks, patients are treated generally for at least 6 months. Patients with more severe forms of the disease may also be treated initially with amphotericin B. Itraconazole may prove to be a superior therapeutic agent to ketoconazole.

Sporotrichosis

• PATHOGENESIS •

Sporotrichosis occurs worldwide in warm temperature and tropical zones. The dimorphic fungus, *Sporothrix schenckii*, lives on plants. Infection, almost always acquired by direct inoculation of skin, occurs most commonly in persons engaged in farming, gardening, or other horticultural activities.

• CLINICAL FEATURES •

Three-quarters of patients with sporotrichosis have lymphocutaneous disease. Weeks or months after inoculation, a painless red papule appears at the site, gradually enlarges, and ulcerates. Pus may exude from the lesion, and a crusted papulonodule eventually forms. The draining lymphatics become red and palpable; small, painless, red-violet nodules arise along their course, which may become ulcerative or suppurative (Figs. 15.22, 15.23). In adults, most disease begins distally on the extremities. Epitrochlear lymphadenopathy is common, but axillary or inguinal nodes are seldom enlarged. In patients with lymphocutaneous disease, symptoms of systemic illness are absent.

One-quarter of patients present with only cutaneous findings and no lymphatic involvement. This so-called "fixed" or "plaque" sporotrichosis is more common in Central and South Americans and in children. The plaque-like lesions are painless and varied in appearance (acneiform, nodular, papillomatous, verrucous, or ulcerative) and there is no lymphatic involvement (Figs. 15.24, 15.25). Among children, equal numbers present with lesions on an extremity versus the face or trunk.

Other types of sporotrichosis include indolent pneumonia, chronic arthritis, and ocular disease with involvement of the eyelids, conjunctivae, or lacrimal glands. Widespread dissemination is rare.

• DIAGNOSIS AND DIFFERENTIAL DIAGNOSIS •

The diagnosis of sporotrichosis can be established by culture of exudate or tissue biopsy on Sabouraud's dextrose agar; growth appears in 3 to 5 days. Yeast forms compatible with *S. schenckii* are rarely seen on smears of exudate; if present, they are cigar-shaped or ovoid and no more than 3 x 6 μm. Biopsy for histopathology should be done, but may not be diagnostic because organisms are not always seen. Pseudoepitheliomatous hyperplasia may simulate squamous epithelial proliferation, and granulomas with microabscesses may be attributed to tuberculosis or blastomycosis. However, asteroid bodies, which are highly characteristic of sporotrichosis, may be seen; these bodies consist of spherical or ovoid cells surrounded by eosinophilic, radial projections spanning a diameter of 30 μm (Fig. 15.26).

The differential diagnosis of lymphocutaneous sporotrichosis includes atypical mycobacteriosis, cutaneous leishmaniasis, primary cutaneous nocardiosis, plus more common considerations, such as bacterial pyoderma, insect bites, and foreign-body granulomas. Fixed sporotrichosis must be differentiated from other mycoses, syphilis, tuberculosis, and leishmaniasis.

• TREATMENT AND CLINICAL COURSE •

Most cases of lymphocutaneous or fixed sporotrichosis can be cured with oral potassium iodide or itraconazole. Extracutaneous disease should be treated with amphotericin B or itraconazole. Skin disease responds well to therapy, which should be continued for at least 1 month after the resolution of all sites of infection.

Rhinosporidiosis

• PATHOGENESIS •

Rhinosporidiosis is endemic in India and Ceylon but also has occurred in many other areas of the world. It is caused by the fungal organism *Rhinosporidium seeberi*. It is not contagious by person-to-person contact.

• CLINICAL FEATURES •

Vascular polyps are the lesions produced by this organism. They occur on any mucosal area, but the nose, nasopharynx, and soft palate are involved in three-fourths of patients. The polyps may grow very large, often extending outward over the lip. Obstruction to breathing is a common symptom. The eye, larynx, vagina, penis, or rectum may also be affected, and the lesions may spread to nearby cutaneous surfaces.

• DIAGNOSIS AND DIFFERENTIAL DIAGNOSIS •

Rhinosporidium seeberi cannot be cultured; therefore, the diagnosis depends on observation of the sporangia of the organism in tissue biopsies. These are spherical, thick-walled structures measuring up to 300 mm in diameter that contain numerous endspores measuring approximately 6 to 7 mm in diameter. Clinical lesions must be differentiated from condylomata of human papillomavirus and rhinoscleroma.

• TREATMENT AND CLINICAL COURSE •

Surgical removal of the papillomatous lesions is the only effective treatment. Chemotherapeutic agents are of no value.

ANNOTATED BIBLIOGRAPHY

Anderson DJ, Schmidt C, Goodman J, Pomeroy C. Cryptococcal disease presenting as cellulitis. Clin Infect Dis 1992;14:666.
> A description of the clinical manifestations, diagnosis, and therapy of cryptococcal cellulitis.

Anderson PC. Cutaneous sporotrichosis. Am Fam Physician 1983;27(3):201.
> A review emphasizing differential diagnosis.

Fader RC, McGinnis MR. Infections caused by dematiaceous fungi: Chromoblastomycosis and phaeohyphomycosis. Infect Dis Clin North Am 1988;2:925.
> A comprehensive review of the clinical syndromes caused by dematiaceous fungi.

Goodwin RA, Jr, et al. Disseminated histoplasmosis: Clinical and pathologic correlations. Medicine 1980;59:1.
> Includes a review of the mucocutaneous manifestations of disseminated disease.

Harvey WC, Greendyke WH. Skin lesions in acute coccidioidomycosis. Am Fam Physician 1970;2(3):81.
> A description of the three types of cutaneous manifestations accompanying primary pulmonary disease.

Lynch PJ, Botero F. Sporotrichosis in children. Am J Dis Child 1971;122:325.
> A comparison of clinical features in children versus adults.

Magana M. Mycetoma. Int J Dermatol 1984;23:221.
> A comprehensive review including many photographs of skin lesions, histopathology, and roentgenograms.

Restrepo A, et al. The gamut of paracoccidioidomycosis. Am J Med 1976;61:33.
> A discussion of the clinical spectrum of disease.

Sellers TF, Jr, Price WN, Jr, Newberry WM, Jr. An epidemic of erythema multiforme and erythema nodosum caused by histoplasmosis. Ann Intern Med 1965;62:1244.
> A description of the cutaneous findings seen with acute pneumonitis associated with histoplasmosis.

Su WPD, Duncan SC, Perry HO. Blastomycosis-like pyoderma. Arch Dermatol 1979;115:170.
> A discussion of the differential diagnosis of the verrucous skin lesions of blastomycosis.

Wilson JW. The importance of the portal of entry in certain microbial infections: The primary cutaneous "chancriform" syndrome. Dis Chest 1968;54(1):43.
> A review of the pathogenesis of primary cutaneous coccidioidomycosis and other mycoses.

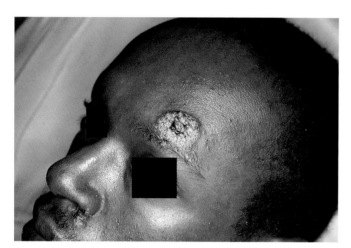

Figure 15.1.   Disseminated blastomycosis in a young man.
Verrucous nodule above the left eyebrow.

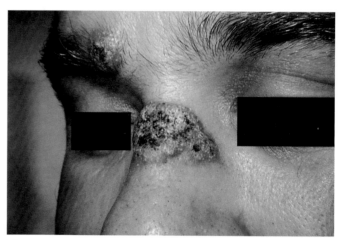

Figure 15.2.   Disseminated blastomycosis. Erythematous
nodules with central crusting.

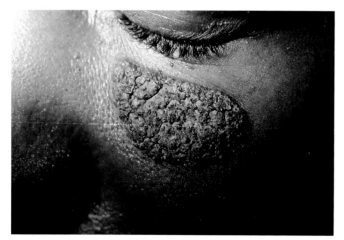

Figure 15.3.   Disseminated blastomycosis. Verrucous plaque
on the upper cheek. (Courtesy of Dr. Charles V. Sanders)

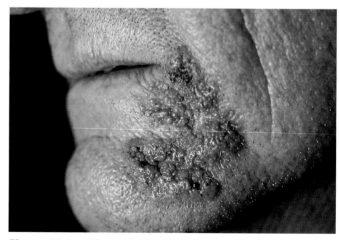

Figure 15.4.   Disseminated blastomycosis. Large erythematous plaque on the lower face. (Courtesy of Dr. Gene Beyt)

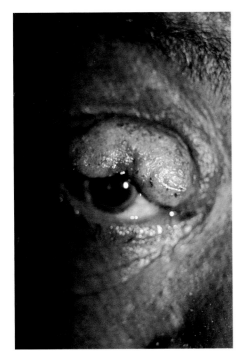

Figure 15.5. Disseminated blastomycosis. Nodular lesion of the left upper eyelid with granular surface. (Courtesy of Dr. Charles V. Sanders)

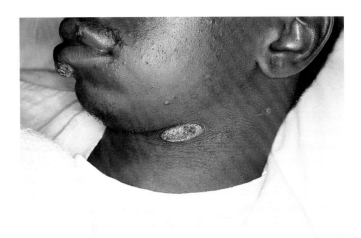

Figure 15.6. Disseminated blastomycosis. Ulcerative and crusted lesions of the neck and lower lip.

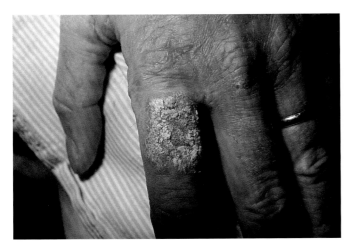

Figure 15.7. Chromoblastomycosis. Early lesion showing verrucous plaque on the dorsum of the fingers. (Courtesy of Dr. Lee T. Nesbitt, Jr.)

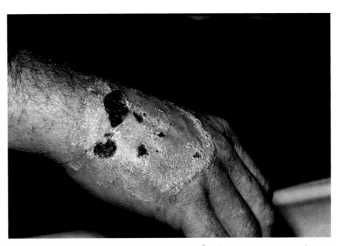

Figure 15.8. Chromoblastomycosis. Large verrucous plaque with ulceration on the dorsum of the hand. (Courtesy of Dr. Lee T. Nesbitt, Jr.)

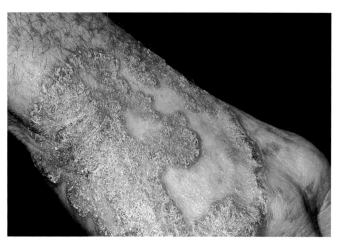

Figure 15.9. Chromoblastomycosis. Large verrucous plaque with sharp margination and irregular border on the dorsum of the hand. (Courtesy of Dr. Lee T. Nesbitt, Jr.)

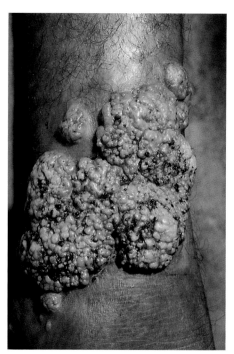

Figure 15.10. Chromoblastomycosis. Verrucoid nodules on the ankle and lower leg. (Courtesy of Dr. Rolando Saenz)

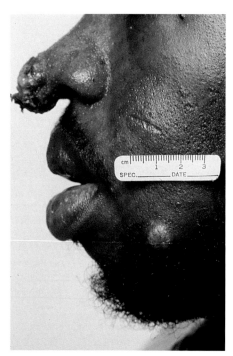

Figure 15.11. Coccidioidomycosis. Raised nodules on the nose and cheek. (Courtesy of Dr. John R. Graybill)

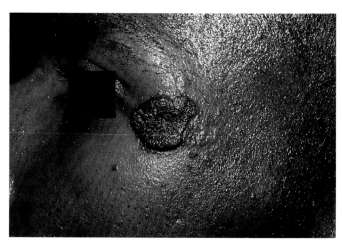

Figure 15.12. Coccidioidomycosis. Hyperpigmented verrucoid plaque of the lateral-to-outer canthus.

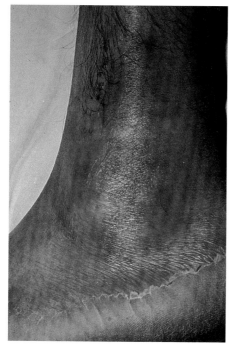

Figure 15.13. Cryptococcal cellulitis. Early well-demarcated erythematous lesions over the ankle in a renal transplant patient. (Courtesy of Dr. Charles V. Sanders)

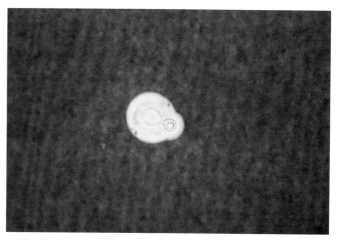

Figure 15.14. *Cryptococcus neoformans.* India ink preparation of cerebrospinal fluid.

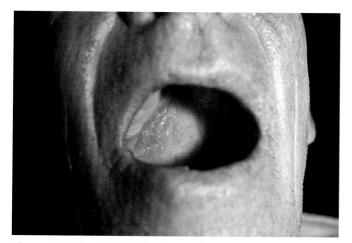

Figure 15.15. Oral histoplasmosis. Erosive lesion on the hard palate due to inoculation by expectoration of the organism. (Courtesy of Dr. Lee T. Nesbitt, Jr.)

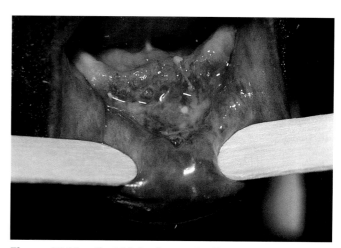

Figure 15.16. Oral histoplasmosis. Erosive ulcerations on the floor of the mouth. (Courtesy of Dr. Lee T. Nesbitt, Jr.)

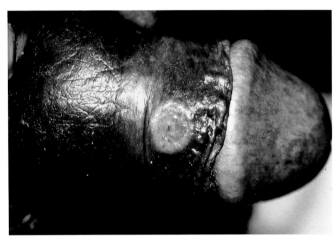

Figure 15.17.   Histoplasmosis. Sharply demarcated ulcerative lesion on the shaft of the penis. (Courtesy of Dr. George H. Karam)

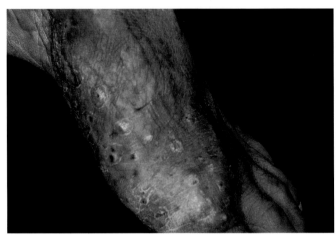

Figure 15.18.   Eumycetoma. Madura foot due to *Pseudallescheria boydii*. Thickened plaque on the side of the foot.

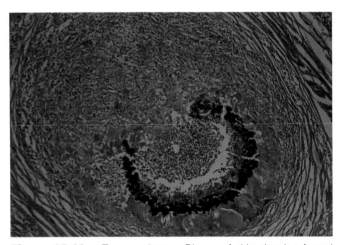

Figure 15.19.   Eumycetoma. Biopsy of skin showing fungal organisms with surrounding giant cell reaction. (Courtesy of Dr. Lee T. Nesbitt, Jr.)

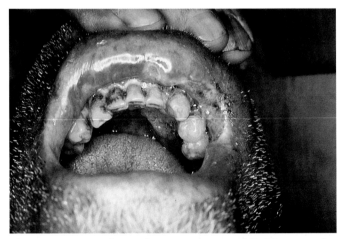

Figure 15.20.   Disseminated paracoccidioidomycosis. Granulomatous raised lesion on the palate and an ulcer on the lip. (Courtesy of Dr. Angela Restrepo)

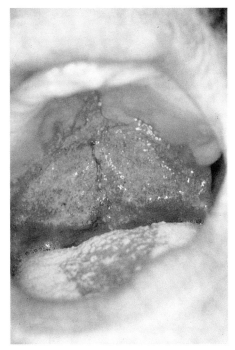

Figure 15.21. Disseminated paracoccidioidomycosis. Involvement of the palate. (Courtesy of Dr. Angela Restrepo)

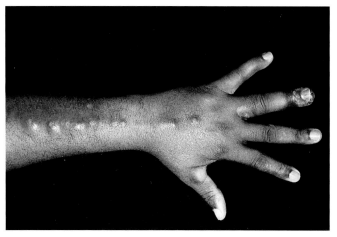

Figure 15.22. Sporotrichosis. Initial inoculation of the 4th finger with ascending nodular lesions of the hand and arm. (Courtesy of Dr. Lee T. Nesbitt, Jr.)

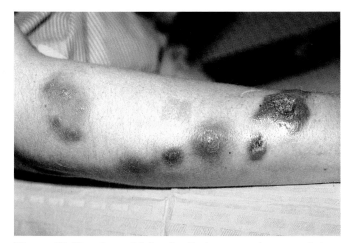

Figure 15.23. Sporotrichosis. Erythematous plaques and ulceration of the forearm.

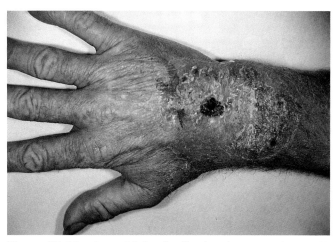

Figure 15.24. Sporotrichosis. Fixed erythematous plaque with ulceration of the wrist. (Courtesy of Dr. Lee T. Nesbitt, Jr.)

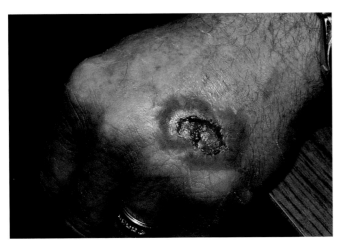

Figure 15.25.   Sporotrichosis. Fixed ulcerative plaque on the dorsum of the hand. (Courtesy of Dr. Charles V. Sanders)

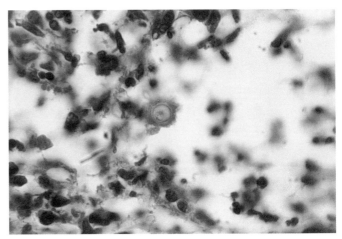

Figure 15.26.   Sporotrichosis. Histopathology specimen showing asteroid bodies.

CHAPTER **16**

Viral Exanthems

WESLEY KING GALEN and STEPHEN E. GELLIS

Patients of all ages, particularly children, may present with generalized erythematous eruptions in association with fever and other symptoms. Such generalized eruptions—which may be composed of macules, papules, vesicles, vesiculopustules, pustules, and/or petechiae—are known as exanthems. Exanthematous eruptions are usually associated with viral illnesses but may occur with bacterial and rickettsial infections or be seen as reactions to drugs.

Differential diagnoses of the viral exanthems are listed in Table 16.1.

This chapter will discuss the following disorders: varicella, rubeola (measles), rubella, enteroviral eruptions, roseola infantum, erythema infectiosum, Colorado tick fever, and eruptions associated with hepatitis and infectious mononucleosis. The tables at the end of the chapter summarize their clinical features, diagnosis, and treatment.

Varicella

The varicella-zoster virus (VZV) is a member of the *Herpesviridae* family. It contains a double-stranded DNA core within its capsid, surrounded by an icosahedral lipid envelope with glycoprotein spikes. It is responsible for two important viral illnesses: varicella (chickenpox), which is its primary infection, and herpes zoster, the reactivation or secondary presentation. A discussion of herpes zoster can be found in Chapter 17.

• PATHOGENESIS •

Chickenpox is extremely contagious. It affects 85% to 90% of the U.S. population by age 15, although 10% to 15% remain uninfected and at risk for primary infection in the adult years. It is estimated to occur in up to 3.5 million persons per year in the United States, prompting about 500,000 to seek medical atten-

Table 16.1. Differential Diagnosis of Common Exanthems by Frequent Lesional Characteristics

Maculopapular	Vesiculopustules	Urticaria	Petechiae
Drug eruption	Drug eruption	Varicella (urticaria around vesicle)	Drug eruption
Secondary lues	Herpes simplex		Bacterial endocarditis
Scarlet fever	Varicella	Coxsackieviruses A5, A9, A16, B4, B5; ECHO 11	Coxsackieviruses A9, A4, B2, B3, B4, B5; ECHO 9, 4, 7, 3
Coxsackieviruses A5, A9, A16, B5	Disseminated zoster	Infectious mononucleosis	Infectious mononucleosis
Reovirus 2	Rickettsialpox	*Mycoplasma pneumoniae*	Rubella
Erythema infectiosum	Coxsackieviruses A5, A16, A8, A10	Hepatitis A, B, C, E	Thrombocytopenia with many acute infections
Gianotti-Crosti	Reovirus 2	Drug eruption	Hepatitis B
Rubella	*Mycoplasma pneumoniae*		Atypical measles
Rubeola	Echovirus 4		Rocky Mountain spotted fever
Hepatitis A	Orf		
Infectious mononucleosis	Milker's nodule		
Arbovirus (dengue)	Rubeola (rare)		
Rickettsioses (Rocky Mountain spotted fever)			

tion. Humans serve as the only reservoir for this illness. Its spread usually occurs by the respiratory route from infected persons or from intimate contact with patients suffering from herpes zoster.

Chickenpox has an incubation period of about 2 weeks or up to 3 weeks in some cases. Epidemics among nonimmune individuals do occur, especially in late winter and early spring. It spreads rapidly to household contacts, affecting almost 90% of susceptible individuals within 3 weeks of exposure. The virus is thought to be particularly contagious during the prodrome (1 to 2 days) before the rash becomes evident. In young, healthy persons, the contagious period persists for about 5 days after the rash is first seen, and the disease is rarely associated with systemic involvement or complications.

The neutralizing antibodies and cellular immunity that are produced limit the infection and its dissemination but do not entirely sterilize the body of the virus. During the infection, VZV gains entry to the dorsal root ganglia of somatic nerves and certain cranial nerves where it may remain latent, only to reemerge years later as a painful localized infection, herpes zoster.

Herpes zoster is discussed in Chapter 17.

• CLINICAL FEATURES •

Varicella often presents with a prodromal illness of fever, malaise, irritability, and, occasionally, mild respiratory symptoms followed by the abrupt onset of rash. The first noticeable lesions are usually red papules on the head or trunk. Each lesion evolves over 24 to 48 hours from a papule to a vesicle to a vesiculopustule that umbilicates and dries to form a crusted papule (Figs. 16.1, 16.2). The lesions occur in crops at almost daily intervals for 3 to 4 days. Thus, lesions in all stages of development may be seen as the illness is fully expressed, aiding in its diagnosis. Bullae may occur when varicella lesions are secondarily infected with *Staphylococcus aureus* strains that cause concurrent bullous impetigo. Lesions spread centripetally but are emphasized on the face, scalp, and trunk. They may be sparse or numerous and may involve the oral mucosa and genitalia. Factors such as sunburn and local skin trauma affect the distribution and increase the density of lesions, even in healthy children, who suffer most from pruritus, irritability, and fever.

As the illness progresses, antibody titers increase; lymphocytic cellular immunity develops; the fever defervesces; and the crusted lesions dry and peel, occasionally leaving slightly depressed scars. Scars are more prominent in traumatized or secondarily infected lesions.

Complications are rare but require recognition. These include: varicella pneumonia, hepatitis, meningoencephalitis, Reye's syndrome, thrombocytopenic purpura, and purpura fulminans.

Adults suffer more pruritus, develop more lesions, and experience a more toxic clinical course characterized by high fever, arthralgias, muscle aches, and profound malaise. Although uncommon among healthy adults, these patients are at greater risk for varicella pneumonia.

Chickenpox is much more severe among children and adults who are immunodeficient, such as those with congenital deficiencies, lymphomas, leukemia, AIDS, and patients receiving chemotherapy and/or corticosteroids. AIDS patients are at great risk for systemic involvement. Varicella occurs in patients with leukemia or lymphoma with much greater frequency; almost one-fourth of such children may develop "progressive varicella," with high fever and cutaneous lesions erupting for twice the usual duration. Lesions may be more numerous, deeper, prominently umbilicated, and more acral in distribution, including the palms and soles. Patients with progressive varicella also tend to have more visceral involvement, including pneumonia, hepatitis, and meningoencephalitis. The mortality rate of this progressive illness can reach 20%.

Varicella infections of pregnant women deserve special attention because maternal-fetal transmission may occur. Infection in the first trimester may result in the fetal varicella syndrome in which affected infants are born with cicatricial, sometimes linear, skin lesions (Fig. 16.3) and, on occasion, limb atrophy. The syndrome may be associated with central nervous system and eye involvement. Fortunately, this severe early intrauterine infection is a very rare occurrence. Varicella infection of the mother late in pregnancy may result in a perinatal infection of variable severity in the newborn. If the maternal illness occurs 2 days before to 5 days after parturition, the baby will be born before the development and transplacental transmission of neutralizing antibody, leaving the neonate vulnerable to severe infection. Speedy recognition and aggressive treatment of the baby is required to reduce morbidity and mortality, which was 30% in years before specific therapy was available.

• DIAGNOSIS AND DIFFERENTIAL DIAGNOSIS •

Chickenpox is usually diagnosed on clinical grounds. Support for the diagnosis may be obtained by Tzank smears from lesions or immunofluorescence stains for VZV. Differential diagnosis includes vesicular enteroviral infections.

• TREATMENT AND CLINICAL COURSE •

Specific treatment of uncomplicated varicella in immunocompetent children is not usually required. Supportive measures, such as drying lotions (calamine, Milk of Magnesia, or pramoxine) and antihistamines (diphenhydramine or hydroxyzine) are helpful. Covering lesions to reduce scratching may also help. Acetaminophen may be used for fever reduction. (Salicylates should be avoided due to their association with varicella-induced Reye's syndrome).

The use of oral acyclovir in healthy children with varicella appears unnecessary. Although it does reduce the number of skin lesions by 25% and the duration of fever by 1 day, acyclovir must be initiated within 24 hours of the first skin lesion to do so. Acyclovir use does not appear to adversely affect the normal immune response, but the benign nature of most chickenpox and the great expense of acyclovir also mitigate against its general use. It is, however, very useful in the treatment of adults and older adolescents, and can be life-saving in immunocompromised patients.

The recent development and licensing of varicella-zoster vaccine is very exciting, particularly for use in immunocompromised patients. It is known to be effective in preventing disease even after exposure to varicella, but its utility in producing lifelong immunity is uncertain and its cost effectiveness in healthy children awaits further study.

Table 16.2 describes the clinical course of varicella, and Table 16.3 lists indications for treatment.

Rubeola (Measles)

Rubeola is an acute childhood illness with a distinctive clinical picture. In most cases, it is a benign illness, but it may produce serious or fatal complications on occasion, mainly in immunocompromised patients. After the measles vaccine was introduced in 1963, the incidence dropped dramatically from between 200,000 to 500,000 cases annually to a low of less than 1500 cases in 1983. Small epidemics, however, continue to occur in unvaccinated young adults and children. In 1989, approximately 18,000 cases were reported in the United States. These statistics encourage physicians to remain vigilant in vaccinating for measles.

Table 16.2. Varicella

Etiology:	Varicella-zoster virus (poxvirus).
Incidence:	Late winter to early spring, but year-round possible. Affects 85%–90% of children by age 15.
Incubation:	10–20 days (mean of 15).
Illness Duration:	7–21 days (until crusts fall); if longer, evaluate for HIV.
Prodrome:	24 hours of fever and malaise.
Enanthem:	Diffusely scattered vesicles or ulcers of 7–10 days duration; may involve mouth, eyes, and genitalia.
Exanthem:	Abrupt onset of red maculopapules followed by a central "dew drop" vesicle that umbilicates within 24 hours, then crusts. Occasionally leaves slightly depressed scars. Crops of vesicles occur over 3–5 days. This accounts for various stages (3–4 crops) being present simultaneously. Centripetal spread to generalized distribution, but central emphasis on face, scalp, and trunk. Rash is photoemphasized.
Clinical Features:	Pruritus, worse in adults than children.
Complications:	Rare. Secondary skin infection, bullous varicella, pneumonitis, hepatitis, meningoencephalitis, progressive varicella, thrombocytopenia purpura, or disseminated intravascular coagulopathy. Fatalities in immunocompromised hosts (purpura fulminans), herpes zoster, Reye's syndrome.
Treatment:	Bed rest, drying lotions, long sleeves and pants to protect from scratching; diphenhydramine or hydroxyzine (antihistamines) for pruritus. Acetaminophen (avoid aspirin) for fever. Acyclovir for adults and older adolescents and for immunodeficient children.

Table 16.3. Acyclovir for Varicella

Varicella in adolescence and adults:
 Treat with acyclovir, if identified within 24 hr of rash.

Varicella in children:
 This is usually "benign" and does not require therapy with acyclovir, although treatment does produce a marginally milder disease if begun within 24 hr of rash. Therapy decreases fever by 1 day and lesions by 20%–25% but does not reduce complications or secondary household spread.

Varicella in atopic patients or patients on corticosteroids:
 Treat with oral acyclovir within 24 hr of rash. Hospitalize and treat with IV acyclovir if infection becomes severe. Any child receiving the equivalent of 1–2 mg/kg/day of prednisone is considered at risk for complications of varicella.

Varicella in pregnancy:
 Appropriate treatment for the mother is the goal. Fetal outcome may not be affected. Varicella's incubation period is 10–21 days. Fetal infection may follow treated infection of the mother. This is a controversial subject pending more data; therefore, consultation with an infectious disease specialist is advised.

• PATHOGENESIS •

The measles virus is an RNA morbillivirus in the paramyxovirus family that is transmitted by oral and nasal secretions. It is a highly contagious virus with an attack rate exceeding 90% in susceptible patients. In prevaccine years, the infection rate was highest among children 5 to 9 years of age. Today, most cases occur in nonimmunized adolescents, inadequately immunized young adults, and very young infants. Measles affects all races and both sexes equally but appears more virulent in certain groups, such as native Americans. Epidemics occur most often in late winter and early spring. The period of communicability begins with the onset of the prodrome and lasts until 4 to 5 days after the onset of the rash.

• CLINICAL FEATURES •

Fever and malaise are the first symptoms of measles, occurring after an incubation period of 10 to 14 days. This is followed by the development of cough, coryza, conjunctivitis (Fig. 16.4), and photophobia. These symptoms peak by the 4th day, with temperature approximately 39.5°C–40.6°C as the rash appears.

The eruption may be seen from 1 to 8 days after the illness begins but usually begins on the 3rd day. Lesions appear as discrete, small, pink macules along the hairline, forehead, upper neck, and behind the ears. The exanthem becomes papular and spreads downward, to involve the face (day 1), trunk (day 2), and, finally, the extremities (day 3) (Fig. 16.5). At areas of initial involvement, especially the face and upper trunk, lesions become confluent and deep red (Fig. 16.6). After 5 to 6 days, the eruption begins to fade in the same order as it appeared, becoming brown and desquamating with a fine scale. Symptoms begin to abate as the lesions disappear.

Koplik's spots, the enanthem that is pathognomonic for measles, appear 2 days after the onset of symptoms and 2 days before the exanthem. They first occur on the buccal mucosa opposite the first lower molars or the inner lip, and they are erythematous, irregular macules with a pinpoint white center. Their number increases until a confluent erythema is formed over the buccal and labial mucosa, with the white specks appearing as grains of salt sprinkled over a red background. The Koplik's spots disappear by the third day of the rash. Similar spots have been noted on the conjunctivae and labia.

Although infection is thought to provide lifelong immunity, cases of recurrent modified or milder measles have been documented on rare occasions.

The complications of measles include viral pneumonia, encephalitis, thrombocytopenia purpura, myocarditis, and secondary bacterial pneumonia or otitis media. Subacute sclerosing panencephalitis is a devastating rare late complication. Children who are immunosuppressed or immunodeficient are at the greatest risk for serious complications and fatal outcome.

An atypical form of measles, summarized in Table 16.4, can occur in persons exposed to natural measles who received the inactivated measles vaccine, used prior to the development of a live attenuated vaccine. Rare cases have also occurred following vaccination with attenuated vaccine. The symptoms begin with high fever, headache, and myalgia. After 2 to 3 days, a rash develops around the ankles and wrists, characterized by petechiae, purpura, papules, and sometimes vesicles (Fig. 16.7). Koplik's spots can occur rarely, as can a form of strawberry tongue. The rash spreads centripetally to the extremities and trunk, producing pruritus. The hallmark of this illness is the development of a pneumonitis that may be severe, with evidence of pulmonary nodules several centimeters in size on X-ray examination. Patients may also complain of abdominal pain and nausea and have associated abnormal liver function.

Table 16.4. Atypical Measles

Etiology:	Paramyxovirus in partially immunized host (killed vaccine)
Incidence:	Summer months
Incubation:	7–14 days
Illness Duration:	14 days or more
Prodrome:	3–5 days of fever, myalgia, coryza, abdominal pain, vomiting, productive cough
Enanthem:	Koplik spots (variable and infrequent); strawberry tongue
Exanthem:	Rash starts on wrists, palms, and soles, then spreads centripetally to extremities and trunk; Lesions are maculopapular and become vesicular, purpuric, and hemorrhagic
Clinical Features:	Pneumonia, transient cardiomegaly, hepatic involvement
Laboratory:	Leukopenia with left shift, thrombocytopenia, raised liver enzymes, rising measles antibody titer
Complications:	Occasional disseminated intravascular coagulopathy
Treatment:	Supportive; prevention with immunization

• DIAGNOSIS AND DIFFERENTIAL DIAGNOSIS •

The diagnosis of measles is usually obvious because of the distinctive clinical picture. Mild forms of measles may be confused with other viral exanthems, such as rubella, or exanthems associated with infectious mononucleosis or *Mycoplasma* and drug eruptions. Diagnosis can be confirmed by immunofluorescent staining of measles antigen in nasal secretions. Confirmation may also be obtained by a 4-fold or greater rise in measles antibody titers, measured by hemagglutination inhibition.

Atypical measles must be differentiated from Rocky Mountain spotted fever, which also has an eruption that starts on the distal extremities.

• TREATMENT AND CLINICAL COURSE •

Supportive care with close observation for potential complications is the primary management. Measles can also be prevented or modified either by active immunization within 3 days of exposure or passively by the administration of pooled gamma globulin 0.25 mL/kg IM within 6 days of exposure. This may be desirable for infants less than a year old, immunocompromised patients, and pregnant women. The latter approach may produce a modified form of measles with a prolonged period of incubation lasting 2 to 3 weeks, or it may entirely prevent the illness.

Prevention can be achieved largely by active immunization with the live attenuated measles virus vaccine. The American Academy of Pediatrics recommends the first vaccination at 12 to 15 months of age along with a vaccine for mumps and rubella (MMR) and a booster dose at 11 to 12 years old. Local epidemics, such as those that have occurred among college students, may dictate immunization needs in select populations.

A summary of measles (rubeola) is presented in Table 16.5.

Rubella (German Measles)

Rubella, or German measles, is usually a mild childhood illness with minimal morbidity. It gains major significance due to its teratogenic effect when acquired during pregnancy.

• PATHOGENESIS •

Rubella is caused by the rubella virus, classified in the *Rubivirus* genus of the *Togaviridae* family. Its only natural hosts and reservoirs are humans, although many primates and laboratory animals have been infected experimentally. Rubella is worldwide in distribution and affects both sexes equally. In prevaccine years, it was highly contagious, affecting some 80% to 90% of the population before the age of 15.

The virus is spread by inhalation of infected respiratory droplets after close contact. The incubation period averages 18 days (range of 12 to 23 days). The period of infectivity stretches from 7 days before the rash until 14 days after its appearance, with maximum viral shedding 5 days before to 6 days after appearance. Before the introduction of immunizations, most

Table 16.5. Rubeola

Etiology:	Measles virus: *Morbillivirus* genus, *Paramyxoviridae* family
Peak Incidence:	Winter and spring
Incubation:	10–14 days
Illness Duration:	9–11 days
Prodrome:	3–4 days of fever with moderate to severe upper respiratory symptoms
Enanthem:	Palatal petechiae, Koplik spots 1–2 days before rash
Exanthem:	Onset is within 3–4 days of prodrome and duration is 3–5 days. Increased fever seen with appearance of rash and catarrh, coryza, distinctive brassy cough, photophobia. Macular to maculopapular intense red-purple to red-to-brown lesions coalesce on the face and upper chest. Distribution is generalized, beginning at the mastoid and occipital neck, spreading to the neck (day 1), face (day 2), arms, trunk, then legs (day 3). Confluent rash on face (day 3). Rash fades with same pattern. A branny postexanthem is common, producing scaly desquamation.
Complications:	Meningoencephalitis, pneumonia, otitis media, mastoiditis, sclerosing panencephalitis, death
Treatment:	Immunization with live attenuated virus is the gold standard (MMR).[a] Supportive treatments include bedrest, fluids, and 60 mg of water-miscible vitamin A.

[a]MMR: measles, mumps, rubella

cases occurred in young children; now, rubella is seen mostly in young adults and adolescents.

• CLINICAL FEATURES •

A mild prodrome characterized by malaise, headache, coryza, low-grade fever, and conjunctivitis may be present. Tender lymphadenopathy involving postauricular, suboccipital, and posterior cervical nodes is an important diagnostic feature. The eruption begins on the face as discrete, fine, pink papules and rapidly spreads centrifugally downward over the trunk. Lesions on the trunk may become confluent, whereas those on the extremities (Fig. 16.8) remain discrete. The exanthem usually persists for 3 to 4 days, disappearing in the order of its appearance.

The complications of rubella are infrequent and consist of arthralgias and arthritis, encephalitis, and thrombocytopenia that is usually reversible. Involvement of joints mainly affects adult women. Encephalitis occurs in 1 per 5000 cases.

Rubella occurring during the first 12 weeks of pregnancy may produce multiple congenital abnormalities in the offspring. Known collectively as the congenital rubella syndrome, the anomalies can be ocular (cataracts, retinopathy, microophthalmia, and congenital glaucoma), auditory (sensorineural deafness), cardiovascular (pulmonary stenosis), and central nervous system problems (congenital meningoencephalitis, microcephaly, and mental retardation).

• DIAGNOSIS AND DIFFERENTIAL DIAGNOSIS •

The diagnosis of rubella may be difficult because of the subtle signs and symptoms. Many mild cases are not diagnosed except in epidemics. Although the gold standard of diagnosis is viral culture, serologic testing should be done, particularly in pregnant patients, because diagnosis is important for epidemiologic reasons. The hemagglutination inhibition test is the most useful because the antibodies are first detected during the presence of the rash and then rise rapidly in 1 to 2 weeks.

• TREATMENT AND CLINICAL COURSE •

Symptomatic care is the mainstay of management for rubella. Pregnant women in the first trimester exposed to rubella should be tested for antibody. If present, the mother is immune and the fetus is protected. If antibodies are absent, the patient should be carefully monitored for any signs or symptoms of rubella and viral cultures obtained promptly if symptoms occur. If the presence of rubella virus confirms maternal infection in the first trimester, the patient should be fully informed of the potential for severe fetal malformations, and termination of the pregnancy may be considered. Inadvertent immunization of pregnant women has been shown on occasion to produce fetal infection, but not teratogenicity.

For a clinical summary of rubella see Table 16.6.

Enteroviral Infections

Enteroviruses are small RNA viruses that form a subgroup in the family of *Picornaviridae*. This subgroup consists of four major viral types: the polioviruses, coxsackievirus group A, coxsackievirus group B, and echoviruses. Only the latter three will be discussed, on the basis that polioviruses do not cause exanthems. Newly discovered serotypes that do not conform to established criteria regarding their effects on animals and tissue cultures are now designated enteroviruses and are numbered 68 through 72. Of interest is the fact that hepatitis A virus is now recognized as enterovirus type 72.

• PATHOGENESIS •

Enteroviruses are found worldwide. Although they have been cultured from a variety of animal species, Mollusca, and even raw sewage, they are generally thought to only infect humans. Enteroviral infections affect both sexes and all races equally but tend to target young, presumably nonimmune persons. Viral transmission is predominantly person-to-person by fecal-oral, respiratory, or oral-to-oral routes. Transmission appears to increase in warm months in temperate climates and may be year-round in tropical and subtropical climates. Transmission by contaminated water or foods is documented in some strains (hepatitis A).

Approximately 30 enteroviruses cause human disease associated with rashes, but the elegance of one virus causing one

Table 16.6. Rubella

Etiology:	*Rubivirus* genus, *Togoviridae* family
Incidence:	Winter and spring, although year-round in dense urban populations
Incubation:	5–28 days (mean of 18 days)
Illness Duration:	3–6 days
Prodrome:	1–5 days of lymphadenopathy, mild fever with respiratory symptoms, malaise, sore throat, headache, eye pain, fever, anorexia, nausea, vomiting. Contagious period ranges from 7 days before to 14 days after onset of rash.
Enanthem:	25% have minute red spots on palate, Forschheimer's sign (petechial enanthem at the junction of the soft and hard palates).
Exanthem:	Begins after 1–5 days of prodrome and lasts 2–3 days; Lesions are nonpruritic, pink macules and papules that coalesce on the face; Generalized distribution begins on cheeks or at hairline and spreads centrifugally to limbs within 24 hours; spares palms, soles, and scalp. Associated with prominent postcervical adenopathy and arthralgia or arthritis. Fades by day 3. Occasionally, a branny post-exanthem occurs.
Complications:	Rare: encephalitis, thrombocytopenia purpura, congenital rubella syndrome
Treatment:	Prevention with immunization (MMR).[a] Supportive therapy including bedrest and acetaminophen or aspirin for fever or arthralgia.

[a] MMR: measles, mumps, rubella

Table 16.7. Enteroviruses

Poliovirus, Coxsackievirus (Cox) Groups A and B, Echovirus (E)[a]

Common Presentations and Etiologies

Morbilliform:	Cox A9, B3, B5; E9 E2, 4, 11, 19, 25 (acral)
Roseola-like:	Cox B1, B5; E11, E16, E25 Persists 2–5 days; may start on face, chest
Vesicular:	Cox A5, A16, B3; E17, E25 Cox A1, A6, A8, A10, A16, A22 (herpangina)

Other Presentations:

Scarlatiniform, zosteriform:	E6; Cox B5
Urticarial:	Cox B5; E25
Petechial and purpuric:	Cox A9, A4, B3, B5; E9
Cherry spots:	E25, E32

[a] Approximately 30 cause rashes, and one virus may cause a variety of rashes. One clinical syndrome (e.g., hand, foot, and mouth disease) may be caused by several enteroviruses.

predominant clinical presentation does not occur. With enteroviral infections, one virus may cause a variety of rashes. Conversely, one clinical syndrome (for instance hand, foot, and mouth disease) may be caused by several enteroviruses. Common presentations are summarized in Table 16.7.

Although illnesses produced by the non-polio enteroviruses are generally not severe, fatalities have occurred due to myocarditis or meningoencephalitis, most often following coxsackievirus group B infections and, rarely, coxsackievirus group A and echovirus infections. Many factors affect the clinical severity of the illness, including the age of the patient, the virulence and tropism of the particular virus, the concentration and route of inoculation, and the immunocompetence of the host. More severe illness is seen in the youngest patients.

• CLINICAL FEATURES •

Infections with enteroviruses are extremely common, and the eruptions they produce are protean. The most common exanthems are macular and maculopapular, which may coalesce to form morbilliform patterns. Such rashes have been documented with numerous enteroviruses, including coxsackievirus groups A6, A9, and A16 and coxsackievirus group B5. Additionally, some of these patients exhibit vesicles as well as purpuric and urticarial eruptions. This demonstrates the complexity of

enteroviral exanthems and the many patterns they may exhibit. Urticarial lesions have been seen with coxsackieviruses A9, A16, B4, and B5, and echovirus 11 infections. Erythema multiforme-like presentations have been reported with infections due to coxsackieviruses A9, A10, A16, B4, B5, and rarely, echoviruses 6 and 11. Hemangioma-like lesions or "cherry spots" have been seen with echoviruses 25 and 32. Pityriasis rosea-like eruptions are reportedly associated with echovirus 6 infections.

Vesiculobullous eruptions mimicking varicella have been reported with echoviruses 5 and 6. Petechiae and purpuric rashes have been seen with coxsackieviruses A4 and A9, coxsackieviruses B2, B3, B4, and B5, and echoviruses 6, 9, 18, 4, 7, and 3. Other patterns reported with some frequency are recognized as hand, foot, and mouth disease; herpangina; roseola; roseola-like illnesses; and exanthems associated with hepatitis A. Some characteristics of enteroviral exanthems are summarized in Table 16.7. These will be further discussed in this chapter.

• DIAGNOSIS AND TREATMENT •

Enteroviral infections should be considered when a patient presents with any combination of fever, headache, meningismus or meningitis, a skin eruption with or without mucosal involvement, and gastrointestinal symptoms.

No specific therapy is available. The majority of patients will be benefited by supportive care, particularly if the above eruptions are associated with nausea, vomiting, diarrhea, myocardiopathy, or evidence of meningismus or encephalitis. Immunization is not available.

Herpangina

• PATHOGENESIS •

Herpangina refers to an acute febrile illness with posterior oral mucosal lesions seen in children most often in the summer and fall in temperate climates. It occurs both sporadically and epidemically and is caused by several enteroviruses. Sporadic cases have been associated with coxsackievirus group A types 7, 9, 16, and 22; coxsackievirus group B types 1, 2, 3, 4, and 5; and echovirus types 6, 9, 11, 16, 17, and 22. Epidemics of herpangina have been traced to coxsackievirus group A types 1, 2, 3, 4, 5, 6, 8, 10, and 22 and group B type 1 as well as echovirus types 16 and 25.

• CLINICAL FEATURES •

Herpangina is defined by the presence of discrete vesicular or eroded lesions on the posterior buccal mucosa, tonsillar pillars, tonsils, pharynx, and soft palate, often following a prodromal phase of listlessness, anorexia, and irritability. The illness begins with the sudden onset of fever (37°C–41.5°C). Older children may complain of associated headaches and backaches. Shortly after the onset of fever, the characteristic mucosal lesions are noted. The vesicular and eroded lesions may measure from 1 to 4 mm in size, generally increasing slowly. They are often surrounded by a red halo and maintain the posterior location in the mouth and throat, in contrast to the more anterior location of herpes simplex lesions. Prominent associated symptoms include drooling, sore throat, coryza, nausea, vomiting, and/or diarrhea, and headache. These symptoms and the fever often resolve over 3 to 6 days. Rare cases are also associated with other eruptions, including maculopapular, roseola-like, petechial, and vesicular lesions. Although most cases resolve fully, rare complications can include myocarditis, aseptic meningitis, and encephalitis.

• DIAGNOSIS AND TREATMENT •

The differential diagnosis includes stomatitis due to herpes simplex or erythema multiforme. Treatment is supportive and aimed at keeping the affected child well hydrated and nourished in spite of the painful mucosal erosions. Analgesics and oral anesthetics such as viscous Xylocaine or Benadryl elixir may help. If oral fluid intake cannot be maintained, then intravenous fluids may be necessary.

Herpangina is summarized in Table 16.8.

Hand, Foot, and Mouth Disease

• PATHOGENESIS •

Hand, foot, and mouth disease has occurred sporadically and epidemically since its recognition over 35 years ago. It is worldwide in distribution and now known to be associated with several strains of coxsackievirus, including types A5, A10, A16, B1, and B3. It predominantly affects children aged 2 to 10 years but exposed adults are not entirely spared. It occurs in the late

Table 16.8. Herpangina

Etiology:	Coxsackievirus A1, 2, 3, 4, 5, 6, 7, 8, 10, 22, and B1 (epidemic) Coxsackievirus B1, 2, 3, 4, and 5 (sporadic) Echovirus A7, 9, 16, 17, 22 (sporadic)
Incidence:	Summer and fall. Affects children, adolescents, adults.
Incubation:	2–9 days
Illness Duration:	3–9 days
Prodrome:	1–2 days. Sudden onset of fever, anorexia, dysphagia, drooling, sore throat, vomiting, and headache.
Enanthem:	Papular, vesicular, or ulcerative lesions on the tonsils, tonsillar pillars, soft palate, and pharyngeal posterior buccal mucosae and pharynx.
Exanthem:	Occasional, consisting of maculopapular, morbilliform, scarlatiniform, or vesicular lesions, or erosions. Shorter duration than herpes simplex.
Complications:	Rare: aseptic meningitis, myocarditis, or encephalitis.
Treatment:	Supportive hydration and nutrition with IV fluids, antiemetics, and pain medications.

spring, summer, and fall in temperate climates and has an incubation period of 3 to 6 days.

• CLINICAL FEATURES •

The early illness is marked by low-grade fever, mild oral discomfort, malaise, abdominal pain, and diarrhea. In 1 to 2 days, oral lesions appear as red maculopapules and develop into vesicles that evolve into shallow erosions over the next few days. These may be 4 to 8 mm in size and are located on the tongue, buccal mucosa, and gingival lateral groove (Figs. 16.9 and 16.10). The associated sore mouth may result in anorexia and occasionally, dehydration. Submandibular lymphadenopathy develops in 20% of affected children.

Skin lesions occur in two-thirds of patients, with papules that evolve into vesicles over the dorsal and volar aspects of the hands (50%) (Fig. 16.11), feet (30%) (Fig. 16.12), and even the buttocks (30%). The lesions, which are surrounded by a halo of erythema, are oval in shape and may number from 10 to 50. They tend to align along creases and cluster in areas of trauma or pressure. They may or may not be tender. In children less than 5 years old, vesicular lesions may be associated with other maculopapular lesions scattered on the buttocks and limbs.

Complications can include pneumonia, myocarditis, aseptic meningitis, paralytic disease, and rarely death.

Table 16.9 summarizes pertinent clinical information.

• DIAGNOSIS AND TREATMENT •

Hand, foot, and mouth disease is usually diagnosed on clinical grounds. It should be differentiated from herpes simplex stomatitis, and erythema multiforme.

Table 16.9. Hand, Foot, and Mouth Disease

Etiology:	Coxsackievirus A16, A5, A10, A7, A9, B1, B3, B5
Incidence:	Late summer and fall
Incubation:	3–6 days
Illness Duration:	7–10 days
Prodrome:	1–2 days of sore mouth (67%); malaise (61%); anorexia (52%); low-grade fever (42%); lymphadenopathy (22%); coryza (11%); cough (11%); diarrhea (10%); and abdominal pain.
Enanthem:	In 90% of patients, tiny vesicles or erosions form in 1–6 days on mucosa and tongue with a halo of erythema.
Exanthem:	In 60% to 70% of patients, oval superficial vesicles, 2–10 mm, form on margin and dorsum of hands, feet, palms, and soles; occasionally scattered on face, limbs, and buttocks (maculopapular); may be tender.
Clinical Features:	Occasional high fever, malaise, diarrhea, joint pain, and lymphadenopathy.
Complications:	Rare aseptic meningitis, myocarditis, meningoencephalitis, or pneumonia. Paralytic disease fatalities rare. Some cases recur for months.
Treatment:	Supportive. Topical oral anesthetics such as viscous xylocaine or diphenhydramine hydrochloride elixir, bed rest; rarely, IV fluids.

The illness tends to resolve over about a week. Rare patients develop a more serious, prolonged, or relapsing course. Treatment is supportive and includes bed rest and fluids to avoid dehydration.

Roseola Infantum

• PATHOGENESIS •

Roseola infantum (exanthem subitum, sixth disease) is a common acute febrile disease of infants that is caused largely by human herpesvirus 6. Many roseola-like illnesses have also been attributed to several enteroviruses, including coxsackievirus A6, A9, B1, B2, B4, and B5, and echovirus 9, 11, 25, 27, and 30. Little is known about the pathogenesis of roseola, its mode of transmission, or the period of communicability. Cases appear year-round, mainly in infants aged 6 months to 2 years.

• CLINICAL FEATURES •

After an incubation period of 5 to 15 days, the illness manifests itself by the sudden onset of fever ranging from 39°C–41°C. Mild coryza, restlessness, and irritability may be seen along with findings of occipital and cervical adenopathy. After 3 to 5 days of fever, the temperature falls abruptly, giving way to blanchable, discrete, rose-pink macules of the trunk and neck, which can spread to the extremities and involve the face. The rash may be evanescent or persist for 1 to 2 days. Usually, the child appears well in spite of the fever and rash. There may

also be mild but definite edema of the eyelids, which may help in establishing the diagnosis. Other associated symptoms include pharyngitis, cough, and coryza in winter cases, and anorexia, vomiting, diarrhea, abdominal pain, headache, and restlessness in summer cases. Febrile seizures occur in about 6% of children. Rare complications of roseola include thrombocytopenic purpura, meningitis, or encephalitis with very rare permanent neurologic sequelae.

• DIAGNOSIS AND TREATMENT •

The diagnosis is made clinically with the hallmark of the disease being the sudden onset of high fever for several days, which resolves suddenly and is followed by the cutaneous eruption. Laboratory studies reveal a leukopenia and lymphocytosis. The differential diagnosis includes other viral exanthems and drug reactions.

Treatment is supportive. If febrile seizures occur, treatment with phenobarbital is recommended.

Table 16.10 summarizes the clinical features of roseola.

Colorado Tick Fever

• PATHOGENESIS •

Colorado tick fever is a lesser known viral exanthem. It is an acute febrile illness caused by a coltivirus that is a member of

Table 16.10. Roseola Infantum and Roseola-Like Illness

Etiology:	
Roseola Infantum:	Human herpesvirus 6
Roseola-like Illness:	Coxsackievirus A6, A9, or B1, B2, B4, B5; Echovirus 9, 11, 16, 25, 27, 30; Rotavirus
Boston Exanthem:	Echovirus 16, Coxsackievirus B5
Incidence:	Year-round; especially summer, late fall, and early spring in infants less than 2 years old.
Incubation:	5–15 days
Illness Duration:	3–7 days
Prodrome:	Sudden high temperature (38°–41°C) for 3–5 days. Usually child looks well in spite of fever, but occasional anorexia, vomiting, diarrhea, restlessness, seizures occur. Periorbital edema; infected pharynx; meningismus; suboccipital lymph nodes; occasional splenomegaly; mild exanthem. Fever resolves by crisis on lysis before or just after the sudden appearance of the rash.
Enanthem:	None.
Exanthem:	Sudden onset with defervescence of other signs and symptoms. Duration 1–2 days; may be evanescent. Lesions are discrete, rose-pink, blanchable macules/papules, 2–3 mm, which begin on neck, trunk, arms, and legs.
Clinical Features:	Leukopenia, relative lymphocytosis (day 3), febrile seizures (6%)
Complications:	Rare
Treatment:	Supportive

the *Reoviridae* family and has a double-stranded DNA core. It occurs in the Rocky Mountain areas of the western United States and Canada, corresponding to the habitat of its vector, the wood tick, *Dermacentor andersoni*. This tick, in its larval form, feeds on the primary hosts and reservoir for the coltivirus, small rodents and rabbits. The tick remains infected until adulthood, when it feeds on larger animals, including man, who becomes an accidental host. The infection, which may occur in spring through fall, is most prevalent in May and June, reflecting increased activity of the adult ticks as well as more human outdoor exposure. A history of tick bite or exposure is elicited in 90% of patients.

• CLINICAL FEATURES •

After an incubation of 1 to 14 days (mean of 3 to 4 days), the patient presents with a flu-like illness. It is abrupt in onset and characterized by fever, chills, malaise, myalgias, headache, retro-orbital and back pain, and hyperesthesia. Less frequently reported symptoms include nausea, vomiting, and abdominal pain. The fever remains high for 3 days, defervesces for 1 to 2 days, and then recurs. The illness may actually have several recurrences.

A rash is reported in approximately 10% of patients. It is described as a pink maculopapular and morbilliform eruption that begins on the face and spreads centrifugally to involve the trunk and extremities. In rare instances, it may be petechial or hemorrhagic. The eruption resolves as the fever abates, only to recur as it returns.

• DIAGNOSIS AND DIFFERENTIAL DIAGNOSIS •

Laboratory abnormalities include either leukocytosis or leukopenia and thrombocytopenia, but these are rarely severe. The morbilliform eruption needs to be differentiated from rubella and enteroviral rashes. Since *Dermacentor andersoni* is also the vector of Rocky Mountain spotted fever, severe cases should be evaluated for this concomitant infection. The diagnosis is supported by serologic studies of acute and convalescent sera, viral culture, and immunofluorescence staining of smears of red blood cells that harbor the virus.

• TREATMENT AND CLINICAL COURSE •

Treatment of Colorado tick fever is supportive, including bed rest, fluid replacement, and fever control. No vaccines are available to date. Uncomplicated recovery is the norm but complications have been reported, including pneumonitis, hepatitis, pericarditis, orchitis, and gastrointestinal bleeding.

Erythema Infectiosum (Fifth Disease)

• PATHOGENESIS •

Erythema infectiosum (fifth disease), an acute infectious disease of childhood, is caused by the human parvovirus B19. Transmission occurs through the inhalation of infected droplets.

Most cases occur during the winter or spring in children 2 to 12 years of age, but adult cases are not rare. The infection is worldwide but more prevalent in temperate climates. It is noted more commonly in girls than boys. Surveys have found 40% to 60% of adults to be seropositive for IgG antibody to human parvovirus B19.

• CLINICAL FEATURES •

After an incubation period of 5 to 20 days (mean 12 to 14 days), a mild prodrome of low-grade fever may develop. This is occasionally associated with malaise, headache, nausea, vomiting, diarrhea, arthralgia (or arthritis), and pruritus, especially in older patients. Young patients may be asymptomatic. The rash, appearing 1 to 2 days later, begins as a deep red, confluent, edematous area over both cheeks, resembling slapped cheeks. The border of the lesions is well-defined, with sparing in the perioral area. The facial rash fades in several days and is followed 1 to 4 days later by a symmetric macular erythema on the extensor aspect of the arms and legs, spreading to the flexural extremities. As some areas fade, the final picture is a net-like reticular erythema (Figs. 16.13–16.15) that may persist for several weeks. It characteristically waxes and wanes with ambient temperature fluctuations, exercise, and sunlight exposure. A rare complication associated with erythema infectiosum is mild arthralgia or arthritis.

Complications of human parvovirus B19 are extremely rare among otherwise healthy children. During the initial prodromal (viremic) period, the rapidly dividing red blood precursor cell is infected and lysed. This produces only a mild transient suppression of red cell production in healthy patients but may result in aplastic crises in children who require high bone marrow output to survive. Such children, especially those with spherocytosis, thalassemia, or sickle cell anemia, suffer severe reticulocytopenia; severe anemia often results, requiring transfusion and bed rest. The illness in immunocompromised children, especially those with acute lymphocytic leukemia, may result in chronic B19 infections with similar severe anemia due to chronic lysis of red cell precursors. Such patients have been helped by the administration of intravenous gamma globulin or transfusions. Because they also have high output marrows, fetuses with intrauterine infection may have severe anemia resulting in hydrops fetalis, fetal death, and miscarriage. The vast majority of the infants with known maternal infections during pregnancy are normal, and there is no evidence to date that the virus is a teratogen.

• DIAGNOSIS AND DIFFERENTIAL DIAGNOSIS •

Erythema infectiosum is usually diagnosed clinically on the basis of its classical presentation characterized by bright erythema of the cheeks and later reticulated erythema of the extremities. If necessary for diagnosis, specific IgM antibody to human parvovirus can be detected in the serum. This antibody is present for up to 2 months following acute infection.

The differential diagnosis includes other viral exanthems and drug eruptions.

Table 16.11. Erythema Infectiosum (Fifth Disease)

Etiology:	Human Parvovirus (B19), spread by respiratory route. Target cell is the red cell precursor of bone marrow. Rash 2–3 weeks after infection is probably secondary to immune complexes.
Incidence:	Affects children, rare in adults; female predominance. More common in temperate climates, winter and spring. Worldwide distribution.
Incubation:	14–20 days
Illness Duration:	1–2 weeks (9–14 days of rash)
Prodrome:	Viremia, low-grade fever; occasionally associated with malaise, myalgia, headache, nausea, vomiting, diarrhea, and/or pruritus, arthritis, arthralgia.
Enanthem:	None; rare reports of associated pharyngitis.
Exanthem:	Classic rash with sudden onset. Malar blush, "slapped cheeks" (day 1); erythematous maculopapular eruption on extensor surface of limbs, spreading to trunk and buttocks (day 2); fading of rash resulting in a lacy and reticulated pattern (day 3). Rash usually fades within 5 days but can recur with activity or heat for weeks. Rash resolves without pigment or peeling. Rare atypical rashes: papular, vesicular, confluent, or purpuric.
Complications:	Rare. Arthritis, arthralgia, pneumonia, hemolytic anemia; transient aplastic crises (TAC) in patients unable to tolerate bone marrow suppression for 7–10 days, i.e., high-output marrows, such as in sickle cell, spherocytosis, and the fetus. Rare chronic infections in immunodeficient patients.
Treatment:	Supportive. IV gamma globulin for TAC and/or immunocompromised patients. Isolate patients with TAC.

• TREATMENT AND CLINICAL COURSE •

Parvovirus B19 viremia in patients with transient aplastic crises or chronic immunodeficiency has been cured with IV gamma globulin. The drug's effectiveness in preventing maternal or fetal infection, however, is unconfirmed. For recognized hydrops fetalis due to B19, fetal transfusions have been successful, although this treatment is experimental. Maternal B19 infection increases the risk of spontaneous fetal loss by 2% to 3%. Therapeutic abortions are not advised since B19 is not thought to be a teratogen.

With known viremic patients, infection control measures should be followed. Unfortunately, transmission among healthy children is difficult to avoid, since the diagnosis is not made until the rash appears following the viremic phase. No vaccination is available.

A summary of the clinical features of fifth disease is presented in Table 16.11.

Infectious Mononucleosis

Infectious mononucleosis was first described by Pheiffer in Germany in 1889 and by West in the United States 6 years later. Although the syndrome's viral etiology, the Epstein-Barr virus,

was recognized 80 years later, another 20 years elapsed before the specific biovar responsible for mononucleosis, the type A Epstein-Barr virus, was elucidated.

• PATHOGENESIS •

Epstein-Barr virus (EBV) is worldwide in distribution and affects both sexes equally. EBV type A (EBV-A) is responsible for symptomatic and asymptomatic mononucleosis. EBV type B (EBV-B) appears to be associated with nasopharyngeal carcinomas in Asians and lymphomas in Africans and HIV patients. In underdeveloped countries, EBV-A causes disease and consequent seroconversion in 90% of children by the age of 2. In more developed countries, some children show evidence of EBV-A infection but a significant number do not develop the illness or seroconvert until adolescence or young adulthood.

EBV has a DNA core within its capsid and outer envelope and belongs to the *Herpesviridae* family. It is spread on rare occasions by transfusion, but most often by means of infected saliva. Oral-to-oral transmission—either indirectly by sharing food, drink, or utensils, or directly by kissing—is the most common means, thus rendering it the label of the "kissing disease." The virus infects B lymphocytes in the oropharynx, then is transmitted hematogenously to the entire body and its reticuloendothelial system, where it infects, lyses, or transforms other lymphocytes. On rare occasions patients may be infected by both EBV-A and EBV-B.

• CLINICAL FEATURES •

The onset of mononucleosis is usually insidious and presents as profound malaise (90%) associated with a sore throat (80%). Other complaints early in its course include fever (90%); lymphadenopathy, especially cervical (80%); pharyngitis (75%); and splenomegaly (40%). Less often reported symptoms include nausea, vomiting, abdominal pain (from mesenteric lymphadenopathy), and jaundice. Tonsillitis is present in 75% and infection with ß-hemolytic streptococci in 25%.

A rash is noted in 10% to 15% of patients. It is present for 3 to 6 days and is usually morbilliform, mimicking rubella, but may become petechial, hemorrhagic, scarlatiniform, urticarial, erythema multiforme-like, or mildly evanescent as in the erythema marginatum seen with rheumatic fever or juvenile rheumatoid arthritis. Treatment with ampicillin or amoxicillin produces a maculopapular or morbilliform cutaneous reaction in all patients (Figs. 16.16–16.17). Eruptions may also occur, although less frequently, with other antibiotics, especially penicillins and cephalosporins. Up to 25% of patients will also have a petechial or red macular lesion of the palatal mucosa. EBV infection in patients with AIDS results in oral hairy leukoplakia.

Mononucleosis causes an unusually long illness as compared to most viral infections. A 4-week course of sore throat, fever, lymphadenopathy, and malaise is common, and many cases persist longer. Symptoms are often most intense for the first week or two, then gradually improve. Severe complications are rare. Streptococcal pharyngitis and tonsillitis require treatment to prevent the rare development of streptococcal sepsis. Another rare but serious complication is splenic rupture, which is suggested by tachycardia, abdominal pain, and a decreasing hematocrit. Rare cases of aplastic anemia and conditions mimicking idiopathic thrombocytopenic purpura have also developed secondary to infectious mononucleosis.

Neurologic symptoms due to aseptic meningitis or encephalitis may occur, as may signs of cranial or peripheral neuropathy, seizures, depression, or psychoses. Respiratory problems may include upper airway obstruction due to enlarged tonsils. Hepatitis is common with elevated liver enzymes (80%), but jaundice is evident in less than 5% of patients. Abdominal pain with nausea and vomiting may also occur due to mesenteric lymphadenitis. Other more rarely reported complications include pancreatitis, orchitis, and renal disease. Finally, lymphoproliferative disorders may occur in patients who are immunocompromised.

• DIAGNOSIS AND DIFFERENTIAL DIAGNOSIS •

Laboratory abnormalities may include atypical lymphocytosis, leukopenia, and thrombocytopenia. Elevated liver enzymes and raised bilirubin are common. Detection of the heterophile antibody will help establish the diagnosis, but specific tests are more precise: the IgM and IgG antiviral capsid antibodies, anti-early antigen (anti-EA), and antibodies to the EBV nuclear antigen. Elevated liver enzymes and raised bilirubin indirectly support the diagnosis.

The differential diagnosis of infectious mononucleosis with an exanthem include illnesses due to HIV, CMV (cytomegalovirus), toxoplasmosis, streptococcal and enteroviral infections, and drug reactions.

• TREATMENT AND CLINICAL COURSE •

Treatment is supportive. The mainstay is bed rest and prevention of splenic rupture through the avoidance of any heavy activity. Abstinence from alcohol may reduce the duration of hepatic dysfunction. Rare and judicious use of systemic steroids may help in severe cases, especially those with upper airway obstruction, thrombocytopenia, aplastic anemia, hemolytic anemia, or severe toxicity. A vaccine for EBV has been developed but awaits further study.

Table 16.12 summarizes the features of infectious mononucleosis.

Hepatitis

Hepatitis is a systemic illness characterized by injury to and necrosis of hepatic cells with resultant inflammation. This illness may be caused by a variety of insults, including chemical exposures, drug reactions, and recently recognized viral agents, especially those now classified as hepatitis A, B, C, D, and E.

Table 16.12. Infectious Mononucleosis

Etiology:	Epstein-Barr virus; Type A herpes (common infection; milder in young patients)
Incidence:	Prevalence high in children in developing countries. In developed countries, primarily affects adolescents and young adults.
Incubation:	30–60 days
Illness Duration:	10–29 days (occasionally prolonged)
Prodrome:	Insidious onset of fatigue and sore throat. Viral capsid antigen.
Enanthem:	Petechial lesions between hard and soft palate in 25% of patients on day 5–7; strep throat (20%–25%).
Exanthem:	Rashes in 10–15% of patients within 4–6 days: maculopapular or morbilliform on the trunk, upper arms, face, proximal limbs; occasionally petechial or hemorrhagic scarlatiniform, urticarial or erythema multiforme-like. Eyelid edema (30%–50%).
Clinical Features:	Insidious onset: fever 37°–41°C (90%) lasting 4–14 days (up to 2 months), headache, malaise (85%), sore throat (80%), generalized lymphadenopathy, especially cervical (80%), membranous tonsillitis, splenomegaly (40%–50%), or hepatitis (5–10%).
Laboratory:	Heterophil>1:112 or a monospot are good screens; atypical lymphocytosis is helpful. More precise tests include anti EA. Other abnormalities can include elevated IgM-VCA, IgG-VCA, leukopenia (20%), neutropenia, thrombocytopenia, and abnormal liver function tests.
Treatment:	Supportive: rest, rare corticosteroids; avoid ampicillin, avoid contact sports to protect spleen. Treat strep throat with antibiotics.
Complications:	Rare: erythema multiforme, persistent lupus erythematosus-like syndromes, hepatitis, upper airway obstruction and pain, splenic rupture, aplastic anemia, encephalitis, aseptic meningitis, seizures, depression, neuropathies, and psychoses.

HEPATITIS A AND E

• PATHOGENESIS •

Hepatitis A, also known as enterovirus 72, and the more recently discovered hepatitis E share significant features and will be considered together. Both viruses are RNA viruses but hepatitis A is classified as an enterovirus, whereas hepatitis E shares many properties with calciviruses. As RNA viruses, both can be waterborne and transmitted enterically through contaminated water sources or food. Hepatitis A virus has a worldwide distribution, whereas hepatitis E has thus far only been reported in India and Southeast Asia. In general, hepatitis E causes a more fulminant illness with higher mortality than hepatitis A; it has a high attack rate in India where overcrowding and poor hygiene result in widespread infection and epidemics. In underdeveloped countries, hepatitis A infects 90% of patients during childhood. In more developed countries, the prevalence of infection is lower in childhood but increases in adolescence and early adulthood.

• CLINICAL FEATURES •

Infections with hepatitis A are frequently asymptomatic: only one in ten infected persons show evidence of disease. Subclinical illness is even more common in children. After an incubation period of 15 to 50 days (mean of 29), the symptomatic infection begins with nausea, vomiting, abdominal discomfort, fever, fatigue, and occasional respiratory complaints. This usually lasts for 3 to 10 days and is followed by jaundice and intense pruritus.

Approximately 5% of patients with hepatitis A will have an exanthem. This may be morbilliform, urticarial, or scarlatiniform. The urticarial eruption of hepatitis A, in contrast to hepatitis B, is rarely if ever associated with joint swelling. It usually precedes the jaundice but, if concurrent, may produce yellow wheals. Complications of hepatitis A are uncommon but include proteinuria, pancreatitis, thrombocytopenia, pleural effusion, myocarditis, and aplastic anemia. Hepatitis A usually resolves over a month's time, but abnormal liver enzymes may persist for a year in some patients. Children appear to heal more rapidly. The prognosis for recovery is good and the mortality rate is less than 1%.

Hepatitis E runs a more fulminant course, particularly in pregnant women and among the poorly nourished. Its signs and symptoms are similar, but complications are more frequent and serious. It has a mortality rate of 10% to 20%.

• DIAGNOSIS AND DIFFERENTIAL DIAGNOSIS •

Diagnosis is made by tests for IgM anti-hepatitis A or anti-hepatitis E antibodies. Abnormal liver enzymes may persist for months.

The differential diagnosis includes other viral causes of hepatitis, such as hepatitis B, C, or D, coxsackievirus, EBV, and CMV; other infectious agents, such as those causing leptospirosis and toxoplasmosis; and hepatic injury due to drugs or chemicals.

• TREATMENT AND PREVENTION •

Treatment is supportive. To reduce further transmission, caretakers and patients should practice careful hand washing. Prophylaxis for those with known exposure includes intramuscular administration of human immune serum globulin in doses of 0.2 mL/kg.

Table 16.13 summarizes the features of hepatitis A and E.

HEPATITIS B, C, AND D

• PATHOGENESIS •

Formerly known as serum hepatitis, hepatitis B (HBV) is worldwide in distribution. Skin manifestations are not uncommonly seen in HBV, which is a DNA virus usually transmitted parenterally by whole blood and its components. The virus is also found and transmitted in other body fluids, such as urine,

Table 16.13. Hepatitis A and E

Etiology:	Hepatitis A (enterovirus 72) and hepatitis E (calcivirus), which are waterborne or enterically transmitted RNA viruses.
Incidence:	Prevalence high in developing countries. In developed countries primarily affects adolescents and young adults. Fecal-oral transmission via contaminated water and food (Mollusca); occasional outbreaks in daycare centers.
Incubation:	15–50 days (mean of 29 days)
Illness Duration:	From 3 to 4 weeks (acute illness, 1 week); children recover more rapidly than adults.
Enanthem:	None
Exanthem:	Rash on presentation in 5% of patients: A. Morbilliform rashes mimicking rubella for 3–5 days B. Urticarial rash before or after the jaundice. The latter results in yellow wheals for 3–5 days, rarely associated with joint swelling. C. Scarlatiniform eruption—generalized and concurrent with icterus.
Clinical Features:	Hepatitis A: Subclinical illness prevalent in 90%. Symptomatic infection characterized by 4–10 days of nausea, vomiting, abdominal discomfort, fever, fatigue and occasionally respiratory symptoms; Scleral and cutaneous jaundice (icterus) and dark urine noted 1–2 days later, often associated with intense pruritus. Hepatitis E: Similar signs and symptoms, more fulminant.
Laboratory:	Abnormal liver function tests may last for 1 year.
Complications:	Proteinuria but rarely renal failure. Pancreatitis, immune thrombocytopenia purpura, myocarditis, pleural effusion, aplastic anemia.
Treatment:	IM-administered prophylaxis with human immunoglobulin given for known exposure (2 mL/kg). Supportive care; infection control.

feces, saliva, and semen, thus it may be a sexually transmitted disease. It is also transmitted perinatally, from mother to child or other intimate family contact, or by tattoos or ritual scarification. Hepatitis C (HCV) and D (HDV) have been recently recognized and are found in many of the same circumstances as HBV. HDV cannot gain entry to hepatocytes unless traveling with hepatitis B, so it is seen in patients with prior or concurrent infection with HBV. It is often associated with severe and chronic hepatitis.

• CLINICAL FEATURES •

Probably 50% of all HBV infections remain subclinical and go undiagnosed. The illness caused by HBV develops after an incubation period of 1 to 3 months. The prodromal and flu-like illness, lasting several days to weeks, is characterized by anorexia, fatigue, weakness, abdominal pain or discomfort, fever, headache, nausea, and vomiting. Other symptoms include cough, sore throat, rhinorrhea, diarrhea, constipation, and myalgia. On physical exam, the liver may be enlarged and tender with associated cervical or generalized lymphadenopathy. Some patients remain anicteric, whereas others develop jaundice that lasts from a few days to weeks. Fulminant hepatitis occurs in fewer than 1% of patients with HBV only, but more often in those patients suffering coinfection with HBV and HDV. In fulminant cases, liver failure occurs with encephalopathy and a high mortality.

Several dermatologic syndromes are associated with hepatitis B infections, including a serum sickness-like syndrome, a polyarteritis nodosa-like syndrome, essential mixed cryoglobulinemia, and papular acrodermatitis of childhood.

The serum sickness-like illness may develop in 15% to 30% of patients with acute hepatitis B infection. It is characterized by urticaria, angioedema, arthralgia, arthritis, proteinuria, and hematuria. Symptoms occur 1 to 6 weeks before the onset of jaundice and may also be present in patients who remain anicteric. The symptoms usually improve in 2 to 3 weeks. Some patients develop a morbilliform eruption that may also be associated with swollen joints.

The polyarteritis nodosa-like illness is estimated to occur once in every 500 patients with hepatitis B. It may develop shortly after a hepatitis infection or years later and is characterized by fever, skin lesions, and neurologic, rheumatologic, and renal symptoms. It may produce neuropathies, hypertension, azotemia, hematuria, and eosinophilia. Histologically, this syndrome is characterized by panarteritis of medium-sized arteries with frequent 1-cm aneurysms.

Some 10% to 15% of patients with hepatitis-associated polyarteritis nodosa develop skin lesions, consisting of livedo reticularis, nodules, and ulcerations. Less frequent manifestations include urticaria, angioedema, and acral gangrene. The nodules are subcutaneous along arteries of the lower extremities; they are painful and they often ulcerate.

Cryoglobulinemia, seen with both hepatitis B and hepatitis C, is characterized by purpura and, in half the patients, arthropathy and renal involvement. The purpura is palpable and is usually seen on the lower extremities (Figs. 16.18–16.19). Raynaud's phenomenon and erythrocyanosis have also been observed. Only one-third of patients have a history of cold sensitivity.

Papular acrodermatitis of childhood (PAC) or Gianotti-Crosti syndrome, a manifestation of hepatitis B, is characterized by a papular rash, lymphadenopathy, and hepatitis. It is usually seen in children aged 2 to 6. The skin lesions are discrete, monomorphic, and nonpruritic papules 2 to 3 mm in size over the face and extremities (Fig. 16.20), which may persist from 3 to 8 weeks. The hepatitis, which is usually anicteric, follows the onset of the skin eruption by 1 to 2 weeks. Thus, liver function tests should be monitored for weeks to months after this diagnosis is suspected. Although children are not usually ill, half have elevated levels of liver enzymes for a prolonged period of time and occasionally develop chronic active hepatitis.

Gianotti-Crosti syndrome needs to be differentiated from the papulovesicular acro-located syndrome (PAS) of childhood, which is usually associated with other viral and bacterial etiologies such as EBV, hepatitis A, CMV, poliovirus, coxsackievirus A16, parainfluenza virus, and ß-hemolytic streptococci.

• DIAGNOSIS AND DIFFERENTIAL DIAGNOSIS •

On biopsy, all the above disorders, other than PAC (which has a nonspecific histology), may show a leukocytoclastic vasculitis. These vasculitic conditions are thought to result from immune complexes, as evidenced by the findings of positive immunofluorescence for IgG and IgM in skin and kidney biopsies. The cryoglobulins are of a mixed pattern with equal amounts of IgG and IgM. Hepatitis virus particles may be found in these precipitates.

• TREATMENT AND PREVENTION •

Alcohol avoidance is necessary for hepatic recovery in all cases of hepatitis. Treatment for hepatitis-associated skin eruptions is primarily supportive. Serum sickness reactions are first

Table 16.14. Gianotti-Crosti Syndrome (PAC) and Papulovesicular Acro-located Syndrome (PAS) [a]

Etiology:	PAC:HBV
	PAS: HBV, EBV, CMV, HAV, respiratory syncytial virus, poliovirus, B-hemolytic streptococcus, coxsackievirus A16, parainfluenza virus
Incidence:	Year-round. Children 3 months to 15 years, especially aged 2–5; males and females equally affected.
Incubation:	Varies with etiology
Illness Duration:	PAC: 15–20 days
	PAS: 7–60 days
Prodrome:	PAC: usually asymptomatic.
	PAS: depends on pathogenesis.
Enanthem:	None
Exanthem:	PAC: Multiple discrete non-pruritic, erythematous papules 2–5 mm located on the face, neck, limbs, palms, and soles. Lesions usually spare the anticubital and popliteal fossa.
	PAS: Lesions may be more papulovesicular and pruritic.
Clinical Features:	Lymphadenopathy and hepatomegaly. Hepatitis may follow rash in 1–2 weeks, is often anicteric, and may lead to chronic liver disease
Laboratory Findings:	Abnormal LFTs (may not be evident until 1–2 weeks after rash appears). Check for HBV, HAV, EBV, CMV, and other obvious infection.
Complications:	Chronic active hepatitis for PAC or PAS.
Treatment:	Supportive.

[a] HBV, hepatitis B virus; EBV, Epstein-Barr-virus; CMV, cytomegalovirus; HAV, hepatitis A virus; LFT, liver function tests.

treated with antihistamines for the urticaria and analgesics for the joint symptoms. The use of steroid and immunosuppressive agents in hepatitis-associated cryoglobulinemia and polyarteritis nodosa is controversial, as their use in chronic active hepatitis could worsen liver disease. Recent use of human recombinant alpha interferon therapy has improved the prognosis and cure rate for some of these patients.

Prevention of infection after exposure is available both in passive and active forms. Administration of hepatitis B immunoglobulin is helpful, although only temporarily. Active immunization with hepatitis B vaccine helps prevent infection and complements the use of immunoglobulin. Both are used for patients with known exposure to HBV. Additionally, vaccination of all children and health care workers and other at-risk populations has greatly reduced the incidence and menace of the illness caused by HBV.

Table 16.14 summarizes information about both PAC and PAS.

ANNOTATED BIBLIOGRAPHY

Chang T, vol ed. Viral exanthems. Clin Dermatol 1989;7(1).
  Practical information from 12 chapters covering a variety of viral disease with cutaneous eruptions.

Cherry JD, Feigin RD. Atypical measles in children previously immunized with attenuated measles virus vaccine. Pediatrics 1972;50:712–717.
  Review of the clinical signs and symptoms of atypical measles occurring in patients who previously received live or killed measles vaccine.
Feigin RD, Cherry JD, eds. Textbook of pediatric infectious diseases. 3rd ed. Philadelphia: WB Saunders, 1992.
  The definitive, two-volume textbook covering all viral infections.
Fenner FJ, White DO, eds. Medical virology. 3rd ed. London: Academic Press, 1986.
  A comprehensive text designed to introduce students to medical virology.
Mandell GL, Douglas RG, Bennet JE, eds. Principles and practice of infectious diseases. New York: John Wiley and Sons, 1985.
  The classic text on infectious diseases.
McElgunn PS. Dermatologic manifestations of hepatitis B virus infection. J Am Acad Dermatol 1983;8:541–548.
  A clinical review of the dermatologic manifestations of hepatitis B virus infection that includes serum sickness, polyarteritis nodosa, essential mixed cryoglobulinemia, and papular acrodermatitis of childhood.
Prose NS, Resnick SD. Cutaneous manifestations of systemic infection in children. In: Current Problems in Dermatology. 5(3):81, 1993.
  Up-to-date evaluation of the child with fever and rash. Highlights of the most characteristic and unique findings of a broad range of infectious illnesses.
Timbury MC. Notes on medical virology. 9th ed. Edinburgh: Churchill Livingstone, 1991.
  Concise summary of medical virology based on a lecture course given to medical students at the University of Glasgow.

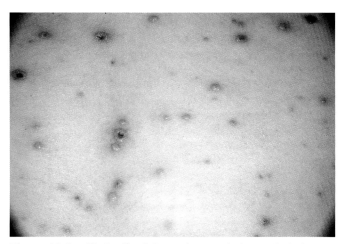

Figure 16.1.   Varicella. Polymorphous vesiculopustular lesions on erythematous bases on the trunk. Some lesions show central necrosis. (Courtesy of Dr. Lee T. Nesbitt, Jr.)

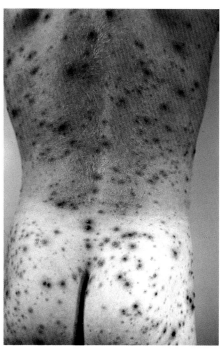

Figure 16.2.   Hemorrhagic varicella. Severe hemorrhagic crusts with surrounding erythema in a young adult. (Courtesy of Dr. Lee T. Nesbitt, Jr.)

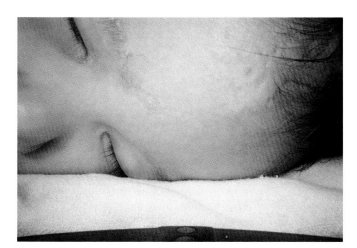

Figure 16.3.   Fetal varicella syndrome. Linear, cicatricial lesions of the forehead.

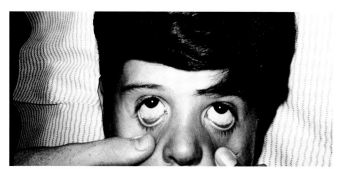

Figure 16.4.   Measles. Conjunctival injection. (Courtesy of Dr. Charles V. Sanders)

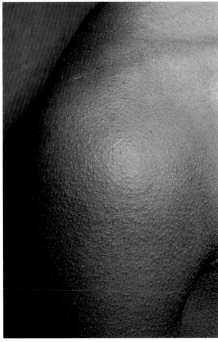

Figure 16.5.   Measles. Maculopapular erythematous eruption. Similar lesions can also be seen with other viral exanthems. (Courtesy of Dr. Lee T. Nesbitt, Jr.)

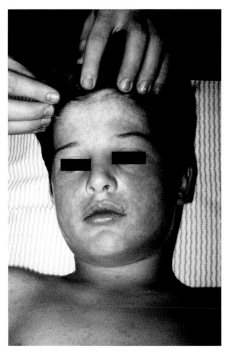

Figure 16.6.   Measles. Maculopapular erythematous eruption of the face and upper trunk in a child. (Courtesy of Dr. Charles V. Sanders)

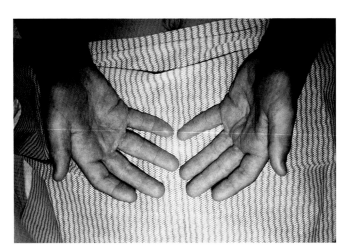

Figure 16.7.   Atypical measles. Petechial and morbilliform erythematous eruption on the hands. (Courtesy of Dr. Charles V. Sanders)

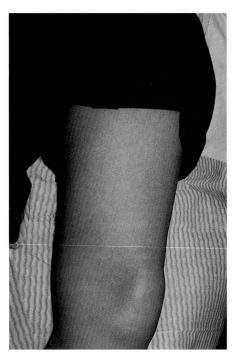

Figure 16.8.   Rubella. Fine erythematous eruption of the anterior thigh. (Courtesy of Dr. Charles V. Sanders)

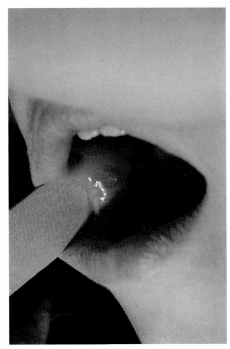

Figure 16.9. Hand, foot, and mouth disease. Ulcerative papules of the buccal mucosa. (Courtesy of Dr. Charles V. Sanders)

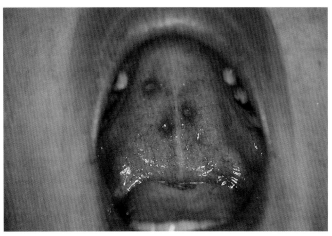

Figure 16.10. Hand, foot, and mouth disease. Papuloulcerative lesions on erythematous bases of the palate. (Courtesy of Dr. Lee T. Nesbitt, Jr.)

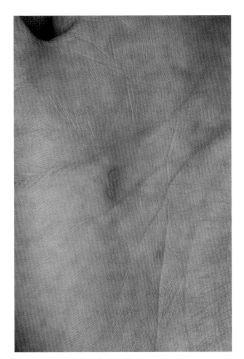

Figure 16.11. Hand, foot, and mouth disease. Two vesicular lesions on erythematous bases on the palm. (Courtesy of Dr. Charles V. Sanders)

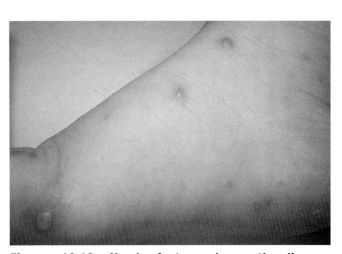

Figure 16.12. Hand, foot, and mouth disease. Vesiculobullous lesions of the medial aspect of the foot. (Courtesy of Dr. Rolando Saenz)

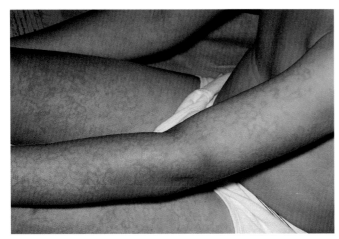

Figure 16.13.   Erythema infectiosum. Erythematous reticulated eruption of the extremities due to parvovirus B19. (Courtesy of Dr. Lee T. Nesbitt, Jr.)

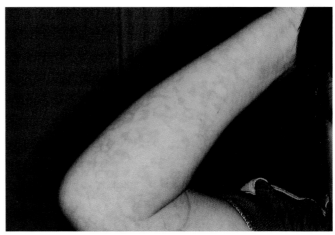

Figure 16.14.   Erythema infectiosum. Reticulated erythematous lesions showing unusual configuration on the forearm. (Courtesy of Dr. Lee T. Nesbitt, Jr.)

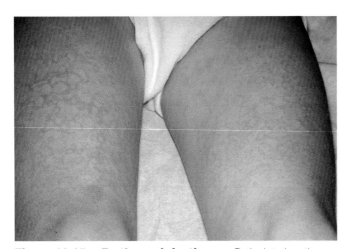

Figure 16.15.   Erythema infectiosum. Reticulated erythematous lesions of the extremities. (Courtesy of Dr. Lee T. Nesbitt, Jr.)

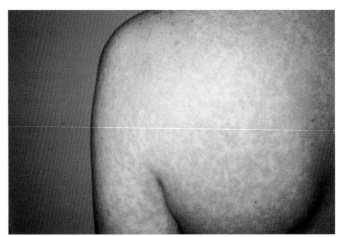

Figure 16.16.   Infectious mononucleosis. Morbilliform maculopapular eruption on the back of a patient who took ampicillin.

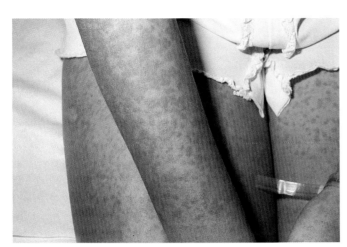

Figure 16.17. Infectious mononucleosis. Generalized erythematous maculopapular eruption characteristic of the association in a patient taking ampicillin. (Courtesy of Dr. Lee T. Nesbitt, Jr.)

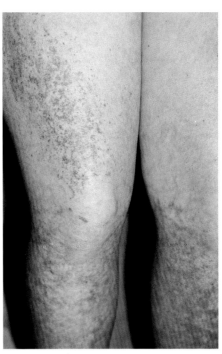

Figure 16.18. Hepatitis C. Petechial eruption of the lower extremities with residual hyperpigmentation.

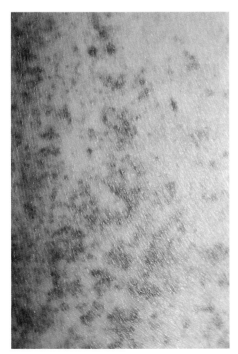

Figure 16.19. Hepatitis C. Close-up view of the patient in Figure 16.8, showing petechial eruption. Patient also had cryoglobulinemia.

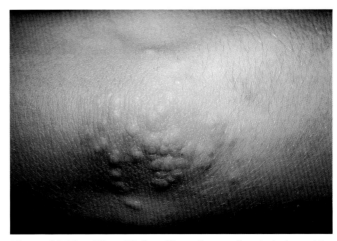

Figure 16.20. Gianotti-Crosti syndrome. Papular lesions of the elbow area. (Courtesy of Dr. Lee T. Nesbitt, Jr.)

CHAPTER 17

Other Viral Infections

JACK L. ARBISER, JO-DAVID FINE, and KENNETH A. ARNDT

Several viruses, most notably those of the herpes virus and human papillomavirus groups, primarily produce skin manifestations. This chapter addresses the infections of primary and recurrent herpes simplex, herpes zoster, extragenital human papillomavirus, cytomegalovirus, Epstein-Barr virus, and hemorrhagic fevers.

Herpes Simplex

• PATHOGENESIS •

Two types of herpes simplex virus (HSV) have been identified serologically: each contains double-stranded DNA. HSV-1 is most often isolated from infected sites, such as the lips (herpes labialis), oral cavity (gingivostomatitis), and external aspect of the eye (herpes keratitis). In contrast, HSV-2 infection is usually confined to the genital areas, although most hand, arm, and buttocks lesions are also caused by this serotype. Serotyping is primarily of importance in epidemiological studies; the course of cutaneous infection with each serotype is similar.

Most HSV infections are subclinical. Symptomatic initial infections are generally reflected in mucocutaneous lesions. The incidence and risk of acquiring an HSV infection depends on the patient's age and the site exposed. For example, herpes gingivostomatitis is almost exclusively seen in infants and children; about 70% of children 10 to 14 years old are seropositive for HSV-1 infection. By contrast, HSV-2 infection is usually acquired through sexual activity; therefore, HSV-2 seropositivity is rarely seen before puberty. Both types of HSV infection are transmitted only by skin-to-skin or skin-to-mucous membrane contact.

The incubation period for HSV infection ranges from 2 to 12 days. Primary herpetic infection frequently lasts from 1 to 3 weeks, with viral shedding for 2 to 6 weeks. Subsequent recurrences have shorter durations (less than 1 week) and shorter detectable periods of virus excretion.

Infection tends to recur in areas of previous primary HSV infection. In some persons, more than one primary infection with different HSV serotypes may occur. Herpes simplex virus rapidly infects those peripheral nerves innervating the areas of exposure, travels to their associated sensory and/or autonomic ganglia, and establishes latent or dormant infection after the active infection has clinically resolved. During this time, intact HSV particles cannot be detected. Clinical recurrence develops after reactivation and retrograde intraneural migration of the virus to the skin; common precipitating events include sunburn, fever, menses, stress, sexual activity, and neurosurgical procedures. Most patients have multiple episodes of recurrence for many years before the disease finally abates.

• CLINICAL FEATURES •

The signs and symptoms in primary HSV infections of the skin are highly characteristic (Fig. 17.1). In primary herpetic gingivostomatitis (Figs. 17.2, 17.3), symptoms include high fever, regional lymphadenopathy, oral pain (sometimes severe enough to interfere with eating), and generalized malaise. Oral findings may include extensive erosions and denudation, as well as severe erythema and induration of the gingivae; occasional intact vesicles may be noted. Primary herpes vulvovaginitis may result in similarly widespread involvement; in severe cases, temporary catheterization may be required because of urinary tract obstruction caused by extensive soft-tissue swelling.

The typical early lesion of recurrent HSV infection (Fig. 17.4–17.7) is a small vesicle; however, because these vesicles are intraepidermal, they tend to be somewhat fragile. As a result, small circular erosions with surrounding erythema and induration may be noted. Such lesions are classically grouped and confined to a localized area of skin. Pain, itching, or paresthesias may precede the appearance of these lesions by several hours. Although the infection is usually not associated with systemic symptoms, some patients have low-grade fever and constitutional symptoms with each recurrence. Within the first day or two of the active infection, the erosions become crusted. Subsequent healing usually occurs without scarring, postinflammatory pigmentary changes, or postherpetic neuralgia.

An uncommon form of primary or recurrent HSV infection, known as Kaposi's varicelliform eruption or eczema herpeticum, usually affects patients with large areas of compromised skin, such as patients with atopic dermatitis, pemphigus, Darier's disease, or epidermolytic hyperkeratosis. This syndrome is characterized by the sudden onset of extensive herpetic lesions, especially on skin involved with the primary disease, and is frequently accompanied by fever, lymphadenopathy, and constitutional symptoms.

In a normal host, HSV infection is generally associated with an acute lytic course, followed by latency. In some immunocompromised persons, HSV infection is associated with chronic ulceration of cutaneous surfaces. This clinical picture should now always arouse suspicion for underlying HIV infection.

Neonates are particularly susceptible to systemic infection with HSV. Intrauterine infection early in embryogenesis is associated with fetal anomalies, while later infection is associated with normal embryogenesis but systemic infection. The incidence of maternal-fetal transmission is approximately 50% from mothers with primary infection, and 5% in recurrent infection. Of interest, primary infection with HSV-2 is often asymptomatic, and reactivation of these initially asymptomatic HSV-2 infections in pregnant women at the time of delivery is common. Fortunately, the rate of asymptomatic shedding is low. Prophylactic acyclovir is sometimes given to infants of infected, but asymptomatic, mothers when a high-risk situation is encountered, such as positive cervical viral cultures, fetal instrumentation, and premature rupture of membranes. The skin is usually the first visible site of infection, but may not be obvious for up to 3 weeks in the newborn.

Disseminated infections may occur in immunocompromised patients, such as those undergoing chemotherapy, those with iatrogenic immunosuppression for transplantation, or persons with acquired or genetic immunodeficiencies, such as AIDS and Wiskott-Aldrich syndrome.

Erythema multiforme has been associated with recurrent HSV infection. Viral proteins and DNA have been detected within active and healed lesions of some patients with erythema multiforme. Prophylactic acyclovir can sometimes be given to prevent future attacks of HSV-related erythema multiforme.

• DIAGNOSIS AND DIFFERENTIAL DIAGNOSIS •

Diagnosis can be definitively established by two methods. Viral culture from early lesions often yields an answer within 1 week. Rapid viral immunofluorescence of cellular material from the base of a lesion can yield an answer within hours and distinguish HSV from varicella-zoster infection (VZV). New techniques, such as the detection of viral DNA through polymerase chain reaction (PCR), are currently under development; however, results using this technique must be cautiously interpreted given its extreme sensitivity.

A rapid and cost-effective method of diagnosing herpes infection is the cytologic (Tzanck) examination of a scraping from the base of an intact vesicle or early erosion. The demonstration of multinucleated giant cells is specific for infection by HSV and VZV infections. Intranuclear inclusions can be seen on biopsy specimens of representative lesions. However,

Tzanck examination or biopsy cannot distinguish HSV infection from VZV infection.

The differential diagnosis of herpetic gingivostomatitis includes aphthous stomatitis, pemphigus vulgaris, and erosive lichen planus. The differential diagnosis of eczema herpeticum includes id reaction and eczema vaccinatum, which is rarely seen today since smallpox vaccination is no longer routinely performed.

• TREATMENT AND CLINICAL COURSE •

Treatment of herpesvirus infection is one of the great triumphs of antiviral therapy. Initially, adenosine arabinoside (vidarabine) was used, but its use has been largely superseded by acyclovir, which is less toxic and more soluble. Other nucleoside antivirals, such as idoxuridine and trifluorothymidine, have been used in treating herpes keratitis.

Acyclovir can be used at doses of 200 mg 3 times daily or 400 mg 2 times daily to decrease the duration of primary or recurrent infection with either HSV-1 or HSV-2. Long-term suppressive therapy with the same dose is effective in patients with frequent or severe recurrences, but this benefit should be measured against the formidable cost of suppressive therapy. Many patients take acyclovir when they experience the herpes prodrome, but this is less effective than constant prophylaxis. New acyclovir-related drugs, such as famciclovir, are becoming available for even superior treatment of herpes infections.

The two targets of antiviral therapy in herpes infections are the viral thymidine kinase and DNA polymerase. Herpes strains resistant to these drugs have been characterized in tissue culture, and, rarely, in AIDS patients on long-term therapy. Many of the thymidine kinase mutants that are acyclovir-resistant are susceptible to phosphonoformate (foscarnet), an inhibitor of viral DNA polymerase.

Supportive measures for herpes infections include mild analgesics, compresses, other drying agents, and topical antibiotics.

Herpes Zoster

Herpes zoster (shingles) and varicella (chickenpox) are both caused by the varicella-zoster virus (VZV), a DNA virus morphologically indistinguishable from other members of the *Herpesviridae* family. To date, only one serotype has been identified.

This chapter focuses on herpes zoster. See Chapter 16 for a discussion of varicella (Figs. 17.8–17.10).

• PATHOGENESIS •

VZV is spread through inhalation of respiratory droplets from viremic patients. Initial infection with VZV results in chickenpox. Herpes zoster most commonly develops in the elderly, when latent VZV infection is reactivated many decades after primary infection (chickenpox). Although varicella is a generalized eruption, herpes zoster is usually localized to a single unilateral dermatome. In immunocompromised persons, however, disseminated infection can occur secondary to hematogenous spread. The inflammation associated with herpes zoster may lead to injury of involved peripheral nerves and resultant postherpetic neuralgia. In contrast to HSV infection, herpes zoster usually does not recur.

• CLINICAL FEATURES •

The incubation of primary VZV infection is 14 to 21 days. In typical herpes zoster, pain or paresthesia along a dermatome is followed within a few days by an eruption beginning on the trunk and, later, spreading centrifugally, evolving from a band of erythema into grouped vesicles, erosions, and crusts (Figs. 17.11–17.14). The eruption evolves over 2 to 3 weeks; postinflammatory pigmentary changes and/or scarring may follow. Some patients continue to experience mild to severe pain after the eruption has completely resolved.

A few lesions (up to about 20) may occur outside of the affected dermatome in localized zoster; such patients do not have increased risk of dissemination or prolonged course of the infection. In contrast, disseminated lesions are not infrequently seen in patients with underlying immunosuppression (Fig. 17.15); associated systemic symptoms represent ongoing viremia.

Prodromal symptoms may be easily misdiagnosed, depending on the dermatome affected. For example, headache, low-back-pain, or bladder discomfort may precede the development of herpes zoster lesions on the scalp or lumbosacral regions respectively. The first division of the trigeminal nerve is a common site. Development of even a solitary lesion on the tip of the nose suggests involvement of the nasociliary branch of this cranial nerve; careful ophthalmological examination is indicated to exclude ocular involvement.

• DIAGNOSIS AND DIFFERENTIAL DIAGNOSIS •

As with HSV infection, both viral culture and rapid viral immunofluorescence confirm a diagnosis of VZV infection. Viral culture may take weeks to yield a positive result, so it is often of limited use in rapid diagnosis. Rapid viral immunofluorescence is especially of value in the evaluation of a herpetic lesion in an immunocompromised host, as the dose of acyclovir used in VSV and HSV infections is quite different.

The Tzanck cytologic examination gives useful confirmatory data in a patient with the clinical expression of herpes zoster (Fig. 17.16). As previously mentioned, the Tzanck examination does not distinguish between HSV and VZV.

• TREATMENT AND CLINICAL COURSE •

Localized herpes zoster can be treated with oral acyclovir, at a dosage of 800 mg 5 times daily for 10 days. Acyclovir therapy is useful only if instituted within the first few days of symptoms. The role of systemic corticosteroids in prevention of postherpetic neuralgia is controversial, and no conclusive claims can be made to its efficacy. Many practitioners give acyclovir and corticosteroids to patients with localized zoster who are at high risk for postherpetic pain, namely, trigeminal distribution

and elderly patients. New antiviral agents, such as bromovinyl uracil arabinoside, are also becoming available for herpes zoster.

Acyclovir has recently been shown to prevent varicella in susceptible family members (1). At doses of 40–80mg/kg/day, acyclovir either prevented symptomatic chickenpox or modified its severity. Most of these patients became seropositive for VZV and are presumably immune to VZV reinfection. However, the status of long-term immunity has not yet been established. Currently, administration of varicella zoster immune globulin is indicated for prophylaxis in immunocompromised patients after exposure to varicella.

Several options exist for the treatment of postherpetic neuralgia, none of them entirely satisfactory. Topical capsaicin has been shown to be of some benefit; however, skin lesions should be completely healed prior to this therapy. A limiting side effect is a burning sensation in some patients. Other options include narcotic analgesics; anticonvulsants, such as phenytoin or carbamazepine; tricyclic antidepressants, such as amitryptiline; or even neurosurgical intervention (i.e., rhizotomy or cordotomy). Transcutaneous electrical nerve stimulation of affected areas has been reported to be successful in some patients. Disseminated herpes zoster is treated with intravenous acyclovir. Impetiginization of skin lesions is treated with warm soaks and topical or systemic antibiotics.

Human papillomavirus

• PATHOGENESIS •

Human papillomaviruses, the causative agent of warts, are small viruses containing a genome of double-stranded DNA, approximately 8 kilobases in length. They are members of a large family of viruses that include SV40, polyoma, and the virus responsible for progressive multifocal leukoencephalopathy. The virus exists as an episome, a circular form of DNA that undergoes autonomous replication in host cells, like a bacterial plasmid.

Approximately 70 papillomavirus types have been characterized. These types differ at the level of DNA sequence. The different clinical manifestations are associated with different clinical types, and some types are associated with malignancy. The progression to cutaneous malignancy involves a complex interplay between the ability of the virus to integrate into the host genome and the immune status of the host.

Human papillomavirus enters the host through direct contact with infected skin or mucous membranes. The viral receptor is not known at present. In recent years, much has been learned about viral gene function in papillomavirus. The virus contains a number of genes necessary for viral replication, called early genes because they are expressed early after infection. The E6 and E7 genes have been intensively studied, because they interact with human oncogenes. The E6 gene of HPV 16 has been demonstrated to immortalize human cells and to interact with the cellular oncogene p53, the most commonly mutated oncogene in human cancer. The p53 gene, which normally acts as a tumor suppressor gene, is destabilized by association with the E6 gene product. E6 genes from low-risk papillomavirus types have less effect on cellular p53. The E7 protein binds to the tumor, suppressing retinoblastoma gene product and inhibiting its effect on cell proliferation.

Immune deficiencies can predispose to squamous cell carcinoma. The autosomal recessive disorder epidermodysplasia verruciformis is associated with malignant transformation of verrucae containing primarily HPV subtypes 5 and 8. Anal squamous cell carcinoma is observed in patients with AIDS and genital warts. Mucosal lesions are commonly associated with HPV 6 and 11, which are common causes of genital verrucae and are associated with verrucous carcinoma. HPV types 16, 18, 31, and 33 are known as "high-risk" types because they are associated with epithelial malignancies, such as cervical and penile cancers.

• CLINICAL FEATURES •

Flat warts are usually small and smooth-surfaced; they are most often found in large numbers on facial skin. Common and plantar warts are usually larger and much more verrucous and are present in fewer numbers than flat warts, except in either immunosuppressed hosts or patients with epidermodysplasia verruciformis. Common and plantar warts are found most often on the hands and plantar surfaces of the feet, respectively (Figs. 17.17–17.19). Filiform warts are solitary, slender, exophytic lesions found especially on the neck and face. Genital warts, usually called condylomata acuminata, appear as moist, verrucoid lesions of the genitalia and surrounding areas (Figs. 17.20–17.22). All types of extragenital warts have a tendency to appear in linear configuration; that is, new warts may develop in adjacent sites secondary to inoculation by minor trauma.

• DIAGNOSIS AND DIFFERENTIAL DIAGNOSIS •

Flat warts may be clinically confused with small dermal nevi, freckles, or appendage tumors such as syringomas. Common warts, especially when large, may occasionally mimic seborrheic keratoses or squamous cell carcinoma. Although the diagnosis of filiform warts is usually obvious, occasionally, lesions may mimic cutaneous horns, necessitating biopsy to differentiate from hypertrophic actinic keratoses or squamous cell carcinoma. Plantar warts may be confused with calluses; demonstration of thrombosed blood vessels at the base of such lesions after careful paring with a scalpel will confirm the diagnosis of a plantar wart. Histologically, characteristic nuclear inclusions can be observed in verrucae.

• TREATMENT AND CLINICAL COURSE •

Isolated warts often spontaneously regress if left untreated for a few years. Additional lesions may, however, develop in the interim by virtue of autoinoculation. Most warts respond well to any of several destructive methods using chemical agents (such as acids) or physical modalities (such as electrodesiccation or cryotherapy). Less frequently used treatments for recalcitrant warts include topical fluorouracil (sometimes in conjunction with topical tretinoin), intralesional injection of bleomycin or fluorouracil, allergic contact sensitization with strong sensitizers such as dinitrochlorobenzene, or CO_2 laser surgery. Individual lesions of epidermodysplasia verruciformis unresponsive to other modalities have recently been shown to respond to intralesional interferon. Extensive warts in immunosuppressed patients tend to respond poorly to any of the therapies currently available.

Epstein-Barr Virus

• PATHOGENESIS •

Epstein-Barr (EBV) virus is a member of the family *Herpesviridae*, and its primary target is B lymphocytes and pharyngeal epithelium. The most common illness associated with EBV is infectious mononucleosis, but EBV is also associated with Burkitt lymphoma and nasopharyngeal carcinoma. High-grade Burkitt lymphomas associated with Epstein-Barr virus rarely arise in, or metastasize to, the skin. Recently, the EBV genome has been found in cells of Hodgkin's lymphoma, but the role of EBV in this tumor has yet to be established.

Oral hairy leukoplakia is an EBV infection of tongue epithelium commonly observed in immunosuppressed patients. These lesions have been shown by immunocytochemistry to express various EBV genes, such as Epstein-Barr nuclear antigen (EBNA). This infection involves the spinous and granular cell layers, but spares the basal cell layer. Expression of EBV proteins appears to be dependent on the differentiation state of the cell.

An interesting model of EBV interaction with the skin has been created by directing expression of the EBV oncogene latent membrane protein to the skin of transgenic mice (2). This resulted in a hyperplastic epidermis and in increased expression of the hyperproliferative keratin K6 in the tongue and skin epidermis.

• CLINICAL FEATURES •

The cutaneous manifestations of EBV infection occur in two forms. The lesions of oral hairy leukoplakia appear as velvety white plaques on the lateral surface of the tongue and cannot be removed by scraping the tongue, in contrast to candidiasis.

The second form is a morbilliform eruption in patients with infectious mononucleosis that almost always occurs when these patients take ampicillin or amoxicillin. The basis for this eruption is not currently understood. Rare manifestations of infectious mononucleosis are leukocytoclastic vasculitis, cold urticaria, and acrocyanosis.

• DIAGNOSIS AND DIFFERENTIAL DIAGNOSIS •

The diagnosis of oral hairy leukoplakia can be made on clinical grounds alone. The presence of an adherent white hairy lesion in the appropriate clinical circumstance is sufficient to establish the diagnosis. If biopsy is performed, the affected epithelium appears hyperparakeratotic and has vacuolated prickle cells. Similarly, the rash associated with ampicillin or amoxicillin in patients with mononucleosis can be diagnosed clinically. The rare case of cutaneous lymphoma in a patient who is immunosuppressed, whether by AIDS, transplant rejection regimens, or genetic immunodeficiency (i.e., X-linked lymphoproliferative disease), can be established by biopsy.

• TREATMENT AND CLINICAL COURSE •

In vitro, EBV transformation and replication can be inhibited by a number of antiviral agents, including acyclovir, ganciclovir, foscarnet, and zidovudine (AZT). In vivo, these drugs have had only transient effects and therefore are not clinically used. These drugs have also not been useful in primary EBV infection of individuals with X-linked proliferative disease. Oral hairy leukoplakia may respond to oral acyclovir but often recurs when the drug is stopped; topical chemotherapy, such as podophyllin in alcohol, may also prove useful for this condition.

Cytomegalovirus

• PATHOGENESIS •

Cytomegalovirus (CMV) is a member of the herpesvirus family, and seropositivity is nearly universal in old age. Cutaneous manifestations of CMV infection are uncommon and tend to be seen only in immunocompromised patients and infants. Cytomegalovirus may cause primary infection of skin cells or may indirectly affect the skin through displacement of hematopoietic elements to the skin or exacerbation of graft-versus-host disease.

• CLINICAL FEATURES •

The most common cutaneous manifestation of CMV infection is perineal ulceration. In infants, this syndrome may present as a severe diaper dermatitis. Congenital CMV infection may lead to the blueberry muffin child, characterized by purpuric papules, which represent dermal hematopoiesis. CMV may also cause an infectious mononucleosis syndrome, an exanthematous eruption associated with ampicillin therapy, and may also be responsible for rare cases of papular acrodermatitis of childhood (Gianotti-Crosti syndrome). CMV has been associated with Kaposi's sarcoma; however, its precise role remains unclear.

• DIAGNOSIS AND DIFFERENTIAL DIAGNOSIS •

Diagnosis of CMV infection may be made by biopsy, which should reveal characteristic "owl-eye" intranuclear inclusions, or by viral cultures of buffy coats. Culture of the virus is slow and laborious, and may require several weeks to obtain a positive result. An antibody test is now available for the rapid detection of CMV-specific proteins, and PCR-based tests may be available soon.

• TREATMENT AND CLINICAL COURSE •

Antiviral agents are available for CMV infection. Ganciclovir is chemically similar to acyclovir but contains an extra hydroxymethyl moiety. This difference allows ganciclovir to be phosphorylated by both viral and cellular kinases, which accounts for both its antiviral activity and toxicity. At present, ganciclovir is only available intravenously, and is indicated for CMV retinitis. Foscarnet (trisodium phosphonoformate) is also effective against CMV retinitis and does not share the myelotoxicity of ganciclovir.

Poxviruses

• PATHOGENESIS •

Poxviruses are the largest of animal viruses and replicate in the cytoplasm, unlike many other viruses, which replicate in the nucleus. These viruses are DNA viruses and are classified on the basis of size and shape. The orthopox viruses, which are the largest, include variola and vaccinia, while the somewhat smaller parapoxviruses include orf and milker's nodule. Molluscum contagiosum, the most common cutaneous poxvirus, falls into a third unclassified category, being intermediate in size between the orthopox and parapoxviruses. The parapoxviruses and molluscum viruses are spread by direct contact with human or animal lesions or by contact with fomites of infected animals.

Molluscum contagiosum causes mitosis of basal keratinocytes and has been found to encode a peptide with remarkable similarity to epidermal growth factor. Orf and milker's nodule both cause vacuolization and epidermal edema.

Molluscum contagiosum is seen in two peak age groups. The first is young children, in whom it may be acquired through close physical contact with lesions, usually through play and, uncommonly, sexual abuse. The second major age group is young adults, who acquire the virus sexually. The incubation period is unknown, and the virus has yet to be cultured.

• CLINICAL FEATURES AND DIAGNOSIS •

Diagnosis is usually made on clinical grounds through the observation of a flesh-colored or pink papule, often with central umbilication (Figs. 17.23–17.25). Staining of crushed papules on a microscope slide reveals distinctive molluscum bodies, which are refractile hyaline bodies that represent virus. These molluscum bodies can also be seen on routine pathology, although biopsy is rarely necessary.

The lesions often are self-resolving after a period of months to years. They may be spread by self-inoculation, such as shaving. Patients with immunosuppressive disorders, such as AIDS, have larger lesions that often do not resolve spontaneously (Fig. 17.26). The differential diagnosis of molluscum contagiosum includes dermal nevi, seborrheic keratosis, appendageal tumor, basal cell carcinoma, epidermal inclusion cyst, acne, pyogenic granuloma, and, in AIDS patients, cutaneous cryptococcus.

Orf is associated with exposure to sheep and goats and is prevalent in farmers, butchers, and veterinarians. Lesions appear after an incubation period of approximately 1 week as hemorrhagic bullae (Fig. 17.27). They may reach several centimeters in diameter and be accompanied by lymphangitis and low-grade fever. The lesions resolve spontaneously after 1 to 2 months. The diagnosis is made clinically, based on physical appearance and a history of animal exposure. When the diagnosis is in doubt, biopsy and/or electron microscopy may be useful. Culture of the lesions is tedious and has a low yield.

Milker's nodule and its close relative, bovine papular stomatitis virus, are diseases of cows and their handlers, and they are similar to orf in their incubation period and clinical appearance (Fig. 17.28). Like orf, the lesions fade spontaneously over several weeks. Since lesions are often difficult to distinguish from orf on microscopic exam, clinical history is most important in distinguishing these two entities.

• TREATMENT AND CLINICAL COURSE •

All of these diseases usually resolve spontaneously. Several therapeutic options are available if the lesions need to be treated, especially for molluscum contagiosum in immunocompromised patients. Cryotherapy is the most commonly employed method, and these lesions are more easily destroyed than warts. Topical therapy with 5-fluorouracil or tretinoin is also of value in destroying numerous molluscum lesions. Orf and milker's nodules are rarely treated except in the case of bacterial superinfection. Treatment of orf lesions with topical idoxuridine has been reported.

Hemorrhagic Fever (Dengue)

• PATHOGENESIS •

Hemorrhagic fevers are caused by a wide variety of arboviruses, RNA viruses that are found in geographically diverse areas and cause a wide variety of clinical syndromes affecting many organs. Many of these syndromes are characterized clinically by hemorrhage of small vessels in many organs, including the skin. One of the most important causes of hemorrhagic fever is the dengue virus, responsible for dengue fever. Since the dengue virus is the primary arbovirus responsible for hemorrhagic fever, this discussion will center on the features of dengue fever, many of which are common to other hemorrhagic fevers. Dengue fever is transmitted by female *Aedes aegypti* or *Aedes albopictus* mosquitoes, and the disease may cause localized or life-threatening hemorrhage. The mosquitoes obtain the virus through the ingestion of viremic blood from infected hosts.

Four serotypes of dengue fever virus exist, known as types 1–4. Type-specific immunity is lifelong but does not confer immunity to other subtypes. In fact, the risk of severe hemorrhage from dengue fever is positively associated with prior infection with a separate serotype. Other factors associated with increased risk for dengue hemorrhagic fever are chronic disease, young age, female sex, and possible differences in virulence between strains.

Virus replication occurs primarily in the macrophage as demonstrated by immunofluorescence of skin biopsy material

from patients with hemorrhagic fever. The petechiae that are characteristic of hemorrhagic fever result from two phenomena: capillary leakage and consumptive coagulopathy. The mechanisms of this are not understood but may involve cytokines, histamine, and depletion of complement.

• CLINICAL FEATURES •

Dengue fever infection ranges from subclinical to life-threatening. The incubation period is from 3 to 15 days after inoculation by a mosquito. The initial clinical signs are high fever and malaise accompanied by retrobulbar pain and congestion of conjunctival capillaries, known as "dengue facies." A second rash is characterized by a macular eruption sparing the bite site. This may be followed by a generalized exanthem, sparing the palms and soles. Dengue hemorrhagic fever is characterized by petechiae, hypotension, thrombocytopenia, mucosal hemorrhage, and a positive tourniquet sign.

• DIAGNOSIS AND DIFFERENTIAL DIAGNOSIS •

The differential of dengue fever is wide, and includes other viral exanthems. The petechiae in dengue hemorrhagic fever may be confused with meningococcemia, Rocky Mountain spotted fever, and other forms of sepsis. A careful history, including travel history, is important in establishing the diagnosis. Paired sera from early and convalescent stages of the illness, demonstrating a rise in dengue antibody titer, confirms the diagnosis. In addition, a high titer of dengue IgM antibody is a rapid diagnostic test.

• TREATMENT AND CLINICAL COURSE •

Therapy for all stages of dengue fever is supportive, with no specific antiviral therapy presently available. Aspirin is avoided, given the potential for hemorrhage. Insect repellents and avoidance of mosquito-prone areas are effective in reducing the risk of infection. Dengue fever vaccines may eventually be available, but all serotypes will need to be covered in order to avoid increasing the risk of hemorrhagic fever.

Other Hemorrhagic Fevers

Several other viruses give rise to hemorrhagic fevers. All of these syndromes, in severe forms, yield cutaneous petechiae. The pathophysiology of hemorrhage in these diseases is similar, resulting from an increase in vascular permeability and moderate consumptive coagulopathy. The salient features of several of the more common hemorrhagic fevers will be discussed.

YELLOW FEVER

Yellow fever is a common viral illness with a spectrum ranging from subclinical infection to prostration and death. It is caused by infection with an RNA-containing flavivirus, is transmitted by *Aedes* and *Haemagogus* mosquitoes, and occurs in South America and central Africa. Prior infection with other flaviviruses is thought to confer partial immunity, resulting in less severe forms of illness. The primary target of the virus appears to be the liver, although yellow fever may be a multisystem disease. Early disease is characterized by fever and paradoxical bradycardia (Faget's sign), while severe illness is characterized by diffuse hemorrhage, dehydration, jaundice, leukopenia, albuminuria, and abnormalities in liver function tests. No specific antiviral drugs are currently available. Diagnosis in the appropriate clinical setting can be made by the detection of a convalescent rise in titers, or detection of antiyellow fever IgM antibodies. Monoclonal antibodies are available for the detection of yellow fever antigens in tissue specimens. Vaccination with the vaccine yellow fever 17d is effective, but it should be given with caution to pregnant women and has been associated with encephalitis in infants.

HANTAVIRUS INFECTION

Infection with this group of RNA-containing bunyaviruses has recently become noteworthy due to a recent outbreak in the southwestern United States. Hantavirus is transmitted by various species of rodents, which appear to be their natural reservoir; human infection apparently occurs through inhalation of aerosolized rodent secretions. The kidney appears to be the primary target of hantavirus, with acute renal failure often ensuing. The pathogenesis of this acute renal failure is incompletely understood, but may involve immune complex deposition. Thrombocytopenia and resulting petechiae are common. Causes of mortality include intracranial hemorrhage and adult respiratory distress syndrome.

Diagnosis can be made by convalescent titers and virus-specific IgM. Isolation of the virus is difficult and requires tissue culture and animal facilities.

Ribavirin is effective in the treatment of hantavirus infection if given before the 4th day of illness. Fluid management is essential in the treatment of severe cases of hantavirus infection.

MISCELLANEOUS SYNDROMES

Other important hemorrhagic fever syndromes include Lassa fever, which is found in West Africa and is treatable and sometimes prevented with ribavirin. Hemorrhagic fevers of South America include Argentine hemorrhagic fever and Bolivian hemorrhagic fever, in addition to the more common dengue and yellow fevers. Ebola and Marburg viral fevers are caused by filoviruses, and result in severe illness in humans. Nosocomial spread of disease is an important mode of Ebola virus infection.

REFERENCES

1. Asano Y, et al. Post-exposure prophylaxis of varicella in family contact by oral acyclovir. Pediatrics 1993;2:219.
2. Wilson JB, et al. Expression of the BNLF-1 oncogene of Epstein-Barr virus in the skin of transgenic mice induces hyperplasia and aberrant expression of keratin 6. Cell 1990;61:1315.

ANNOTATED BIBLIOGRAPHY

Androphy EJ. Human papillomavirus infection and its relationship to cancer: From molecular biology to cure? Progress in Dermatology: Dermatology Foundation 1993;27:1.

   A review of the molecular biology of papillomavirus infection.

Asano Y, et al. Post-exposure prophylaxis of varicella in family contact by oral acyclovir. Pediatrics 1993;2:219.

   A study describing the effective use of acyclovir in prophylaxis after exposure to patients with varicella infection.

Frenkel LM, et al. Clinical reactivation of herpes simplex virus type 2 infection in seropositive pregnant women with no history of genital herpes. Ann Intern Med 1993;118:414.

   A study describing a relatively high seropositivity rate for HSV-2 in women with no clinical history of infection, noting a high rate of clinical reactivation late in pregnancy.

Halstead SB. Antibody, macrophages, dengue virus infection, shock, and hemorrhage: A pathogenetic cascade. Rev Infect Dis 1989;4:S830.

   A review of the pathogenesis of dengue fever.

Highet AS, Kurtz J. Viral Infections. In: Champion RW, Burton JL, Ebling FJG, eds. Rook's Textbook of Dermatology. Boston: Blackwell Scientific Publications, 1992:867.

   A thorough review of cutaneous poxvirus infections.

Lange WR, Beall B, Denny SC. Dengue fever: A resurgent risk for the international traveler. Am Fam Physician 1992;45:1161.

   A good clinical and epidemiological description of dengue virus infection.

Lesher JL. Cytomegalovirus and the skin. J Am Acad Dermatol 1988;18:1333.

   A summary of the various clinical situations in which CMV can play a role.

Monath TP, Fisher-Hoch SP, McCormick JB. In: Strickland GT, ed. Hunter's Tropical Medicine. 7th ed. Philadelphia: WB Saunders, 1991:233.

   An extensive review of the clinical features of hemorrhagic fevers.

Schinazi RF, Prusoff WH. Antiviral agents. Pediatr Clin North Am 1983;30:77.

   A review of many of the nucleoside antivirals in current use.

Straus SE, Cohen JI, Tosato G, Meier J. Epstein-Barr virus infections: Biology, pathogenesis, and management. Ann Intern Med 1993;118:45.

   An excellent review of the clinical and molecular aspects of Epstein-Barr virus infection.

Wilson JB, et al. Expression of the BNLF-1 oncogene of Epstein-Barr virus in the skin of transgenic mice induces hyperplasia and aberrant expression of keratin 6. Cell 1990;61:1315.

   A description of the phenotypic consequences of BNLF-1 expression in the skin of transgenic mice.

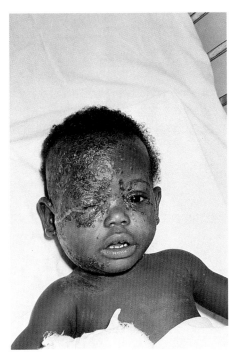

Figure 17.1.   Primary herpes simplex. Numerous vesicles, erosions, and crusts on the face. This eruption simulated varicella-zoster. (Courtesy of Dr. Lee T. Nesbitt, Jr.)

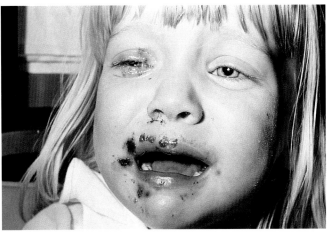

Figure 17.2.   Primary herpes simplex. Vesicles and crusting on the lips and around the right eye. (Courtesy of Dr. Lee T. Nesbitt, Jr.)

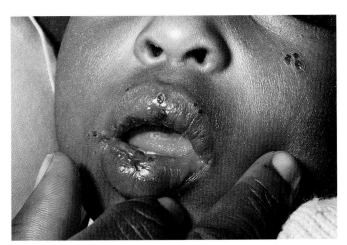

Figure 17.3.   Herpes simplex gingivostomatitis. Multiple vesicles, erosions, and crusts on the mouth and cheeks. (Courtesy of Dr. Lee T. Nesbitt, Jr.)

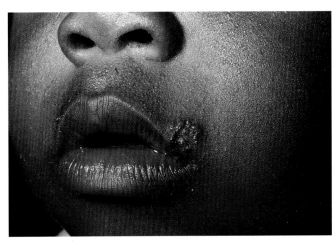

Figure 17.4.   Herpes simplex type 1. Grouped vesicles on erythematous bases on the upper lip. (Courtesy of Dr. Lee T. Nesbitt, Jr.)

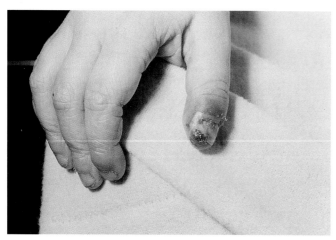

Figure 17.5.   Herpetic whitlow due to herpes simplex virus. Erythema surrounding a vesiculopustular lesion of the thumb. Same patient as in Fig. 17.2. (Courtesy of Dr. Lee T. Nesbitt, Jr.)

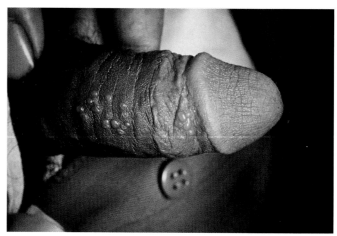

Figure 17.6.   Herpes simplex type 2. Grouped vesicles on erythematous bases on the shaft of the penis. (Courtesy of Dr. Lee T. Nesbitt, Jr.)

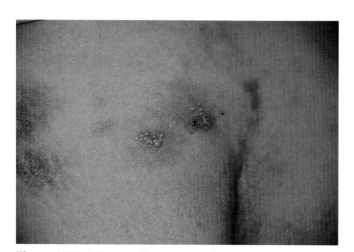

Figure 17.7.   Herpes simplex type 2. Recurrent grouped vesicles on erythematous bases on the buttocks of a female patient (Courtesy of Dr. Lee T. Nesbitt, Jr.)

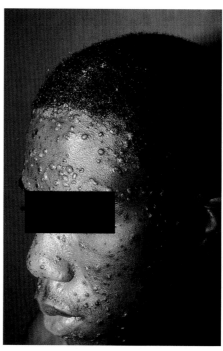

Figure 17.8.   Varicella. Multiple vesiculopustular lesions of the face.

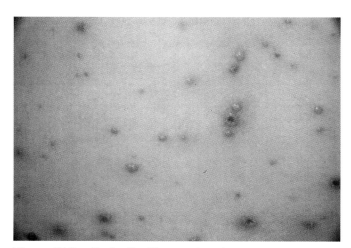

Figure 17.9.   Varicella. Close-up view of primary lesions showing vesiculopustules. (Courtesy of Dr. Lee T. Nesbitt, Jr.)

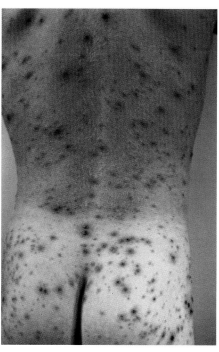

Figure 17.10.   Varicella. Severe hemorrhagic type of infection showing large vesicles with crusting and hemorrhage. (Courtesy of Dr. Lee T. Nesbitt, Jr.)

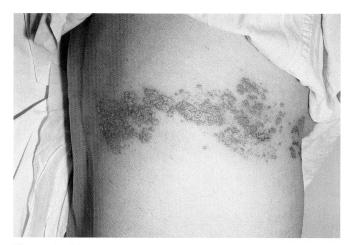

Figure 17.11.   Herpes zoster. Grouped vesicles on erythematous bases in a typical dermatomal pattern on the back and abdomen. (Courtesy of Dr. Lee T. Nesbitt, Jr.)

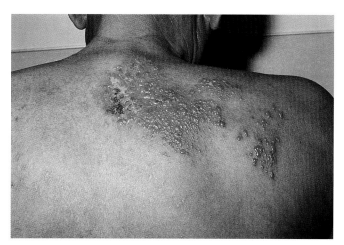

Figure 17.12.   Herpes zoster. Grouped vesicles on erythematous bases on the upper back. Lesions stop abruptly at the midline. (Courtesy of Dr. Lee T. Nesbitt, Jr.)

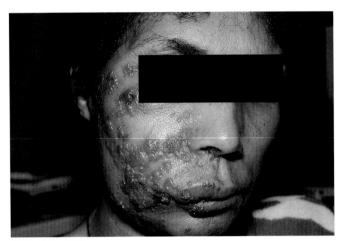

Figure 17.13.   Herpes zoster. Large vesicles with facial swelling corresponding to branches 2 and 3 of the trigeminal nerves. (Courtesy of Dr. Lee T. Nesbitt, Jr.)

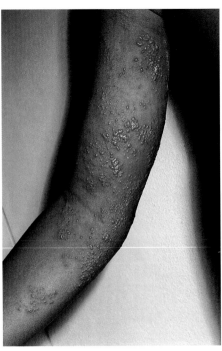

Figure 17.14.   Herpes zoster. Severe erythema surrounding grouped vesicles on the arm. (Courtesy of Dr. Lee T. Nesbitt, Jr.)

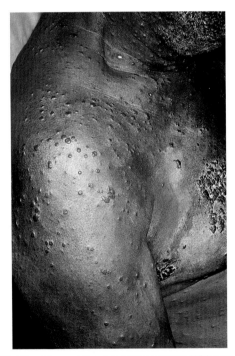

Figure 17.15.   Generalized herpes zoster. Widespread lesions simulating varicella. (Courtesy of Dr. Lee T. Nesbitt, Jr.)

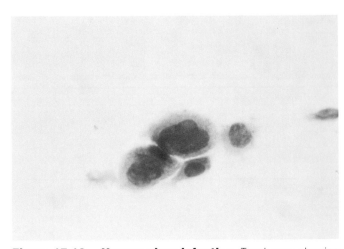

Figure 17.16.   Herpes virus infection. Tzank prep showing multinucleated giant cells.

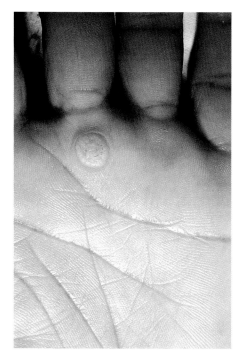

Figure 17.17. Verruca vulgaris (common warts). Translucent papular lesion on the palm. (Courtesy of Dr. Lee T. Nesbitt, Jr.)

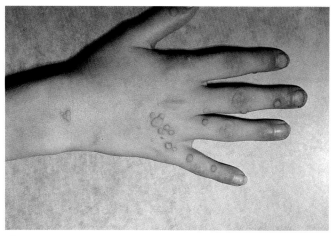

Figure 17.18. Verruca vulgaris (common warts). Multiple papules on the back of the hand and wrist. (Courtesy of Dr. Lee T. Nesbitt, Jr.)

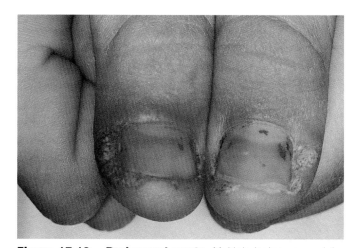

Figure 17.19. Periungual warts. Multiple lesions around the thumbnails. (Courtesy of Dr. Lee T. Nesbitt, Jr.)

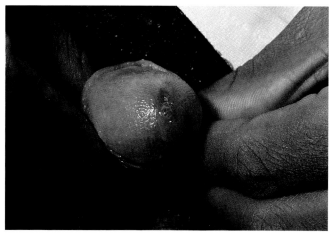

Figure 17.20. Condylomata acuminata. Exuberant erythematous growths from the urethra in a patient who had lesions extending to the bladder. (Courtesy of Dr. Lee T. Nesbitt, Jr.)

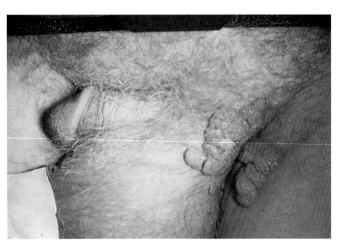

Figure 17.21.   Condylomata acuminata. Multiple verrucous plaques of the inguinal fold. (Courtesy of Dr. Lee T. Nesbitt, Jr.)

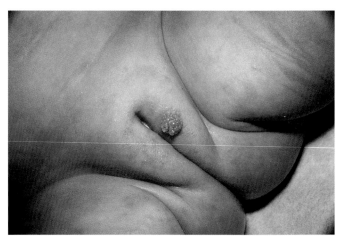

Figure 17.22.   Verruca vulgaris (common warts) of the external genitalia in an infant. Lesions such as this should raise the suspicion of child abuse. (Courtesy of Dr. Lee T. Nesbitt, Jr.)

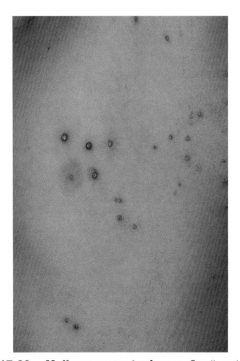

Figure 17.23.   Molluscum contagiosum. Small erythematous papules with umbilicated centers on the chest. (Courtesy of Dr. Lee T. Nesbitt, Jr.)

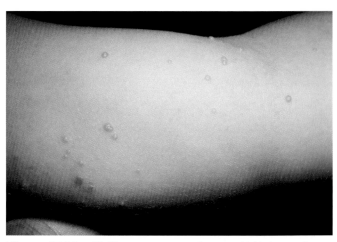

Figure 17.24.   Molluscum contagiosum. Multiple translucent papules on the arm. (Courtesy of Dr. Lee T. Nesbitt, Jr.)

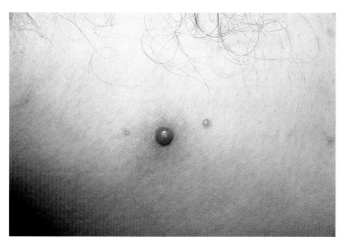

Figure 17.25.   Molluscum contagiosum, inflamed. Two typical papules and one central lesion with marked inflammation and enlargement. (Courtesy of Dr. Lee T. Nesbitt, Jr.)

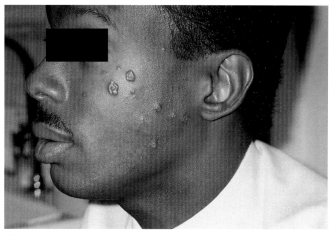

Figure 17.26.   Giant molluscum contagiosum. Giant molluscum contagiosum of the face in an HIV-positive patient. (Courtesy of Dr. Lee T. Nesbitt, Jr.)

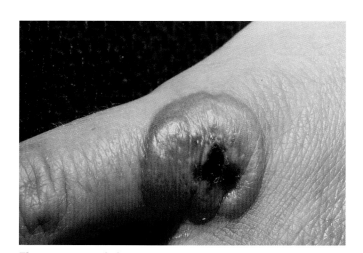

Figure 17.27.   Orf. Indurated hemorrhagic bullous plaque with central crusting on the finger. (Courtesy of Dr. Lee T. Nesbitt, Jr.)

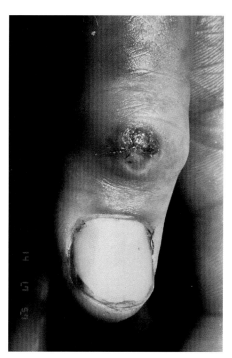

Figure 17.28.   Milker's nodule. Indurated plaque with crusting of the thumb.

CHAPTER 18

Protozoan and Helminth Infections

JOY D. JESTER, ROLANDO E. SAENZ, LEE T. NESBITT, JR.,
and W. A. KROTOSKI

Protozoal Diseases

Protozoa are single-cell organisms that have the capacity for metabolism and reproduction. The protozoa are extremely variable as to biology and are classified morphologically as *Mastigophora* (flagellates, tissue, or luminal parasites), *Sporozoa* (organisms that have sexual and asexual cycles), *Sarcodina* (amoebas, primarily lumen dwellers), and *Ciliata* (a rare cause of human disease). Some of the diseases caused by these organisms have long been present in temperate climates; others are becoming more prevalent because of increasing world travel and predisposing illnesses, such as AIDS.

AMERICAN TRYPANOSOMIASIS (CHAGAS' DISEASE)

Chagas' disease, or American trypanosomiasis, is one of the most important zoonoses in the Western hemisphere. It is endemic in South and Central America, where more than 16 million are infected, approximately 30% of whom will develop Chagas' cardiac disease.

• PATHOGENESIS •

The parasite, *Trypanosoma cruzi*, is a flagellated protozoan of the family Trypanosomatidae, which passes through different morphological stages. In Chagas' disease, the trypomastigote form of *T. cruzi* ultimately migrates to the insect's hind gut and is excreted with feces following a bite. The trypomastigote is also an infective form of the parasite and is found in the peripheral blood.

Worldwide, there are more than 100 species of triatomine blood-sucking insect vectors of Chagas' disease, but the most important are those preferring human blood. Many other animals also serve as reservoirs of infection. In the United States, *T. cruzi* usually circulates between opossums and armadillos, but environmental conditions and vector habits are not favorable for human infection. There are only three recorded cases of indigenous transmission of Chagas' disease in the U.S., and two instances of transmission by blood transfusion (1).

The pathogenetic mechanisms depend on both the parasite and the host. Parasite factors include virulence, size of inoculum, cell

tropism and polymorphism. Most strains are myotropic and invade primarily smooth, skeletal, and heart muscle (Fig. 18.1). Different strains are associated with different clinical syndromes.

In the acute stage of the infection, a local inflammatory response produces a lesion at the site of entry in the conjunctiva or skin. The parasites replicate at this site, disseminate widely, and establish intracellular infection. Lesions may also develop in the esophagus, gastrointestinal tract, and sympathetic and parasympathetic nervous systems. The acute phase is followed by an asymptomatic period that may last for decades before signs of the chronic phase appear.

Trypanosoma cruzi can be transmitted to the fetus transplacentally at any stage of the infection in the mother.

• CLINICAL FEATURES •

Although the acute phase of the disease is often asymptomatic, the chagoma, the first manifestation of infection in 20% of cases, appears at the cutaneous inoculation site as an indurated area of erythema and swelling accompanied by regional lymph node involvement. When the parasites enter through the periorbital skin or ocular conjunctiva (80% of cases), palpebral edema, conjunctivitis, and preauricular lymphadenopathy may be observed. This complex, called Romaña's sign, can be useful in the diagnosis of acute infection (Figs. 18.2, 18.3).

The local reaction is followed by fever, malaise, lymphadenopathy, hepatosplenomegaly and generalized edema, myocarditis in some patients, and, rarely, meningoencephalitis. The majority of acute cases of Chagas' disease resolve within 2 to 30 months to an indeterminate stage characterized by asymptomatic parasitemia, but with the presence of antibodies to a variety of *T. cruzi* antigens. Whereas most chronically infected persons continue in this stage for life, approximately 30% develop chronic cardiomyopathy, megaesophagus, or megacolon.

• DIAGNOSIS AND DIFFERENTIAL DIAGNOSIS •

During the acute phase, the diagnosis can be made by finding the trypomastigote in wet mounts of Giemsa-stained thin and thick smears of blood or buffy coat. Hemocultures employing NNN, Bonacci, Warren, LIT, and other culture media are positive 5 to 15 days after inoculation.

Serologic diagnosis can also be very helpful, particularly with the detection of IgM antibodies to *T. cruzi* by indirect immunofluorescence or with indirect enzyme immunoassay. Seroconversion of IgG antibodies from negative to positive is also a valid indication of recent infection.

During the chronic phase, parasitemia is absent or extremely low, and diagnosis depends on serologic tests. The most sensitive and specific assays for IgG antibodies to *T. cruzi* are the complement fixation (Machado-Guerreiro), indirect hemagglutination, indirect immunofluorescence, and more recently, ELISA (enzyme-linked immunoadsorbent) assays. All of these can cross-react with serum from patients with leishmaniasis, *T. rangeli* infection, tuberculosis, leprosy, and syphilis. Xenodiagnosis is another useful procedure, allowing the isolation of *T. cruzi* in half of such patients with positive serology. New techniques for the diagnosis of Chagas' disease include the detection of *T. cruzi* by DNA amplification, using the polymerase chain reaction, and competitive antibody enzyme immunoassay, using *T. cruzi* species-specific monoclonal antibody.

During the acute stage of the infection, the differential diagnosis includes typhoid fever, kala-azar, brucellosis, infectious mononucleosis, malaria, and glomerulonephritis.

• TREATMENT AND CLINICAL COURSE •

Only two drugs have shown activity in suppressing parasitemia and clinical manifestations in the acute stage. These are nifurtimox, which is available in the U.S. from the Centers for Disease Control and Prevention (CDCP), and benznidazole. Therapeutic response seems to depend on the geographic location, particularly in regard to the sensitivity of the *T. cruzi* strain. There is no evidence that chronic disease can be reversed by these drugs.

Nifurtimox is given orally in doses of 8 to 10 mg/kg/day to adults and 15 mg/kg/day to children, in 4 doses daily for 60 to 120 days. The recommended oral dosage of benznidazole is 5 mg/kg/day for 60 days in adults and 10 mg/kg/day in children. A favorable response to treatment is indicated by the remission of signs and symptoms and the elimination of parasitemia. Allopurinol has recently proved useful for the treatment of chronic Chagas' disease in oral dosages of 600 to 900 mg daily for 60 days.

AFRICAN TRYPANOSOMIASIS

African trypanosomiasis (sleeping sickness) is seen only in equatorial Africa. It usually shows a raised, red, tender lesion at the site of the tsetse fly bite and often an erythematous, urticarial, or hemorrhagic eruption during the acute phase of the illness. It will not be discussed further in this text.

CUTANEOUS LEISHMANIASIS

Cutaneous leishmaniasis is endemic in Central and South America, Southern Europe, Asia, and Africa. According to the World Health Organization, there are 400,000 new cases of cutaneous leishmaniasis each year and an estimated prevalence of 12 million cases. It is caused by a hemoflagellate protozoan of the genus *Leishmania* and is transmitted by phlebotomine sandflies (Fig. 18.4). The principal reservoirs are sloths, rodents, and anteaters. Domestic animals are secondary hosts, and humans are incidental hosts.

Cutaneous leishmaniasis is commonly divided into Old World and New World forms, produced by different leishmania organisms (Table 18.1) and with different sandfly vectors. New World disease differs in that mucosal lesions are much more common—some organisms produce lesions in 40% of patients—whereas these lesions are uncommon in Old World disease. Strictly cutaneous forms are clinically similar in both parts of the world. Visceral leishmaniasis (kala-azar) has no skin lesions and will not be considered in this discussion, although post-kala-azar dermal lesions may occur in 5% of patients in East Africa and 20% of those in India.

Table 18.1 Geographic Specificity and Clinical Manifestations of *Leishmania* Species[a]

Species	Geographic Location	Clinical Manifestation
Leishmania major	Northern and Western Africa, Iran, Iraq, India, southern former USSR	OWCL
Leishmania tropica	Mediterranean, India, Afghanistan	OWCL, kala-azar
Leishmania aethiopica	Ethiopia, Kenya	OWCL, DCL, MCL
Leishmania donovani	India, China, East Africa	kala-azar
Leishmania donovani Infantum	India, China, Mediterranean, Southern Europe, Sudan, Sub-Saharan Africa	kala-azar, MCL
Leishmania donovani chagasi	Central and South America	kala-azar
Leishmania mexicana amazonensis	Central and South America	NWCL, DCL, kala-azar
Leishmania mexicana mexicana	Mexico, Central America	NWCL
Leishmania mexicana pifanoi	Venezuela	DCL, MCL
Leishmania mexicana garnhami	Venezuela	NWCL
Leishmania braziliensis braziliensis	South America	NWCL, MCL
Leishmania braziliensis panamensis	Central America, Columbia	NWCL, MCL

[a]OWCL: Old World cutaneous leishmaniasis; NWCL: New World cutaneous leishmaniasis; MCL: Mucocutaneous leishmaniasis; DCL: Diffuse cutaneous leishmaniasis.

• PATHOGENESIS •

There are four major clinicopathological entities of leishmaniasis: cutaneous leishmaniasis, mucocutaneous leishmaniasis, disseminated anergic cutaneous leishmaniasis, and visceral leishmaniasis.

The basic histopathological features of cutaneous leishmaniasis (tropical sore) are the presence of intracellular organisms or amastigotes within macrophages and histiocytes with an associated infiltrate of lymphocytes, monocytes, and plasma cells. In mucocutaneous leishmaniasis, the histopathological findings are similar, but the number of amastigotes is more scarce, especially in older lesions. In contrast, disseminated anergic cutaneous leishmaniasis shows a large number of parasites in foamy macrophages and a minimal infiltrate of lymphocytes and plasma cells. In visceral leishmaniasis, parasites infect cells of the reticuloendothelial system of virtually any organ, especially spleen, liver, and bone marrow.

• CLINICAL FEATURES •

Manifestations of cutaneous leishmaniasis range from small, dry, crusted lesions to large, deep, ulcerative lesions. Lesions may be single or multiple on the exposed areas of the body. The initial lesion, an erythematous papule (Fig. 18.5), appears 2 to 8 weeks after the sandfly bite and progresses to ulceration and crusting. The typical leishmania ulcer is round with raised borders and a granulating base (Figs. 18.6–18.9). Regional adenitis is common, and, occasionally, a chain of multiple nodules develops along the lymphatic vessels and mimics sporotrichosis (Fig. 18.10). The ulcer may resolve spontaneously within 3 to 6 months or may persist for several months. After therapy with pentavalent antimony, the ulcers heal in a period of 4 to 6 weeks, leaving a depressed and hyperpigmented scar.

Relapsing chronic cutaneous leishmaniasis, or leishmaniasis recidivans, is characterized by partial healing of the ulcer with persistent activity along the edges (Fig. 18.11) or by the presence of satellite lesions surrounding the scar of the initial ulceration.

Reinfection is marked by the appearance of a new lesion in a different area of the body in an immunocompetent host. It could be due to exogenous reinfection or reactivation of a latent infection.

Diffuse or disseminated cutaneous leishmaniasis, which is rare, is characterized by nodular rather than ulcerative lesions affecting multiple areas of the body (Figs. 18.12, 18.13). There is loss of skin reactivity to leishmanin but to no other antigens, and there is poor or absent response to antileishmanial drugs.

In mucocutaneous leishmaniasis, the oronasopharyngeal mucosa may be affected by contiguous or lymphatic spread of the parasites when the face is infected (Fig. 18.14) or by hematogenous dissemination when other sites are infected. The mucosal involvement usually appears months or years after primary infection and is considered a late manifestation of a latent infection.

The lesion in the nose may begin as a diffuse erythema, small ulceration, or nodule located on the nasal septum or the inferior turbinate. The most common symptoms are epistaxis, nasal obstruction, rhinorrhea, and itching. The infection may progress to produce turbinate atrophy, perforation of the nasal septum, and, later, destruction of the nasal bridge, which may give rise to the so-called tapir nose deformity (Fig. 18.15). The oral mucosa may also be involved (Fig. 18.16), and the lip and palatal lesions may extend to the pharynx and trachea, causing dysphagia and dysphonia. Spontaneous healing of mucosal leishmaniasis has not been reported.

• DIAGNOSIS AND DIFFERENTIAL DIAGNOSIS •

Leishmaniasis should be considered in the differential diagnosis of chronic ulcerative lesions of the skin or the nasooropharyngeal mucosa of patients who reside in or have traveled to an endemic area. The most important direct means of diagnosis is the identification of amastigotes in Giemsa-stained smears, the isolation of the parasite by culture procedures (diphasic NNN medium, Schneider's medium), or inoculation of the organism in hamsters. Scrapings, aspirates, or punch biopsy specimens should be taken from the edge of the ulcer. Speciation of the isolates by isoenzyme electrophoresis or by DNA probes is very useful because of the marked differences in clinical course and therapeutic response.

Leishmaniasis cannot be reliably diagnosed by serological tests alone. In mucosal leishmaniasis, the yield of positive smears and cultures is very low but may be increased by hamster inoculation. In the absence of a positive smear or culture, the diagnosis of mucocutaneous leishmaniasis is based on the characteristic mucosal involvement, the presence of a scar suggestive of previous cutaneous leishmaniasis, a strong skin test to the leishmanin antigen (more than 5 mm induration), positive serology, and a negative biopsy for other pathological conditions.

The differential diagnosis of cutaneous leishmaniasis includes mycobacterial infections, leprosy, blastomycosis, paracoccidioidomycosis, sporotrichosis, lupus vulgaris, simple tropical ulcer, and rhinosporidiosis.

• TREATMENT AND CLINICAL COURSE •

Treatment of cutaneous leishmaniasis varies tremendously due to the difference in species' response to chemotherapy. For example, the Oriental sore due to *Leishmania major* and the chiclero's ulcer due to *L. mexicana* heal spontaneously in 90% of cases. Treatment, therefore, is unnecessary except to prevent or limit scar formation from facial lesions. In infections caused by species capable of producing mucocutaneous complications, such as *L. braziliensis* var. *braziliensis* and *L. braziliensis* var. *panamensis*, systemic therapy with pentavalent antimony is recommended (Figs. 18.17, 18.18). These drugs, sodium antimony gluconate and antimony *N*-methylglucamine, are the treatment of choice for all of the leishmaniases, and may be given IM or IV. The CDCP recommends 20 mg/kg/day given subcutaneously for 20 days in cutaneous disease and a minimum of 28 days in mucocutaneous disease. In Old World cutaneous leishmaniasis, intralesional injection with sodium antimony gluconate may produce good results. Paromomycin-based ointments topically applied for 10 to 30 days have successfully cured patients infected with *L. major, L. tropica*, and *L. aethiopica.*

Treatment alternatives to these antimonial drugs, such as pentamidine or amphotericin B, are far from ideal. Ketoconazole, however, appears promising against *L. brasiliensis* var. *panamensis* with a cure rate of 70%, a rate similar to that obtained with pentavalent antimony. However, these results cannot be extrapolated to cutaneous leishmaniasis caused by other species or strains of *Leishmania.*

Chemotherapy for diffuse cutaneous leishmaniasis is generally disappointing, and multiple relapses are common. Local heat treatment may be effective in some of these patients.

MALARIA

About 270 million people worldwide are infected with the causative organisms, sporozoa of the genus *Plasmodium*. The majority of the 2 million deaths per year are of children aged 1 to 5 years in hyperendemic areas. Older children acquire partial immunity, but later immunity may lapse with pregnancy or immunosuppression. Approximately 1100 cases per year, virtually all imported, occur in the United States.

Four species of *Plasmodium* are pathogenic to humans: *P. falciparum, P. vivax, P. malariae,* and *P. ovale.* Of these species, two—*P. vivax* and *P. ovale*—can produce long-term or delayed relapses. In the United States and Europe, malaria is seen predominantly in immigrants, in persons with congenital disease or blood transfusion-associated disease, and in airport personnel infected by stowaway mosquitoes. Small epidemics have occurred in the United States through mosquito transmission. Certain genetic factors appear protective against infection.

• PATHOGENESIS •

The obligate intracellular parasite is transmitted to humans via bites of infected female *Anopheles* mosquitoes. Sporozoites from the mosquito's salivary glands enter subcutaneous capillaries, migrate to the liver, and invade parenchymal cells. They eventually evolve into numerous merozoites that invade erythrocytes, producing systemic clinical findings. The life cycle of the organism continues through bites of infected persons by other mosquitoes.

• CLINICAL FEATURES •

The hallmark of acute malaria is the triad of high fever, chills, and rigor. Hepatosplenomegaly and jaundice are rare in children but common in adults, and patients are often diagnosed as having hepatitis. Anemia is commonly present.

Cutaneous manifestations are uncommon and lymphadenopathy is absent. *Plasmodium falciparum* cases have as much as a 4% incidence of urticaria that responds rapidly to antimalarials. Rarely, petechiae or purpura are present. An occasional patient with severe *P. falciparum* malaria may present with purpura fulminans and spontaneous bleeding of the gums.

Peripheral vasculitis with gangrene has also been described in children with chronic malaria.

• DIAGNOSIS AND DIFFERENTIAL DIAGNOSIS •

Diagnosis can be confirmed when parasites are demonstrated in peripheral blood smears. Because the density is highly variable, smears should be obtained every 6 to 8 hours for several days. The differential diagnosis is broad. Patients with early *P. falciparum* are most commonly misdiagnosed as having influenza or hepatitis. Also in the differential are meningitis, enteric fever, septicemia, leptospirosis, hemorrhagic fever, and relapsing fever. A travel history is very important.

• TREATMENT AND CLINICAL COURSE •

Treatment, empiric if necessary, must be started immediately, if *P. falciparum* is suspected. In severe illness, quinine may be given first, since all chloroquine-resistant strains currently respond to it, at least initially. All other types respond readily to chloroquine. Newer antimalarials include mefloquine and halofantrine.

TOXOPLASMOSIS

Toxoplasmosis is caused by *Toxoplasma gondii*, an obligate intracellular protozoan that is ubiquitous in nature. Cats are the definitive hosts, producing the transmissible oocyst. In the United States, 20% to 70% of healthy adults are seropositive. The major modes of transmission are ingestion and congenital. Transmission to the fetus occurs if the mother becomes infected during pregnancy.

• PATHOGENESIS •

Toxoplasma may be found in three forms: tachyzoites, tissue cysts, and oocysts. Tachyzoites are the actively invasive form—they can invade every mammalian cell except erythrocytes and tend to disseminate via the bloodstream and lymphatics. The tachyzoite multiplies in the host cell until either a cyst is formed or the host cell lyses. The proliferative tachyzoites tend to produce foci of necrosis with surrounding inflammation. Tissue destruction ceases with development of humoral and cellular immunity, but since antibodies cannot penetrate the eye and central nervous system, the organisms multiply unchecked, causing wide destruction.

After superficial lymphatics, the skin is the most frequent initial target organ; organisms have been found in clinically normal skin of asymptomatic individuals. Within a week of infection, tissue cysts can be found in any organ, especially the brain, heart, and skeletal muscle. Cysts vary in size, containing up to 3000 organisms that remain viable for years and are sources of chronic infection. These cysts elicit little inflammatory response but can lead to reactivated acute disease, especially with immunosuppression.

Tissue cysts are a common source of infection through the ingestion of raw or undercooked meat. Gastric enzymes release viable organisms, which invade gastrointestinal mucosa and disseminate. Freezing and thawing, heating above 60° C, and desiccation all destroy tissue cysts. Oocysts, an essential part of the organism's life cycle formed in cat intestines and shed in their feces, can also be ingested in contaminated foods and water.

Host response depends on the organ involved and the stage of the organism. Toxoplasmic lymphadenitis tends to exhibit a distinctive reactive pattern without granulomas, abscesses, or necrosis. Within the central nervous system, in contrast, widespread vasculitis and necrosis follow the invasion of vessel walls by tachyzoites, and necrotic abscesses may coalesce or calcify. Chorioretinitis is characterized by granulomatous inflammation and neovascularization of the vitreous, sometimes revealing tachyzoites and cysts in the retina. Skeletal muscle may exhibit little inflammation or widespread myositis.

• CLINICAL FEATURES •

Clinical manifestations can generally be divided into four categories: acquired infection in immunocompetent hosts, acute disease in immunocompromised hosts, ocular disease, and congenital infection. The clinical presentations tend to be nonspecific.

Only 10% to 20% of infections in immunocompetent adults are symptomatic; cervical lymphadenopathy is usually the only expression of disease. Younger patients tend to have more clinical symptoms—usually, a mononucleosis-like syndrome that may uncommonly include a maculopapular rash. This eruption is usually diffuse, initially involving palmar and plantar surfaces and spreading centripetally with an erythematous to cyanotic color and, usually, sparing of mucous membranes. Rarely, some cases have lichenoid, purpuric/telangiectatic, vesiculobullous, or urticarial eruptions. Elderly patients may have peculiar chronic lesions that are nodular and which may ulcerate or suppurate. Biopsies in these cases reveal a mixed dermal infiltrate with large foci of necrosis and trophozoites free in the dermis or in macrophages.

Of special interest are cases of toxoplasmosis mimicking dermatomyositis. Earlier reports of high *Toxoplasma* serologies in patients with dermatomyositis had been attributed to coincidental disease, given the high prevalence of toxoplasma infection. However, an occasional case with clinical signs of dermatomyositis may completely resolve with treatment for toxoplasmosis; muscle biopsies should be performed to demonstrate tachyzoites in suspected cases.

Patients with AIDS or those on immunosuppressive drugs are at risk for severe and often fatal toxoplasmosis with encephalitis, either as a newly acquired infection or as recrudescent disease. Cutaneous manifestations can include a diffuse erythematous maculopapular eruption, sometimes with neutrophilic infiltrates or subcutaneous purpuric nodules.

Congenital disease follows an acute, usually asymptomatic, infection acquired by the mother during gestation. Clinical manifestations can be severe and progressive. More than 90% of infected infants eventually develop some sequelae. Cutaneous eruptions are described as papular/hemorrhagic, nodular, bullous, necrotic, erythrodermic, or with calcinosis.

• DIAGNOSIS AND DIFFERENTIAL DIAGNOSIS •

Acute infection may be diagnosed by isolation of the organism from blood or body fluids, demonstration of tachyzoites on histological sections, characteristic lymph node histology, demonstration of tissue cysts in the placenta, fetus, or neonate, or serological tests. Serological tests for antibodies are most commonly utilized in diagnosis. Limitations include the high prevalence of antibodies in most populations, the persistence of high titers, and the finding of low titers in patients who are immunosuppressed or have ocular disease. Since maternal IgG is transferred to the fetus, either a rising IgG titer or a positive specific IgM titer is considered diagnostic in neonates.

In the usual presentations of toxoplasmosis, the broad differential diagnosis includes mononucleosis, cytomegalovirus infection, lymphoma, sarcoidosis, cat-scratch disease, tuberculosis, tularemia, and metastatic carcinoma. The differential diagnosis in congenital infection includes the other members of the TORCH syndrome (rubella, CMV, HSV), as well as syphilis, erythroblastosis fetalis, and sepsis.

• TREATMENT AND CLINICAL COURSE •

Pyrimethamine and sulfadiazine are active against tachyzoites and are synergistic. Tissue cysts are resistant to all available agents. Immunocompetent adults are only treated if there is visceral disease such as ocular involvement, but immunosuppressed hosts are treated for 4 to 6 weeks after all symptoms have resolved. Treatment of pregnant women reduces but does not eliminate fetal infection. Treatment of neonates is believed to prevent some later sequelae. Please see chapter 21 for the treatment of toxoplasmosis in AIDS patients.

Crucial in the containment of disease are preventive measures, including proper cooking and storage of meats, avoidance of unpasteurized milk, and careful handling of cat feces in litter boxes and sandboxes.

AMEBIASIS

Entamoeba histolytica, the causative organism, infects about 10% of the world's population, and over 50% in some locales. Amebiasis causes considerable morbidity, although fewer than 10% of infected persons have invasive disease. Behind malaria and schistosomiasis, amebiasis is the third most common fatal parasitic disease.

Rates of infection are highest in areas of crowding and poor sanitation. In the United States, the overall prevalence is about 4%, but certain groups of immigrants are commonly infected, and institutionalized mentally retarded patients have high rates of colonization and invasive disease. Invasive disease is seen more in patients who are immunosuppressed, malnourished, or have hemochromatosis.

• PATHOGENESIS •

Entamoeba has a relatively simple lifestyle involving encystment of a trophozoite within the bowel and maturation within the lumen or in other moist surroundings. Trophozoites are relatively fragile, but cysts are resistant to gastric acid and survive for months in a moist environment. Trophozoites invade the intestinal wall and can also destroy leukocytes. Inflammatory cells, therefore, are found only at the periphery of the granular, eosinophilic material that surrounds trophozoites. Cell-mediated rather than humoral immunity protects against invasive disease.

• CLINICAL FEATURES •

Most infected individuals have asymptomatic luminal infection only. Gastrointestinal symptoms can range from diarrhea to fulminant colitis, the latter seen mostly in children. Liver disease may develop days to years after the onset of dysentery, but over 60% of patients with hepatic abscess have no prior symptoms of intestinal disease.

Cutaneous disease is uncommon, the most common form being disease secondary to direct inoculation, especially the extension of the abdominal wall or perineal abscesses to the skin. These are usually serpiginous ulcers with red/violet, heaped-up, sometimes verrucous borders, and a purulent base. Extreme pain and a rapid increase in size are characteristic. Penile lesions occur secondary to genital-rectal contact.

• DIAGNOSIS AND DIFFERENTIAL DIAGNOSIS •

The diagnosis is usually made by identifying trophozoites or cysts in the stool. Intestinal scrapings or biopsy may be helpful. Skin biopsies of primary inoculation lesions show ulceration or acanthosis with an infiltrate of lymphocytes, plasma cells, eosinophils, and trophozoites with the typical central karyosome in an eccentric nucleus.

The gastrointestinal differential diagnosis includes *Shigella, Salmonella, Campylobacter, Vibrio* or *Yersinia*, invasive *Escherichia coli*, carcinoma, and inflammatory bowel disease. For cutaneous lesions, the differential includes pyoderma gangrenosum, cutaneous Crohn's disease, carcinoma, syphilis, granuloma inguinale, lymphogranuloma venereum, tuberculosis, deep fungal infections, and leishmaniasis.

• TREATMENT AND CLINICAL COURSE •

Asymptomatic carriers may be treated with tetracycline or the luminal agents, diloxanide and iodoquinol. Metronidazole is the treatment of choice for colitis or liver abscess. Emetine may be added.

Prevention of disease can be accomplished by eradicating fecal contamination of food and water.

Helminth Infections

Helminths, or worms, are macroparasites with highly variable biology found worldwide. They are divided into three major groups: the two groups of flatworms—trematodes (flukes) and cestodes (tapeworms)—and the roundworms (nematodes). Only those helminths producing skin lesions will be covered in this text.

INTESTINAL NEMATODES

Infections with intestinal nematodes are the most common types of human parasitic disease. Those that cause skin lesions include hookworm infections and strongyloidiasis.

Hookworm Disease

Two species of hookworms, *Ancylostoma duodenale* and *Necator americanus*, affect an estimated quarter of the world's population. Infections occur primarily in tropical and subtropical climates, and in the southeastern United States. The spread of hookworms is controlled by proper disposal of fecal waste and avoidance of walking barefoot over contaminated soil.

• PATHOGENESIS •

Adult worms live in the jejunum, attached to the mucosa and feeding on villi. The eggs are excreted in feces and develop into infective larvae in shaded, moist soil. About 5 to 10 minutes' contact with contaminated soil is required for skin penetration, often through follicles. Larvae then migrate in 1 to 2 days via the blood stream to the lungs, pass up the bronchial tree, are swallowed, and reach the duodenal and jejunal mucosa where they mature to complete the life cycle.

Most of the clinical effects can be explained by the parasites' feeding habits. Hookworms feed on intestinal villi and actively suck blood from the gut wall. They also secrete an anticoagulant, which is responsible for continued blood loss after the parasite has moved on.

• CLINICAL FEATURES •

At the time of cutaneous penetration a pruritic, erythematous, vesicular rash ("ground itch") occurs, most commonly on the feet and lasting 7 to 10 days. The larvae leave the subcutaneous tissue rapidly, and serpentine rashes are rarely seen. Dyspnea, wheezing, and cough can occur when larvae pass through the lungs. The major clinical manifestations are anemia and hypoalbuminemia secondary to intestinal blood loss. Pallor, koilonychia, angular stomatitis, and cheilosis are cutaneous findings associated with toxemia. Patients commonly have a kwashiorkor-like hypopigmentation of the face, extremities, and perineum that may persist.

• DIAGNOSIS AND DIFFERENTIAL DIAGNOSIS •

Direct smear of feces reveals eggs. The differential includes infection with *Strongyloides, Trichostrongylus*, and *Rhabditis*.

• TREATMENT AND CLINICAL COURSE •

Mebendazole or pyrantel palliate are effective. Patients respond readily to antihelminthic agents but reinfection is common.

Strongyloidiasis

Strongyloidiasis due to the roundworm *Strongyloides stercoralis* is widespread in the tropics. In the United States, the prevalence is 0.4% to 4% in Southern states but 1.8% to 7.4% in institutions.

• PATHOGENESIS •

The worms can live and reproduce as parasites within the intestines or as free-living organisms in the soil. Especially if constipation and other factors prolong the passage of noninfectious larvae through feces, the larvae may transform into infective filariform larvae, which penetrate the colon or perianal tissue to initiate "autoinfection." Larvae that have been excreted into the soil can penetrate human skin through abrasions or follicles, rapidly entering the circulation to be carried ultimately to the small intestine.

• CLINICAL FEATURES •

Up to half of infected humans are asymptomatic. Early stages of the disease may present with an acute papulovesicular eruption and/or Loeffler-like pneumonitis very similar to hookworm disease. More characteristic are the gastrointestinal symptoms of chronic disease.

Most patients with chronic disease have cutaneous manifestations that are, most commonly, recurrent maculopapular or urticarial eruptions. Some patients, especially in Southeast Asia, have larva currens or "racing larva," a peculiar form of cutaneous larva migrans (CLM), discussed in a later section in this chapter. In contrast to the slow rate of typical CLM, *Strongyloides* larvae migrate at rates of several centimeters per hour. The rash most frequently appears over the buttocks, perineum, and thighs, secondary to cutaneous penetration by larvae from the patient's own feces. Attacks of larva currens generally last a few hours, and patients often can remain asymptomatic for weeks or months between attacks.

Strongyloides "hyperinfection" refers to a massive increase in parasite load with invasion of lungs and other tissues seen in immunocompromised hosts, especially patients on corticosteroids. Patients present with severe generalized abdominal pain, diffuse pulmonary infiltrates, ileus, and, sometimes, secondary Gram-negative sepsis. Some have a peculiar cutaneous syndrome of periumbilical purpura, with purpura sometimes appearing elsewhere on the body. Mortality from hyperinfection is high in patients with periumbilical purpura.

• DIAGNOSIS AND DIFFERENTIAL DIAGNOSIS •

In the usual patient, feces or abdominal fluid are examined for larvae; eggs are virtually never seen. A jejunal swab or biopsy specimen via endoscopy or the "string test" may be necessary to detect the parasite. ELISA (enzyme-linked immunoadsorbent assay) has a sensitivity of over 80% but is not widely available.

The differential diagnosis includes infections with hookworms, *Ascaris*, and other intestinal parasites. Cutaneous larva migrans can usually be distinguished from hookworm varieties by the speed of migration.

• TREATMENT AND CLINICAL COURSE •

Thiabendazole or ivermectin is given for 3 days or for 1 week in cases of hyperinfection. All patients suspected of hyperinfection require Gram-negative coverage because of mucosal disruption. Patients with a history of strongyloidiasis should be examined carefully before immunosuppressive or corticosteroid therapy is instituted.

TISSUE NEMATODES

These diseases, affecting millions of people worldwide, are predominantly seen in the tropics, but some, such as trichinosis, are prevalent in temperate climates. Those causing skin lesions include filariasis, loiasis, onchocerciasis, and trichinosis.

Trichinosis

Trichinosis follows ingestion of undercooked meat, usually pork, that is contaminated with *Trichinella spiralis*. The parasite is found throughout most of the world in numerous carnivores; humans are incidental hosts. Currently, most United States swine are grain-fed and uninfected; only swine feeding on meat scraps or animal carcasses acquire infection. Fewer than 100 cases are reported per year now in the United States, mostly within ethnic groups who eat raw pork. Infections may be asymptomatic but a heavy parasite load can be associated with significant symptoms and even death.

• PATHOGENESIS •

Larvae enter the gastrointestinal tract through undercooked meat, develop into adult worms in the small intestine, and produce hundreds of larvae. Larvae migrate to skeletal muscle, where they burrow into muscle fibers, "encysting" and maturing. A lymphocytic and eosinophilic infiltrate occurs and leads to myositis, transient myocarditis, and possible brain or other organ damage from larva migration.

• CLINICAL FEATURES •

Infections tend to be subclinical except with a heavy parasitic load. Symptoms, which usually begin in the 2nd week after larvae have begun to migrate, include fever, marked eosinophilia, headache, dyspnea, cough, hoarseness, myositis, and dysphagia. Periorbital edema, subconjunctival hemorrhage, and subungual petechiae can also be seen. Up to 10% of patients exhibit a transient maculopapular or petechial eruption. Symptoms peak at 2 to 3 weeks, then gradually subside.

• DIAGNOSIS AND DIFFERENTIAL DIAGNOSIS •

The diagnosis should be considered in a patient with fever, eosinophilia, periorbital edema, and myositis. Muscle biopsy may demonstrate larvae. Antibodies only appear 3 weeks after infection. The differential diagnosis includes influenza, dermatomyositis, sinusitis, glomerulonephritis, angioedema, and typhoid. The eruption may resemble scarlet fever, measles, or typhus.

• TREATMENT AND CLINICAL COURSE •

The antihelminthic drugs have little effect on muscle larvae but corticosteroids may help patients with severe allergic symptoms. The average clinical course is one of chronic asymptomatic disease; rarely do inflammatory effects lead to morbidity or death. Proper cooking of pork and other meat is preventive.

Dracunculiasis

Dracunculiasis, or guinea worm disease, develops after drinking water containing copepods infected with *Dracunculus medinensis*. The disease affects about 50 million people in the tropics, especially Africa and India where people bathe and wade in water also used for drinking.

• PATHOGENESIS •

When water containing infected copepods (water fleas) is ingested, larvae are released into the intestine, ultimately migrating to the retroperitoneum where they mature and mate. The gravid female migrates to subcutaneous tissue about 1 year later. The overlying skin ulcerates with a portion of the worm visible. On contact with water, larvae are released and are ingested by copepods.

• CLINICAL FEATURES •

Patients are asymptomatic until the worm migrates downward to reach the skin surface, usually on the lower extremity, at which time a stinging papule develops. Some individuals experience urticaria, diarrhea, and fever. The lesion vesiculates, then ulcerates. Discharge of larvae-containing milky fluid from the female worm occurs intermittently on contact with water until the worm is absorbed or extruded (Fig. 18.19). Secondary bacterial infections and resulting disability are common.

• DIAGNOSIS AND TREATMENT •

The clinical findings are diagnostic. Antihelminthic agents do not affect the worm but do decrease inflammation to permit easy removal of the worm by gradually rolling it onto a small stick (Fig. 18.20). (This is the origin of the medical symbol, the caduceus.) Surgical resection may increase allergic responses. The infection is prevented when drinking water is treated by boiling or chlorination.

Filariasis

The filariases are a group of diseases involving nematodes that live in the host as adult pairs, mating and shedding microfilaria. Humans are infected through various arthropod vectors, which ingest larvae and transmit them through biting.

Bancroftian and brugian filariasis are clinically similar conditions caused by *Wuchereria bancrofti*, *Brugia malayi* (Malayan filariasis), and *Brugia timori* through mosquito vectors. Over 90 million individuals worldwide are infected with these organisms, with 90% being infected by *Wuchereria bancrofti*, which is endemic in the tropics and subtropics but not seen natively in the United States since the 1930s. Symptomatic disease often requires repeated exposure to the organism, sometimes by many thousands of bites.

• PATHOGENESIS •

Infective larvae migrate to lymphatics where they mature into adult worms that can cause lymphatic obstruction. Once in the humans, they can reproduce for many years.

• CLINICAL FEATURES •

Many infected persons have few or no symptoms despite having microfilaremia. Symptoms can include scrotal enlargement (Fig. 18.21), recurrent orchitis and epididymitis, chronic unilateral hydrocele, and lymphedema with elephantiasis of the extremities (Fig. 18.22). In elephantiasis, the longstanding edema is followed by lichenified, often warty thickening of the skin commonly accompanied by ulceration and secondary infection.

• DIAGNOSIS AND DIFFERENTIAL DIAGNOSIS •

The diagnosis is generally based on clinical and travel history, identification of microfilariae in the blood, especially at night (Fig. 18.23), or by lymph node biopsy. Serological tests cannot distinguish different types of filariasis. The differential diagnosis includes loiasis, onchocerciasis, and elephantiasis nostras verrucosum.

• TREATMENT AND CLINICAL COURSE •

Preventive measures involving control of mosquitoes are very important because treatment is not satisfactory. Diethylcarbamazine citrate (DEC) may reduce microfilaremia but has dubious effects on adult worms. Ivermectin has also been shown to clear microfilaremia. Death of microfilaria may be associated with systemic symptoms, such as fever, arthralgias, and hypotension.

Loiasis

Loiasis is caused by the nematode *Loa loa*, which is transmitted to humans by tabanid (horse) flies of the genus *Chrysops*. The disease is limited to the rain forests of western and central Africa.

• PATHOGENESIS •

Long threadlike adult worms wander through the deep connective tissue causing surrounding inflammation and edema and subsequently giving rise to microfilariae in the blood.

• CLINICAL FEATURES •

Most native patients are asymptomatic except for occasional migrating subconjunctival worms producing transient conjunctivitis. Nonnatives more commonly exhibit the characteristic "Calabar" swellings, which are transient areas of localized, painless subcutaneous edema that are often preceded by itching. They are mostly seen on the arms or hands, near the eyes, or over joints, and tend to persist for several days. Nonnatives may have frequent, profound angioedema, urticaria, myalgias, arthralgias, and peripheral eosinophilia.

• DIAGNOSIS AND DIFFERENTIAL DIAGNOSIS •

The diagnosis is made based on clinical and residential history and identification of microfilaria in a daytime blood sample. The swellings of loiasis are typically seen near the orbit or on the hands and forearms in contrast to the truncal nodules of onchocerciasis. The differential diagnosis includes onchocerciasis and nonparasitic urticaria and angioedema.

• TREATMENT AND CLINICAL COURSE •

Diethylcarbamazine kills microfilariae and probably adult worms as well, but treatment may be followed by encephalitis, arthritis, retinitis, and other signs of an inflammatory response. Steroids may need to be administered concomitantly with diethylcarbamazine. The clinical course is usually benign, but, occasionally, patients develop renal disease.

Onchocerciasis

Onchocerciasis is caused by *Onchocerca volvulus*, a nematode transmitted by the blackfly, *Simulium*, mostly in Africa and Central America. The disease takes the form of ocular disease and/or dermatitis, partly depending on the strain of parasite and the locale. About 40 million people worldwide are infected, many of them blinded from the disease. No animal reservoir has been identified, although other *Onchocerca* species are seen in cattle.

• PATHOGENESIS •

After transmission by blackfly bites, larvae penetrate the skin and travel widely through connective tissue, eventually developing into adult worms that are often found, even years later, within nodules of fibrous tissue. The severity of the disease correlates with heavy parasitic loads and repeated infections.

• CLINICAL FEATURES •

Granulomatous inflammation and fibrosis eventually surround adult worms in tissue or nodules to produce the firm, mobile, subcutaneous nodules seen in most patients, usually corresponding to bite sites (Fig. 18.24). Pruritus is the earliest and, sometimes, the only sign of disease. Transiently there may be a papular eruption (Fig. 18.25) with pigmentary alteration in the same regions; these papules contain degenerated microfilariae with eosinophils, microabscesses, and occasional transepidermal elimination. The legs especially tend to develop mottled depigmentation. Lichenification and atrophy are late cutaneous changes. About a third of patients in Africa develop severe lymphedema with secondary leathery elephantiasis of the groin.

• DIAGNOSIS AND DIFFERENTIAL DIAGNOSIS •

The diagnosis is usually made with skin snips of the scapular or gluteal skin. When the snips are placed in saline or tissue cul-

ture media, microfilariae can be seen in the fluid within hours (Fig. 18.26). Biopsy of a nodule demonstrates adult worms, but biopsies of dermatitis exhibit few organisms. A positive Mazzotti test is considered diagnostic (Fig. 18.27); the test involves the acute exacerbation of skin disease after a trial of diethylcarbamazine (DEC). Slit chamber examination of the anterior chamber of the eye may reveal microfilariae. The differential diagnosis includes filariasis and loiasis.

• TREATMENT AND CLINICAL COURSE •

DEC and suramin are standard, although risky, treatments. DEC kills microfilariae and suramin kills some adult worms. For skin disease, they can be administered together; for ocular disease, DEC is given first, then suramin. Ivermectin has recently proved very helpful, significantly reducing microfilarial counts and rendering patients less infective to vectors for 6 months. Nodulectomy may be helpful.

ABERRANT NEMATODE INFECTIONS

A variety of nematodes may accidentally infect humans but are unable to mature and complete their life cycles because their definitive hosts are other animals. These parasites, therefore, do not persist indefinitely in the human host but do provoke inflammatory responses of varying severity. Cutaneous and visceral larva migrans are the most notable of these conditions.

Cutaneous Larva Migrans

Cutaneous larva migrans (CLM), or creeping eruption, is a syndrome of migratory, serpiginous, pruritic skin lesions caused by various larvae in patients in tropical and subtropical climates. In the United States, it is usually seen in the southeast, particularly the Gulf Coast. It is also common in the Caribbean, South America, Africa, and the Orient.

The most common agent of CLM is *Ancylostoma braziliense* (dog and cat hookworm), but other nematodes include: *A. caninum* (dog hookworm), *Uncinaria stenocephala* (dog hookworm), *Bunostomum phlebotomum* (cow hookworm), *Gnathostoma spinigerum, G. hispidium*. The human pathogens *Ancylostoma duodenale, Necator americanus*, and *Strongyloides stercoralis* have also been included, but they are usually distinguishable because *Ancylostoma duodenale* and *Necator americanus* migrate through the skin only briefly before entering the circulation and do not tend to form serpiginous patterns. *Strongyloides stercoralis*, as discussed earlier in this chapter, migrates very rapidly, producing larva currens. *Strongyloides myopotami* is another agent that occurs in Louisiana bayous, is intermediate in the speed of its migration pattern, and produces an eruption known as "nutria itch" (Fig. 18.28).

• PATHOGENESIS •

Most cases of CLM are acquired through prolonged contact with contaminated soil. Warm, moist soil or sand allows rhabditiform larvae to develop into infectious filariform organisms. In *Ancylostoma braziliense* infections, the larvae burrow through the epidermis (resulting in spongiotic dermatitis) because they lack the ability to penetrate the human basement membrane. *Ancylostoma caninum* can penetrate into the dermis, creating a granulomatous tissue response.

Gnathostomiasis, most common in the Orient and South America, involves a different mechanism. The definitive hosts are dogs, cats, tigers, leopards, and pigs with fresh water fish being the intermediate host. When humans eat raw fish (in "sashimi" or "ceviche"), the parasite migrates from the stomach to the liver and, finally, to the subcutaneous tissue and skeletal muscle where its enzymes can cause destruction.

• CLINICAL FEATURES •

When larvae penetrate the skin, patients may report a tingling sensation. Because the parasites commonly invade the skin via hair follicles, one expression of CLM is "hookworm folliculitis" with numerous larvae coiled in follicles and an occasional granuloma. Larvae migrate within days to weeks, producing an intense pruritus followed by development of bullae along raised, erythematous, serpiginous tracks (Figs. 18.29–18.31), expanding at a rate of about 1 to 2 cm per day. The track may disappear for a few days, reappear, and advance repetitively until it disappears (Figs. 18.32, 18.33). Moderate eosinophilia may be seen.

Gnathostomiasis is characterized by intermittent migratory deep edema. In Ecuador and Southeast Asia, the parasite is responsible for nodular migratory eosinophilic panniculitis, sometimes with vasculitis. *Gnathostoma spinigerum* may persist for years; *G. hispidium* and *G. doloresi* may self-resolve in a few months.

• DIAGNOSIS AND TREATMENT •

The diagnosis is made clinically. Larvae should be present 1 to 2 cm from the proximal advancing edge, but in one survey, only 8 of 300 biopsies demonstrated the parasite (2).

Cutaneous larva migrans with *Ancylostoma braziliense* is best treated with occlusive topical thiabendazole suspension. The human parasites *A. duodenale, Necator americanus,* and *Strongyloides stercoralis* are readily distinguishable clinically, and all require systemic treatment. Gnathostomiasis, involving deeper tissues, does not respond to known antihelminthic drugs. Surgical removal of the worm is the treatment of choice. Albendazole 400 mg b.i.d. for 3 to 7 days has shown promise.

Toxocariasis (Visceral Larva Migrans)

Texocariasis is a syndrome resulting from infection with one of several animal ascarids, usually *Toxocara canis* (dog nematodes), but also *T. cati* (cat) and *T. leonensis* (dog and cat). The disease is seen worldwide in both temperate and tropical climates, especially affecting young children who ingest contaminated soil or water.

• PATHOGENESIS •

After ingestion as eggs, second-stage larvae hatch in the upper small bowel, penetrate the mucosa, and begin somatic migration

mainly to the liver but also to lungs, muscles, kidney, heart, and central nervous system. During migration, the larvae secrete proteolytic enzymes that are also responsible for damage. The host response comprises both immediate and delayed hypersensitivity.

• CLINICAL FEATURES •

Clinical symptoms vary from mild inflammation with peripheral eosinophilia to profound infection with multiorgan involvement and blindness. Nodular skin lesions and urticaria may be seen. Serum gamma globulin is greatly elevated and eosinophilia is usually marked.

• DIAGNOSIS AND DIFFERENTIAL DIAGNOSIS •

The characteristic pathological finding is a granulomatous nodule with numerous eosinophils around a degenerating larva. Stool specimens are not helpful and liver biopsies are rarely diagnostic. ELISA is both sensitive and specific for *T. canis.*

The differential includes schistosomiasis, hookworm and filarial disease, trichinosis, and strongyloidiasis.

• TREATMENT AND CLINICAL COURSE •

Usually the disease is self-limited, subsiding after 1 to 3 months. Antihelminthic drugs are variably successful.

Dirofilariasis

Humans are not the definitive hosts of *Dirofilaria.* Organisms enter accidentally through bites from infected mosquitoes but undergo only partial development. *Dirofilaria immitis* is the dog heartworm parasite, infecting up to 60% of dogs in the United States, *Dirofilaria tenuis* is found in raccoons and opossums, and *D. ursi* in bears.

• PATHOGENESIS AND CLINICAL FEATURES •

In cases of *D. immitis,* the filarial larvae partially mature in subcutaneous tissue, then enter the circulation and subsequently die, embolizing to the lung or subcutaneous tissue and producing granulomatous nodules. Many infected patients are asymptomatic while some have cough or chest pain.

The parasite *D. tenuis* normally resides in the subcutaneous tissue of raccoons. It localizes similarly in humans, resulting in subcutaneous nodules most commonly on the face (especially near the eye), trunk, and arms. In the United States, the majority of cases have been described in Florida.

• DIAGNOSIS AND TREATMENT •

The diagnosis is usually made at the time of surgery, demonstrating the parasite surrounded by granulomatous inflammation. Surgical resection is the treatment of choice for symptomatic disease. Serology is usually not helpful.

TREMATODES

There are two orders of trematodes but only the order Digenea contain parasites of medical importance: blood flukes, intestinal flukes, and tissue flukes. These are diseases of tropical and subtropical climates and are rarely seen in temperate zones except in immigrants and in cases of "swimmer's itch," the accidental infection of humans by schistosomes whose definitive hosts are usually avian. Endemic zones for flukes are geographically limited because specific snails are necessary as intermediate hosts.

SCHISTOSOMIASIS (VISCERAL SCHISTOSOMIASIS)

The three human blood flukes, *Schistosoma mansoni*, *S. japonicum*, and *S. haematobium*, infect more than 200 million people worldwide. In the United States, infection can be seen in immigrants from Puerto Rico, Brazil, the Philippines, and the Middle East. Species are geographically specific.

• PATHOGENESIS •

Humans are the definitive hosts for these species. Adult worms live in the venous system, where they mate. Gravid females attach to the endothelial surface of pelvic veins and release fully embryonated eggs that can penetrate the vessel wall. Depending on the species, some eventually break into gastrointestinal or genitourinary tract lumina and are excreted in urine or feces.

Eggs of *S. haematobium* are passed in urine while the eggs of *S. mansoni* and *S. japonicum* are passed in feces. The excreted eggs hatch in fresh water, where the organism enters its intermediate host, the snail; 4 to 6 weeks later free-swimming cercariae are released, capable of penetrating human skin. Once penetration is achieved, they quickly migrate hematogenously to the liver where they mature, mate, and descend via the venous system to their final habitat to again deposit ova.

• CLINICAL FEATURES •

Disease symptoms correlate with the stage of development of the parasite. A papular rash, similar to, but not as severe as, swimmer's itch occurs with cutaneous penetration and lasts longer in sensitized individuals. Acute schistosomiasis, or Katayama fever, is a serum sickness-like illness that occurs 4 to 6 weeks after penetration, seen most commonly with *S. japonicum* and caused by immune complexes involving ova antigens.

Host response to ova in tissues can be intense, especially with *S. haematobium* in adolescents, producing granulomatous lesions in the genital and perigenital regions. The vulva may develop exuberant granulomas that progress to fibrosis and sometimes pseudoelephantiasis. Other genital and perianal lesions produce warty nodules, or vitiligo-like depigmentation. Periumbilical lesions are common, and involvement of other ectopic sites in the skin or other organs, such as the eye, lung, and central nervous system (CNS) can be seen.

• DIAGNOSIS AND DIFFERENTIAL DIAGNOSIS •

The diagnosis is suspected on the basis of travel history and contact with water, plus a typical eruption or systemic response. Definitive diagnosis is achieved by finding ova in feces or urine or in biopsy specimens within granulomas or abscesses. Eosinophils are also prominent in biopsies. Serology is predominantly useful in cases of CNS or ectopic disease without demonstrable parasites in feces, urine, or biopsy specimens.

The differential diagnosis is broad. Gastrointestinal symptoms simulate a variety of diseases, including dysentery, typhoid, and trichinosis. Cutaneous lesions must be differentiated from various pruritic dermatoses, other parasitic infections, venereal infections, granulomas, and carcinoma.

• TREATMENT AND CLINICAL COURSE •

Praziquantel is a broad-spectrum antihelminthic agent effective against all three species. The clinical course varies from asymptomatic chronic disease to fatal disease resulting from liver or renal failure.

Cercarial Dermatitis (Swimmer's Itch)

"Swimmer's itch" and "clam digger's itch" are pruritic skin diseases caused by cutaneous penetration of schistosomes whose definitive hosts are birds or small mammals. The disease is seen worldwide and can be associated with sea water or fresh water contact, such as lakes or rice paddies. In the United States, humans contract the diseases swimming, wading, or digging for clams, especially in the lakes and coastal areas of the north central and Atlantic seaboard states. These parasites are avian schistosomes, and disease follows the migration patterns of sea birds, such as ducks and geese.

• PATHOGENESIS •

As with other schistosomes, larvae infect mollusks and reproduce to release motile cercariae. On penetrating human skin, the parasites live only a short time, evoking an intense hypersensitivity reaction, which self-resolves.

• CLINICAL FEATURES •

Patients experience pruritus and occasional brief urticaria at penetration. Usually within hours, a pruritic papular eruption appears that may become swollen, or bullous if severe. The reaction peaks at about 72 hours, then gradually resolves. Repeated exposure leads to acceleration and intensification of symptoms.

• DIAGNOSIS AND DIFFERENTIAL DIAGNOSIS •

Diagnosis is made on clinical history. The differential includes chigger and other insect bites, mosquito bites, and "sea bather's eruption" from contact with other marine life and scabies.

• TREATMENT AND CLINICAL COURSE •

Treatment is symptomatic, only requiring antipruritic agents. The condition usually resolves within 10 days.

CESTODES (TAPEWORMS)

Tapeworms, or segmented worms, are noteworthy because of their length (up to 30 feet) and the visible cysts of the larval stage that give meat a "measled" appearance. The most common human tapeworms—*Taenia saginata, T. solium, Diphyllobothrium latum,* and *Hymenolepis nana*—can involve humans as a definitive host (i.e., adult worms reside in the intestines) and present primarily with gastrointestinal symptoms. Larval tapeworm disease involves humans as an intermediate dead-end host. These diseases usually become more symptomatic as larval forms migrate into other tissues.

Taenia solium (Pork Tapeworm)

Humans acquire this gastrointestinal disease by ingesting uncooked pork containing the encysted larval form. The infection is most common in Eastern Europe, Central and South America, Spain, Portugal, Africa, China, and Southeast Asia but rare in North Americans who have not travelled to endemic areas. The adult worm may reach 20 feet, but clinical symptoms are mild. The disease is diagnosed by identifying proglottids in the stool and is treated with niclosamide or praziquantel.

Cysticercosis is the larval form of infection with *T. solium*, which occurs when humans ingest eggs to become accidental intermediate hosts.

• PATHOGENESIS •

Usually the source of infection is food or water that is contaminated with human feces. Rarely, an individual with existing intestinal *T. solium* acquires cysticercosis either by fecal-oral autoinfection or reverse peristalsis. After penetrating the human intestinal mucosa, the oncosphere is a fully infective larva that becomes encysted within weeks. The cyst is viable for a few years, after which it degenerates, leading to an intensification of the host immune response.

• CLINICAL FEATURES •

Cysticerci may develop in almost any organ. Some cysts occur in muscle, but more significant is the potential for ocular and CNS involvement, including a mass lesion with its usual symptoms. In the skin, subcutaneous nodules are firm and painless, measuring about 1 to 2 cm in diameter.

• DIAGNOSIS AND TREATMENT •

The diagnosis is usually made by radiological studies, especially CT (computed tomography) scans. Serological tests have some cross reactions. Stools are examined for the characteristic operculated eggs and proglottids. Often, the diagnosis is made at the time of surgery.

Treatment is largely surgical. Albendazole or praziquantel are also used.

Sparganosis

Sparganosis is an infection with plerocercoid larvae (spargana) of tapeworms of the genus *Spirometra*, especially *S. mansonoides*. It is harbored by cats and dogs. A rare, severe form called proliferative sparganosis is caused by *S. proliferum.*

• PATHOGENESIS •

Humans are infected with the plerocercoid form of the organism by drinking contaminated water, eating raw meat, or applying raw frog poultices to wounds (a tradition in the Orient). Plerocercoids migrate to various organs.

• CLINICAL FEATURES •

A slow-growing subcutaneous nodule that may be migratory is typical; it may or may not be tender (Fig. 18.34). The larvae may infect other organs as well. In proliferative sparganosis, the parasite proliferates diffusely, primarily in the subcutaneous tissue.

• DIAGNOSIS AND TREATMENT •

The diagnosis is established at the time of surgery. Surgical treatment is curative in the usual sparganosis, but proliferative sparganosis produces a severe systemic illness that is often fatal.

REFERENCES

1. Deneris J, Marshall NA. Biological characterization of a strain of *Trypanosoma cruzi* isolated from a human case of trypanosomiasis in California. Am J Trop Med Hyg 1989;41(4):422.
2. Miller AC, et al. Hookworm folliculitis. Arch Dermatol 1991;127(4):547.

ANNOTATED BIBLIOGRAPHY

American Trypanosomiasis (Chagas' disease)

Bittencourt AL. Congenital Chagas' disease. Am J Dis Child 1976;130:97.
    Complete review on the obstetrical, clinical, and pathological findings, diagnosis, and treatment of congenital Chagas' disease.
Gallerano RH, Marr JJ, Sosa RR. Therapeutic efficacy of allopurinol in patients with chronic Chagas' disease. Am J Trop Med Hyg 1990;43:159.
    A comparison of allopurinol with benznidazole for the treatment of chronic Chagas' disease showed similar efficacy and less toxicity.
Gluckstein D, Ciferri F, Ruskin J. Chagas' disease: Another cause of cerebral mass in the acquired immunodeficiency syndrome. Am J Med 1992;92:429.
    A description of the first case of Chagas' disease causing an intracranial mass in AIDS patients.
Hagar JM, Rahimtoola SH. Chagas' heart disease in the United States. N Engl J Med 1991;325:763.
    Description of disease presentation in the United States; occurrence among immigrants from endemic areas and similarity to coronary artery disease or idiopathic dilated cardiomyopathy.
Marsden PD. Selective primary health care: Strategies for control of disease in the developing world. XVI. Chagas' disease. Rev Infect Dis 1984;6:855.
    Description of methods to reduce the risk of transmission of *Trypanosoma cruzi* infection in endemic areas.
Morris SA, Tanowitz HB, Wittner M, Bilezikina JP. Pathophysiological insights into the cardiomyopathy of Chagas' disease. Circulation 1990;82:1900.
    Review of recent studies offering new hypotheses to explain the pathology and clinical course of chagasic cardiomyopathy.

Cutaneous Leishmaniasis

Berman JD. Chemotherapy for leishmaniasis: Biochemical mechanisms, clinical efficacy, and future strategies. Rev Infect Dis 1988;10:560.
    Extensive review on the chemotherapy of leishmaniasis, with emphasis on biochemical mechanisms and the role of purines and sterol inhibitors as potential oral agents.
Herwaldt BL, Berman JD. Recommendations for treating leishmaniasis with sodium stibogluconate (Pentostam®) and review of pertinent clinical studies. Am J Trop Med Hyg 1992;46:296.

Current CDCP recommendations for the treatment of leishmaniasis.

Kubba R, Al-Gindan Y. Leishmaniasis. Dermatol Clin 1989;7:331.

Review article with emphasis on the different clinical patterns of cutaneous leishmaniasis.

Magill AJ, et al. Visceral infection caused by *Leishmania tropica* in veterans of Operation Desert Storm. N Engl J Med 1993;328:1383.

Report of 8 cases of visceral leishmaniasis due to *L. tropica* in soldiers returning from an endemic area.

Report of WHO Expert Committee Technical Report Series 701. The Leishmaniases. World Health Organization, Geneva, 1984.

Complete review of parasitic, clinical, and epidemiological factors, public health issues, and control methods.

Other Protozoal and Helminth Infections

Binazzi M. Profile of cutaneous toxoplasmosis. Int J Dermatol 1986;25(6):357.

A detailed review of clinical and laboratory features of the different categories of toxoplasmosis.

Chandry AZ, Longworth DL. Cutaneous manifestations of intestinal helminth infections. Dermatol Clin 1989;7(2):275.

A complete review of intestinal helminths as manifested by dermatological disease.

Davis BR. Filariases. Dermatol Clin 1989;7(2):313.

A detailed discussion of various manifestations of filarial diseases, concentrating on cutaneous disease.

Gonzalez E. Schistosomiasis, cercarial dermatitis and marine dermatitis. Dermatol Clin 1989;7(2):291.

A discussion of schistosome-associated disease with emphasis on cutaneous features.

Katz M, Despommier DD, Gwadz RW. Parasitic Diseases. New York: Springer-Verlag, 1989.

A general reference for parasitic infections, including life cycles and detailed pathogenesis.

Mandell GL, Douglas RG, Bennet JE, eds. Principles and practice of infectious diseases. New York: John Wiley and Sons, 1985.

A general reference for parasitic disease focusing on visceral manifestations.

Richman TB, Kerdel FA. Amebiasis and trypanosomiasis. Dermatol Clin 1989;7(2):301.

A review of amebiasis and trypanosomiasis focusing on cutaneous manifestations.

Saenz RE, Paz H, Berman JD. Efficacy of ketoconazole against *Leishmania braziliensis panamensis* cutaneous leishmaniasis. Am J Med 1990;89:147.

Ketoconazole and stibogluconate sodium (Pentostam®) were more effective than placebo in cutaneous leishmaniasis. Ketoconazole was as effective as Pentostam®, producing cure in 76%.

Visvesvara GS, Stehr-Green JK. Epidemiology of free-living ameba infections. J Protozool 1990;37(4):25S.

A complete review of infections with free-living amebas, including epidemiology of the organisms and descriptions and incidences of disease syndromes worldwide.

Warrell DA, Molyneaux ME, Beales PF, eds. Severe and complicated malaria. Trans R Soc Trop Med Hyg 1990;84(2):1.

A comprehensive text developed by participants of a World Health Organization meeting in 1988.

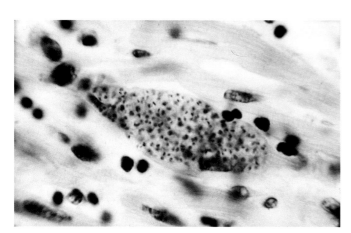

Figure 18.1.   American trypanosomiasis. *Trypanosoma cruzi* pseudocyst of amastigotes in the cardiac muscle of a patient with acute disease.

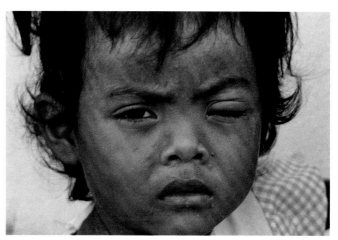

Figure 18.2.   American trypanosomiasis. Romaña's sign with periorbital edema. Patient also had multiple papules elsewhere on the face.

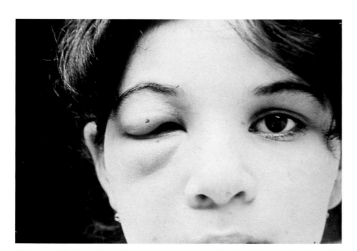

Figure 18.3.   American trypanosomiasis. Romaña's sign with periorbital edema.

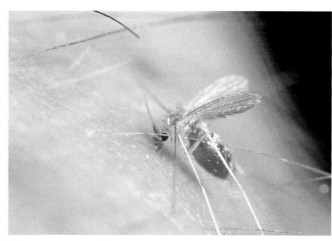

Figure 18.4.   Leishmaniasis. Sandfly of the genus *Lutzomyia*, vector of leishmaniasis.

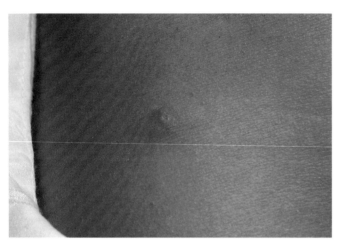

Figure 18.5.   Cutaneous leishmaniasis. Early papular lesion.

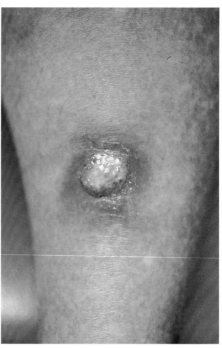

Figure 18.6.   Cutaneous leishmaniasis. Punched-out ulcer on the lower leg in a missionary in southernmost Venezuela.

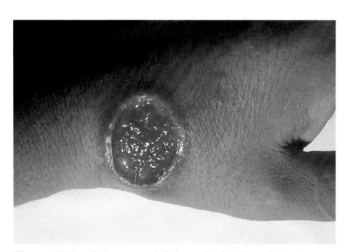

Figure 18.7.   Cutaneous leishmaniasis. Ulcerative lesion.

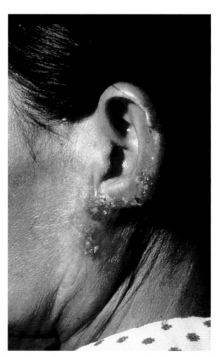

Figure 18.8.   American cutaneous leishmaniasis. Chiclero's ulcer with ulceration and scarring of the earlobe and neck.

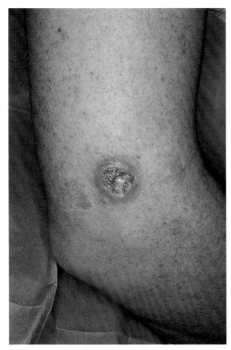

Figure 18.9.   Cutaneous leishmaniasis. Nodular lesion with central ulceration of the arm. (Courtesy of Dr. Charles V. Sanders)

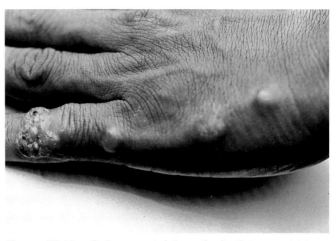

Figure 18.10.   Cutaneous leishmaniasis. Cutaneous leishmaniasis with lymphangitic spread.

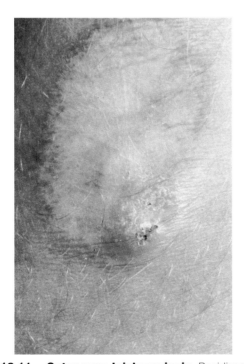

Figure 18.11.   Cutaneous leishmaniasis. Recidivans type of lesions surrounding scar of previous disease.

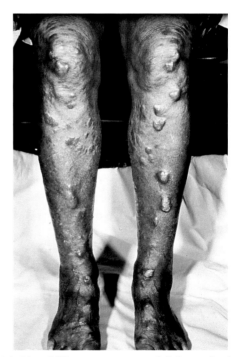

Figure 18.12.   Diffuse cutaneous leishmaniasis. Multiple nodular lesions of the legs.

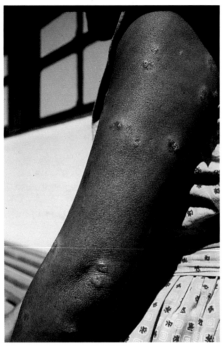

Figure 18.13.   Diffuse cutaneous leishmaniasis. Multiple papular nodules of the arm.

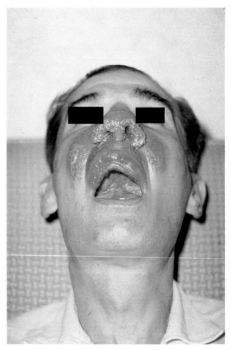

Figure 18.14.   Mucocutaneous leishmaniasis. Upper lip, nose, and cheek involvement.

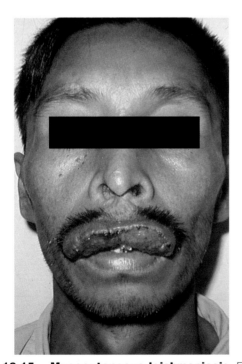

Figure 18.15.   Mucocutaneous leishmaniasis. Extensive upper lip involvement and tapir nose deformity.

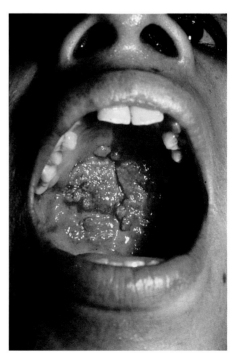

Figure 18.16.   Mucocutaneous leishmaniasis. Extensive upper lip involvement of the hard and soft palates.

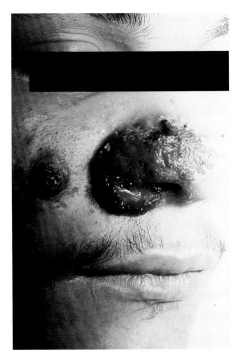

Figure 18.17. Mucocutaneous leishmaniasis. Mucocutaneous leishmaniasis before treatment.

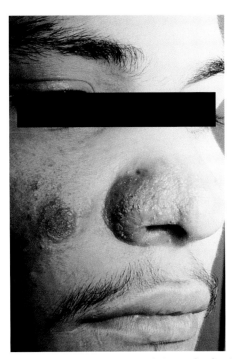

Figure 18.18. Mucocutaneous leishmaniasis. Mucocutaneous leishmaniasis after treatment with pentavalent antimony (same patient as Figure 18.17).

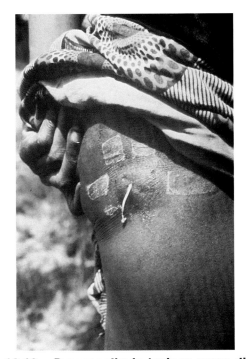

Figure 18.19. Dracunculiasis (guinea worm disease). Nodular swelling of the upper thigh with extruded female worm. (Courtesy of Dr. Joy Barrett, United States Peace Corps)

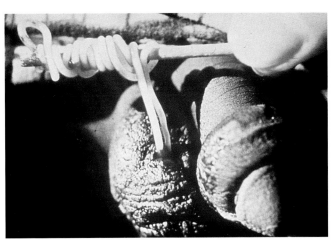

Figure 18.20. Dracunculiasis (guinea worm disease). Extraction of the female worm by rolling onto a small stick. (Courtesy of Dr. Joy Barrett, United States Peace Corps)

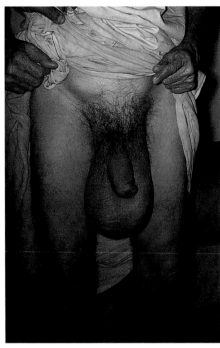

Figure 18.21.   Scrotal elephantiasis (lymphatic filariasis). Scrotal elephantiasis due to *Wucheria bancrofti* in a male in Calcutta, India.

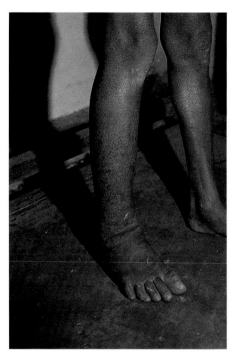

Figure 18.22.   Elephantiasis (lymphatic filariasis). Elephantiasis of the lower leg due to *Wucheria bancrofti* in a male in Calcutta, India.

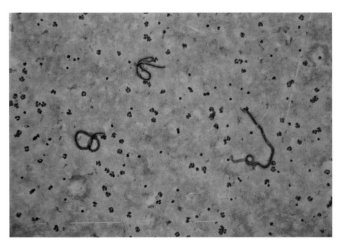

Figure 18.23.   Filariasis. Stained thick blood smear showing the characteristic sheathed microfilariae of *Wuchereria bancrofti*.

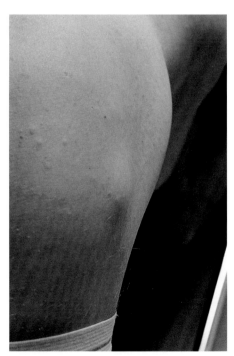

Figure 18.24.   Onchocerciasis. Subcutaneous nodule inhabited by the adult filarial worms of *Onchocerca volvulus*. These give rise to the microfilariae that produce the dermal and ocular manifestations of onchocerciasis.

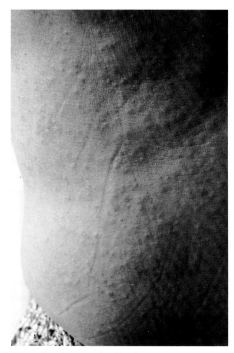

Figure 18.25. Onchocerciasis. Onchocerciasis due to the micro-filariae of *Onchocerca volvulus* in a missionary in southernmost Venezuela. Lower trunk shows accompanying dermal edema.

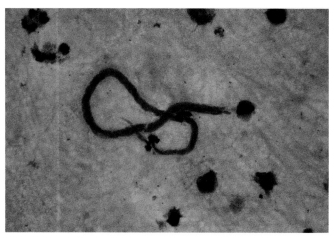

Figure 18.26. Onchocerciasis. Microfilariae of *Onchocerca volvulus* in Giemsa-stained dermal scraping. Note the absence of a microfilarial sheath.

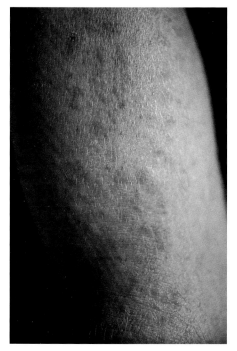

Figure 18.27. Onchocerciasis. Mazzotti reaction provoked by diethylcarbamazine. The reaction is considered confirmatory of onchocerciasis in individuals from endemic areas.

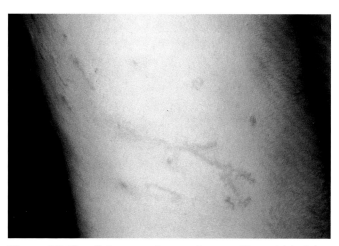

Figure 18.28. Cutaneous larva migrans. *Strongyloides* infection (nutria itch), showing serpiginous, erythematous tracks on the trunk, indicating more rapid migration of the organism.

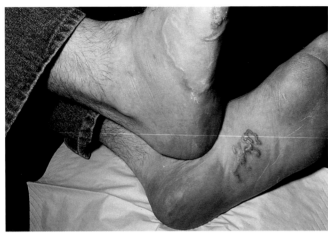

Figure 18.29.   Cutaneous larva migrans. Multiple larval tracks of both feet in a patient who walked barefoot in Mexico.

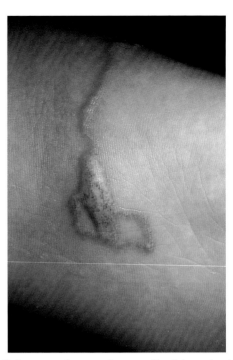

18.30.   Cutaneous larva migrans. Serpiginous track with bulla formation on the sole of the foot.

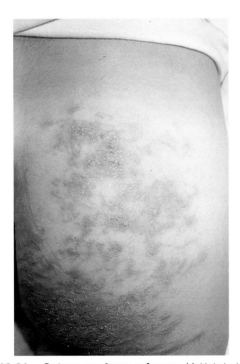

Figure 18.31.   Cutaneous larva migrans. Multiple lesions of the buttocks that developed after the patient sat on a Caribbean beach.

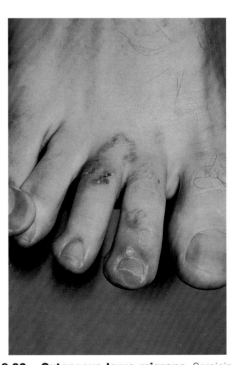

Figure 18.32.   Cutaneous larva migrans. Serpiginous tracks on the toes, mimicking tinea infection.

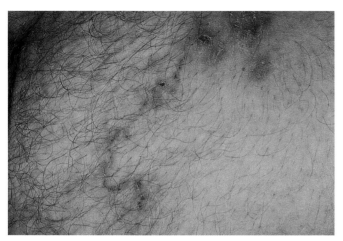

Figure 18.33. Cutaneous larva migrans. Serpiginous track with excoriations and small ulcers of the buttocks after the patient sat on contaminated soil.

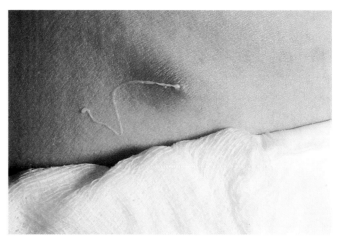

Figure 18.34. Cestode infection. Sparganosis. Long, slender larval worm (*Sparganum*) being discharged from a cutaneous nodule.

CHAPTER 19

Bites, Stings, and Infestations

MERVYN L. ELGART

Arthropods and ectoparasites—insects and mites—transmit disease to humans through bites and infestations, which involve different mechanisms of damaging the skin. The injection of substances into the skin by insects may cause disease by producing toxicity, as in the case of fire ant sting, or through allergic responses to the insect, which occurs with flea bites. Few organisms actually penetrate the epidermis, and fewer still set up housekeeping within the dermis and deeper tissues. While arthropods and ectoparasites are dreaded mostly for their filth, few actually carry disease. Those that do carry disease are listed in Table 19.1.

Bites and Injections

BEES, WASPS, AND HORNETS

These members of the class Hymenoptera are responsible for approximately 40 cases of anaphylaxis in the United States per year. Much more common than these systemic reactions are local reactions, such as pain and swelling.

Most bees in the United States are the relatively harmless *Apis mellifera*, or honeybee. These feed on flowering plants and differ from wasps and hornets (Vespidae) by being wider and having no sharp distinction between the thorax and abdomen. Honeybees sting by leaving stinger and venom sac with their victim, therefore killing itself in the process. It is important to avoid squeezing the venom sac in removing the stinger by laterally moving a knife or scalpel across the stinger, parallel to the skin. *Apis mellifera scutellata*, the African or "killer" bee of Mexico and Central America, is a more aggressive, swarming insect that has been implicated in several deaths.

Vespidae have a thinner body, with a distinct thorax and abdomen. Hornets are more colorful than wasps. Both attack other insects and worms, do not leave their stinger, and are free to sting again.

• PATHOGENESIS •

The reaction depends on the components of the venom, which are listed in Table 19.2.

Table 19.1. Transmission of Disease by Insects

DISEASE	AGENT OF TRANSMISSION
Bacterial Diseases	
Anthrax	*Tabanus* species
Tularemia	*Dermacentor andersoni* and *Tabanus* species
Lyme disease	Ticks, especially *Ioxides scapularis (dammini)* and *Ioxides pacificus*
Bubonic plague	*Xenopsylla cheopis* and *Pulex irritans*
Bartonellosis	*Lutzomyia* species
Rickettsial Diseases	
Typhus, epidemic	*Pediculus humanus corporis* (can be transmitted by ticks as well)
Typhus, endemic	*Ornithonyssus bacoti* and *Dermanyssus gallinae*
Typhus, murine	*Xenopsylla cheopis*
Typhus, Queensland tick	*Ioxides holocyclus*
Trench fever	*Pediculus humanus corporis*
Rickettsialpox	*Liponyssoides sanguineus* and *Ornithonyssus bacoti*
Rocky Mountain spotted fever	*Dermacentor andersoni* and other ticks
Ehrlichia infections	*Dermacentor variabolis* and *Amblyomma americanum*
Viral Diseases	
Viral encephalitis	*Chrysops* species
Colorado tick-fever	*Dermacentor andersoni* and *Dermacentor occidentalis*
Louping ill	*Ixodes ricinus*

Table 19.1. Transmission of Disease by Insects

DISEASE	AGENT OF TRANSMISSION
Central Europe tick-borne encephalitis	*Ixodes ricinus*
Japanese encephalitis	*Dermacentor, Ixodes* and *Haemaphysalis* species
Western equine encephalitis	*Ornithonyssus bacoti, Ornithonyssus sylviarum* and *Ornithonyssus bursa*
St. Louis encephalitis	*Ornithonyssus bacoti* and *Ornithonyssus sylviarum*
Yellow fever	*Aedes aegypti*

Parasitic Diseases

Leishmaniasis, Old World	*Phlebotomus* species
Leishmaniasis, South American	*Lutzomyia* species
Trypanosomiasis, East African	*Glossina* species
Trypanosomiasis, West African	*Glossina* species
Chagas Disease	*Trypanosoma cruzi*
Malaria	*Anopheles* species
Filariasis	*Culex* species
Onchocerciasis	*Onchocerca* species
Dracunculosis	*Dracunculus medinensis*
Loa Loa	*Chrysops* species
Dermatobia hominis eggs	*Psorophora* species

Table 19.2. Components of Hymenoptera Venoms

Biochemical Group	Bee	Wasp	Hornet
Biologic amines	Histamine Dopamine Noradrenaline	Histamine Dopamine Noradrenaline Serotonin	Histamine Serotonin Acetylcholine
Peptides and small protines	Apamin Melitin MCD peptide Protease inhibitor	Wasp kinin	Hornet kinin
Enzymes	Phospholipase A Hyaluronidase Esterases Phosphatases	Phospholipase A Phospholipase B Hyaluronidase	Phospholipase A Phospholipase B Hyaluronidase

From Elgart GW. Ant, bee, and wasp stings. Dermatol Clin 1990, 8(2):231.

reactions require antihistamines and, if severe, rapid injections of epinephrine. Anaphylaxis may require IV fluids, maintenance of airway, shock trousers, and so forth.

To diminish future reactions, immunotherapy (hyposensitization) may be helpful in those who are repeatedly exposed. Others may benefit from carrying epinephrine syringes ready for instant use.

ANTS

Although ant bites and stings are generally harmless, the fire ant of the American southeast has become a major problem, producing serious local and, occasionally, systemic, reactions. The two species differ primarily in color: *Solenopsis richteri* is black, while *S. invicta* is red. Fire ants live on the ground, in dense mounds of interconnecting tunnels.

• CLINICAL FEATURES •

Local reactions consist of erythema and edema, sometimes with a central puncta, and rarely last more than an hour. Systemic reactions may begin within minutes, starting first with itching or urticaria and progressing to shock and anaphylaxis, with death due to respiratory failure. Most deaths occur in patients who delay treatment for an hour or more. Multiple stings, such as with the African honeybee, may produce direct toxic effects that simulate anaphylaxis.

• DIAGNOSIS AND TREATMENT •

The identification of the involved insect depends on the history given by the patient. The appearance of the local sting, except in the case of the honeybee, is not distinctive. Patients suffering systemic reactions warrant careful diagnostic testing to identify the insect. Skin testing may be done, but RAST (radioallergosorbent tests) may be more specific.

Local reactions are treated with cool compresses and antihistamines. Occasionally, topical steroids are of value. Systemic

• PATHOGENESIS •

Fire ants bite in a two-part process. First, the insect grabs the skin with its powerful jaws. It then twists its body beneath it and stings the skin, releasing venom. The insect may swivel its body around to produce a circle of stings around a central pair of puncta from the bite.

The fire ant's venom differs from that of other Hymenoptera. About 90% consists of 6-N-alkyl (or alkenyl), 2-methyl piperidines. These alkaloids are responsible for the local reaction, causing pain and a papule that rapidly evolves to a characteristic pustule. The remainder of the toxin contains proteins and peptides, which represents the allergenic fraction of the venom. Proteins of the two *Solenopsis* species display a high degree of cross-reactivity (1). These proteins are responsible for venom hypersensitivity, which may result in serious systemic allergic reactions, including anaphylaxis.

• CLINICAL FEATURES •

The initial bite and sting is usually painful. The characteristic toxic reaction is the formation of a pustule within 24 hours, which may be confused with local infection, folliculitis, etc. (Fig. 19.1). The local reaction may be intense, especially with multiple stings. Cellulitis and secondary infection may result.

About 2% of the stings may result in severe, life-threatening allergic reactions, including urticaria, shock, restricted airway, and even cardiac arrest. Positive IgE antibodies may be found in up to 60% of victims.

• DIAGNOSIS AND TREATMENT •

No bacteria are present in the pustule. The contents are mostly neutrophils, although eosinophils may be present in up to 13% of "reactors," individuals prone to systemic reactions (2).

The treatment of local reactions includes topical or oral corticosteroids, antihistamines, and local measures such as cool compresses. Systemic reactions require epinephrine, antihistamines, and measures to combat shock. Individuals who have suffered systemic symptoms and who must come in future contact with the fire ant may be tried on immunotherapy, although efficacy has not been validated.

MOSQUITOS

Mosquitos belong to the family Culicidae and the blood-sucking order Diptera. They include the *Culex* (the house mosquito), the *Aedes* complex (vectors of yellow fever and dengue), the *Psorophora* (carry *Dermatobia hominis* eggs), and *Anopheles* (carry malaria). All require water for development.

• PATHOGENESIS •

According to Mellanby, reactions to mosquito bites vary with repeated exposure (3). In his study, there was no immediate reaction with the initial bite, but there was a delayed reaction, consisting of a papule, that appeared within 24 hours (stage 1). Subsequent bites (stages 2 and 3) produced an immediate reaction in the form of a wheal, but by the final exposure neither type of reaction was seen. The disappearance of all reactions is the reason why endemic populations show little reaction to mosquito bites. This pattern of immunity, the so-called "papular urticaria," is probably also operative in other bites, such as those of the bedbug and flea.

• CLINICAL FEATURES •

Mosquito bites may produce papules, wheels, or puncta in hemorrhagic macules. In severe allergic situations, there may be bullae or confluent hives. Anaphylaxis is rare.

• DIAGNOSIS AND TREATMENT •

The bites are not specific and therefore cannot be differentiated from many other bites of similar appearance.

Symptomatic therapy with cool compresses is helpful. Antihistamines or topical steroids usually suffice as medical treatment, but in severe cases systemic corticosteroids may be necessary. Severe local reactions may subside faster after the intralesional injection of 0.1 cc of triamcinolone acetonide, 3 to 5 mg/cc.

DEET (N,N-diethyl-m-toluamide) is the recommended insect repellent, although a much more effective product is now available. Permethrin, a synthetic pyrethrin, is well-known to physicians as a treatment for lice and scabies. It is really a toxicant rather than a repellent, but is being widely used because it remains active on the skin for several days. In addition, it can be incorporated into clothing, where it may withstand several washings. Control of stagnant water will diminish breeding sites.

FLIES

There are several large families of flies, described briefly here.

Psychodidae contain the Phlebotomus and Lutzomyia flies, transmitters of leishmaniasis in Africa and the Americas, respectively. These are very small (2 to 3 mm) with characteristically erect wings. Eggs are laid in moist soil.

Simuliidae comprise the black flies or buffalo flies. *S. damnosum* is the vector of onchocerciasis. They breed in running water and bite on exposed surfaces.

Ceratopogonidae includes gnats and midges, which attack in swarms. They are very small, 1 to 4 mm in length. Eggs are laid in water or mud.

Tabanidae include the deer flies and horse flies. They are large, up to 2.5 cm in length. The females are blood feeders, and the bites are deep and painful.

Glossinidae include the Tsetse fly, vector of human and animal trypanosomiasis. They are up to 15 mm in length and viviparous. Their bite is minimal.

The most notable member of the Muscidae is the house fly, *Musca domestica*, which cannot bite.

• PATHOGENESIS •

Reaction to the bites of most flies will vary with the immune status, as is the case with mosquitos. The actual bites are usually minimal, except in the case of the Tabanid flies (see below). Very little is written about the actual bites of many of these organisms; attention is more often devoted to the diseases they carry.

• CLINICAL FEATURES •

For most of these flies, the bites are not characteristic. There may be puncta or minimal hemorrhage, or occasionally a small vesicle (Fig. 19.2). The exception is the Tabanid flies, which produce deep, painful bites. The attention of the victim interrupts feeding, which is then often repeated, leading to multiple open tears in the skin. Secondary infection is common.

• DIAGNOSIS AND TREATMENT •

Treatment for simple bites is symptomatic—calamine lotion will suffice. When secondary infection appears, antibiotics will be necessary.

BITING BUGS

The most important organism of this group is the bedbug, *Cimex lectularius.* The kissing bug, or reduviid bug, is another common member.

• PATHOGENESIS •

All biting bugs require blood meals, often between molts. Most parasitize animals. Bedbugs tend to be nocturnal feeders and often bite again if disturbed, producing the characteristic grouped bites. The bugs often defecate after biting; those that carry Chagas disease can therefore directly inoculate their bites with contaminated feces.

• CLINICAL FEATURES •

The bites may present as papules with a central punctum, grouped in a linear fashion. Clusters of vesicles or bullae, urticaria, or hemorrhagic nodules can be seen (Fig. 19.3). Although most of the reactions are local, systemic responses, such as anaphylaxis, can occur.

• DIAGNOSIS AND TREATMENT •

Diagnosis is usually difficult unless the bug has been seen. Multiple bites in a row suggest bedbugs or flea bites. Treatment is the same as for mosquitos.

FLEAS

Only a few fleas are of medical significance. Although *Pulex irritans* is the human flea, animals are more often victimized. Dog and cat fleas (*Ctenocephalides canis, C. felis*) often bite humans when their primary host is unavailable. *Xenopsylla cheopis,* the Oriental rat flea, is the historical vector of bubonic plague and endemic typhus.

• PATHOGENESIS •

Fleas mate on their host animal, but the female then requires a blood meal each time she produces fertile eggs. These eggs may be deposited in rugs or upholstered furniture, or in the nests or baskets of its host animal.

• CLINICAL FEATURES •

Small papular lesions, often in groups, are seen mostly on the legs of adults but anywhere on the body in children (Fig. 19.4). The allergic changes in papular urticaria (see section on mosquitos) are also seen frequently with flea bites (Fig. 19.5).

• DIAGNOSIS AND TREATMENT •

The suggestive features are the grouped bites and the locations. There are no diagnostic findings. Treatment is the same as for mosquito bites.

MOTHS, BUTTERFLIES, AND CATERPILLARS

These organisms cause cutaneous human problems by contact with hairs in their caterpillar stages. The condition may be referred to as cutaneous lepidopterism. In the United States, the most reported sting is from the *Megalopyge opercularis* (thought by some to be the "asp" that poisoned Cleopatra), but other caterpillars of lesser significance also sting.

• PATHOGENESIS •

Poison hairs are found on the dorsal and lateral surfaces of the caterpillar. These may inject or ooze venom. Some of the tissue damage is caused mechanically by the spines.

• CLINICAL FEATURES •

Reaction to caterpillars generally begins with an itch, followed by erythema, then by maculopapules 2 to 5 mm wide that sometimes are superimposed with vesicles (Fig. 19.6). Reaction may be delayed by up to a week.

In *Megalopyge* contacts, there is immediate, intensifying pain. Lymphangitis and lymphadenopathy may develop rapidly. Local lesions may persist for days, and systemic reaction may develop, consisting of nausea, vomiting, headache, numbness, convulsions, and even shock.

• DIAGNOSIS AND TREATMENT •

History is usually the most helpful feature in diagnosis. Treatment is aimed at relieving symptoms. Topical steroids and antihistamines are rarely helpful. Cellophane tape stripping may remove residual poison hairs. Severe pain from *Megalopyge* may require intravenous calcium gluconate; the shock syndrome is treated with epinephrine.

CHIGGERS

These are the six-legged larvae of the Trombiculid mites, or harvest mites. There are many species worldwide. *Eutrombicula alfreddugesi* is the most common species in the United States.

• PATHOGENESIS •

The newly hatched larvae congregate on low-lying vegetation until they can attach to a host, generally on an area of the body where the skin is soft and where a constriction in clothing prohibits migration. Here they bite, feed, and fall off without burrowing into the skin. After feeding, they return to the ground where they continue their maturation, emerging as nymphs in about a month.

• CLINICAL FEATURES •

Multiple erythematous bites are seen near a belt or other constricted area 2 to 4 hours after exposure. Lesions may be papular or vesicular. Ankles, thighs, genitalia, axillae, and breasts are common target areas (Figs. 19.7, 19.8).

• DIAGNOSIS AND TREATMENT •

The appearance of groups of lesions in these locations is helpful in diagnosis. The individual lesions cannot be distinguished from other bites. Differential diagnosis includes scabies, lice, and other mite infestations.

Local treatment with antipruritics and topical corticosteroids is helpful. Secondary infection should be treated with antibiotics. Wearing tight clothing and using insect repellent may prevent attacks.

SPIDERS

Although several spiders can cause bites in humans, the most destructive are the *Loxosceles reclusa* (the brown recluse spider (Fig. 19.9), and the *Latrodectus mactans* (the black widow). Each can produce severe necrosis because of envenomation.

• PATHOGENESIS •

The venom of *Loxosceles reclusa* contains proteases, alkaline phosphatase, lipase, sphingomyelinase D, and hyaluronidase. The necrosis depends on complement and polymorphonuclear leukocytes. The venom of *Latrodectus mactans* is a neurotoxin, known as alpha-latrotoxin. Its effect is mediated by a massive release of acetylcholine.

• CLINICAL FEATURES •

Reaction to the brown recluse bite falls into three categories. The first is a mild local reaction (Fig. 19.10). The second is a severe reaction, with pain, erythema, and edema, occasional blister formation, and, sometimes, necrosis and extensive local tissue destruction (Fig. 19.11). The third category is systemic reaction, with fever, chills, weakness, nausea, vomiting, petechia, convulsions, and hemolysis (4).

Cutaneous reaction to the black widow bite may be obvious in the presence of other symptoms that begin within 30 minutes, peak within 6 hours, and last 24 to 48 hours: pain, cramps, muscle contractions, fatigue, restlessness, and anxiety. The bite itself shows slight erythema, local piloerection, mild edema, or urtication.

• DIAGNOSIS AND TREATMENT •

Complete diagnosis is difficult without finding the spider. The diagnosis is usually made on the basis of a characteristic necrotic lesion that occurs after a spider bite in an endemic area. Treatment of brown recluse bites includes local therapy with cool compresses and surgical debridement as needed. Early therapy with dapsone, 50 to 100 mg once or twice a day may help (5).

Diagnosis of the black widow bite depends on a consistent clinical picture described above. Treatment focuses on the relief of cramping and pain with calcium gluconate or narcotics. The use of *Latrodectus* antivenom should be reserved for the most severe cases, since there is a risk of anaphylaxis in the use of horse serum.

TICKS

These are arthropods with eight legs and an unsegmented body. There are hard ticks, or Ixodidae, and soft ticks, or Argasidae. The hard ticks have a more chitinous (shell-like) body, and the mouth parts protrude from the front end of the body (Fig. 19.12). The mouth parts of the soft ticks are hidden by the anterior edge of the animal (Fig. 19.13).

• PATHOGENESIS •

The tick attaches itself by a tearing motion into the skin, and then secretes a cementing substance that holds it in place while feeding. In hard ticks, feeding may take several days, after which it often pulls free and falls to the ground.

• CLINICAL FEATURES •

The bite may appear as an erythematous papule, sometimes with numbness. Occasionally, the tick remains in place, enlarging, and the patient presents with a "rapidly enlarging mole." Ticks may carry disease, the most notable of which is Lyme disease, but may also cause tick bite paralysis or alopecia.

Tick bite paralysis is an acute ascending lower motor neuron paralysis. It leads to flaccid paralysis, which can progress to bulbar paralysis and death. Removal of the tick produces rapid recovery. The diagnosis depends on finding the tick: in the absence of this evidence, the mistaken diagnosis is frequently polio. The cause of the paralysis is unclear, but is thought to be a toxin secreted by the tick.

Several accounts of tick bite alopecia have been described. It seems to be associated with toxin-induced tissue necrosis (scarring alopecia) secondary to inflammation (6).

• DIAGNOSIS AND TREATMENT •

Diagnosis of tick bite may be difficult when the tick is no longer present. A central punctum with a surrounding erythematous ring (erythema chronicum migrans) suggests a tick bite and the potential for subsequent Lyme disease. In instances of tick bite paralysis or tick bite fever, a very careful examination of the total body, including the scalp, the axillae, the pudendal area, and skin between the toes, may be needed to find the offending tick.

Removal of ticks must be done so as not to leave attached mouth parts behind. This is done by applying chloroform or ether to the tick, then gently exerting pressure. Surgical removal with a punch biopsy is always satisfactory.

For information on Lyme disease and Rocky Mountain spotted fever, see Chapters 9 and 10.

Infestations

SCABIES (HUMAN)

Sarcoptes scabiei var. *hominis* has been known to cause disease since the 17th century. Although mites are merely an annoyance in this country, secondary pyoderma, glomerulonephritis, and death are not unknown in developing countries.

• PATHOGENESIS •

Infestation with *Sarcoptes scabiei* var. *hominis* requires an incubation period of about 30 days from the time of exposure. During this period, the mites mate, burrow, and lay eggs without producing pruritus in the host. After the incubation period, however, itching becomes quite severe and is related to an immune response to some fragment of the mites' growth, possibly the scybala (mite feces) or saliva. Once the itching has begun, the patient may excoriate sufficiently to remove most of the mites.

The precipitating event is not always the same. In young adults, sexual contact seems to be the most common method of transmission, although touching and hand-shaking may be sufficient. In children, simple touching may transmit the organism. In nursing homes, infestation may spread to nursing personnel and other patients (7). In immunocompromised persons, the organism may proliferate to such an extent that large numbers of mites and eggs are noted in a thickened keratin. Although the infected host may be asymptomatic, those around the patient—medical personnel, relatives, friends, and other patients—may all develop itching.

• CLINICAL FEATURES •

The presenting symptom is usually pruritus, often described as severe, disturbing, and worse at night. The clinical signs include the burrow and excoriations. Normally mild-mannered individuals scratch with such vigor that the skin is lined with deep scratches, serum crusts, and even impetigo. But these findings can be seen in many patients who itch for other reasons.

The diagnostic finding is the burrow. This is a lesion in which the gravid female mite burrows into the skin, depositing eggs and scybala in her path. The burrow appears as a small line, perhaps 2 to 5 mm in length, at the top of a papule. These lesions are usually found on the nipples, the head of the penis, the scrotum, the labia majora, between the fingers, and in the axillae (Figs. 19.14, 19.15). Mites rarely burrow in other areas, although papules, pustules, and excoriations may be present (Fig. 19.16).

In immunocompromised patients, a severe form of disease, Norwegian scabies, may be seen. There is no initial response, and, therefore, no itching. Mites proliferate in huge numbers, and many caregivers may become infested. When itching finally appears, it may be intense. By that time, there may be thickening of the epidermis to accommodate the mite population (Figs. 19.17–19.19). Response to the usual treatment (permethrin) is rapid.

An interesting finding is the involvement of the face and scalp in prepubescent children, but not in adults. This curious phenomenon can be a valuable clue. In infants and children, the disease affects all areas and presents as infected eczema, particularly of the hands and feet.

• DIAGNOSIS AND TREATMENT •

The demonstration of the mite, an egg, or a newly hatched nymph (Fig. 19.20) confirms the diagnosis. This is done by scraping the burrow onto a slide, adding a drop of microscope oil, and examining under low power. The mite is 300 microns in diameter and sometimes contains an egg ready for hatching. The nymph forms are notable in that they have only one pair of hind legs. If mites are not identified, scybala may be found. This material is dissolved by KOH (potassium hydroxide), hence the use of the microscope oil in the examination.

The presence of a mite confirms the diagnosis. If no mite is found, the differential diagnosis includes exposure to other mites that do not burrow on humans (*Cheyletiella, Ornithonyssus, Dermonyssus,* and animal scabies), other insect bites, systemic causes of itching, and dermatologic causes of itching.

The treatment of choice is permethrin, a synthetic pyrethrin (8), or lindane. The latter product has been used for years, but has come under recent attack because of a few cases of seizures in small children (9). Either product should be applied at bedtime, from the neck down, and left on for 8 hours. It is washed off in the morning, and the patient is instructed to change bed sheets and clothing. The process is repeated in 48 hours (for lindane) and, if necessary, again in 1 week. Permethrin remains active on the skin, so repeating treatment before 1 week is unnecessary.

Clothing can be washed or dry cleaned. Although Mellanby's World War II studies found that mites did not survive well off the body (10), others have worried about survival of the mites in homes under conditions of moisture and warmth. Clearly, they survive better on inanimate objects in tropical climates.

SCABIES (ANIMAL)

Every warm-blooded animal species attracts a different variety of scabies. The disease produced in the animal requires that the animal develop a sensitivity to the mite, as in humans. The clinical picture in the animal is usually "mange," missing hair, crusts, and scales.

• PATHOGENESIS •

Humans develop irritation as soon as they are in contact with the mites. Therefore, irritant dermatitis occurs rather than contact allergy, which requires the development of sensitivity. An infected dog will cause itching in virtually all persons in contact with it. The itching diminishes or ceases when the dog is removed.

• CLINICAL FEATURES •

Itching and/or excoriations are present in areas exposed to the affected animal. If the animal is a horse (cavalryman's itch), the itching is on the inner thighs and groin. There may be papules (bites) but no burrows.

• DIAGNOSIS AND TREATMENT •

Diagnosis requires finding the mite on the animal. In the absence of this, the occurrence of itching in several exposed individuals is very suggestive. For differential diagnosis, see the section on human scabies.

The affected animal must be treated adequately. Human contacts need only symptomatic treatment (antihistamines, soothing lotions, antibiotics if secondarily infected).

CHEYLETIELLA

Cheyletiellae are mites, not unlike the scabies mite, seen on cats and rabbits. They produce all the signs and symptoms of animal scabies but differ in one respect: they do not produce mange on the affected animal. For this reason, the pet may not be suspected as a cause of the infestation.

• PATHOGENESIS •

In human disease, mites that do not usually involve themselves with humans attack humans because of the death or absence of the usual primary host. Overwhelming infestation may also provoke human attacks. The human presents with many small papular lesions, the result of bites in several areas. Sometimes the mites appear in sufficient numbers to be found on windowsills or bedding, and the diagnosis is made.

• CLINICAL FEATURES •

Clinical features in humans are the same as for animal scabies (see previous section). Patients may have multiple erythematous pruritic papules, generally on anterior surfaces.

• DIAGNOSIS AND TREATMENT •

When the mite is present, the diagnosis is obvious. In the absence of the offending mite, the condition is often called "itchy red bump disease"—thought to be due to insects, but unproven. Treatment involves removal of the source of the mites, and symptomatic relief with antihistamines and soothing lotions.

Diagnosis requires demonstration of the organism on the animal. Since the parasite produces only slight scaling on the animal, this disease has been called "walking dandruff." What appears to be dandruff on an animal may be material that contains mites, which can be demonstrated by brushing the animal over a dark piece of paper.

ORNITHONYSSUS AND DERMANYSSUS

These mites produce itching on humans by biting. While they prefer animal hosts, they will attack man when the animal host is not available.

• PATHOGENESIS •

The Ornithonyssus mites are present on the bodies of rats, mice, and birds. If the animal dies, the mite will seek another warm-blooded host and may invade man if he is nearby. The Dermanyssus mites are different from Ornithonyssus in that they feed at night and spend the day in the nest or chicken coop. If the bird does not return to the nest, they will seek other hosts. Often people afflicted by these mites have found numerous examples on a windowsill or near a chimney. Most problems occur in the late spring, when birds leave their nests.

• CLINICAL FEATURES •

Most patients present with small erythematous papules, most often on exposed areas of the arms of legs. Sometimes puncta may be present. The pruritic nature of the bite means that excoriation will be a prominent feature and puncta may be obscured and difficult to distinguish.

• DIAGNOSIS AND TREATMENT •

Without a good history, these bites are not easily distinguished from others. A definitive diagnosis can be made only when the mite is found. Sometimes this can be accomplished by placing tape in strategic areas with the sticky side out.

Treatment of the bites is symptomatic—cool compresses, topical steroids, and antihistamines. Demonstration of the mite and removal of the source is optimal.

Lice

PEDICULUS HUMANUS (BODY LOUSE AND HEAD LOUSE)

These organisms, Pediculus humanus var. corporis and P. humanus var. capitis, are variants of each other. They are virtually identical, differing only in that the body louse is larger than the head louse (Fig. 19.21). They mate with each other, and they assume the other's behavior when placed in the alternate body site.

• PATHOGENESIS •

Pediculus causes problems by biting in order to feed. Head lice set up housekeeping in the scalp. Few organisms are usually present, but once impregnated, the female can continue to lay eggs for life at the base of the hair. Each egg is oval-shaped, with an operculum, or lid, on one end and adheres to the hair in an asymmetrical manner. As the hair grows, the egg, or nit, is carried from the level of the scalp outward. The disease may be transmitted by wearing the hats or using the combs of infested persons.

Body lice live in the seams of clothing, leaving only to feed on the individual. The nits are attached to the clothing. The mode of transmission is unclear but is most likely by body contact.

• CLINICAL FEATURES •

The clinical feature of head lice is nits in the scalp (Fig. 19.22). Lice are also present but are more difficult to locate. Lice and nits are often found where the hair is moist and warm, such as the underside of the hair near the ears and over the occiput. Itching may be related to bites along the back of the neck.

Body lice also produce bites and itching. Poor hygiene and lack of bathing usually lead to secondary infection of the bites, with pyoderma and cellulitis. While head lice usually carry no disease, body lice may carry typhus and, under extremely unsanitary conditions, trench fever.

• DIAGNOSIS AND TREATMENT •

Diagnosis requires the finding of lice or live nits. Unless specifically removed, the nits will remain on the hair shaft after treatment. Differential diagnosis of head lice nits includes white piedra, dandruff, and hair casts (keratin from skin attached to the hair).

Head lice may best be treated with a pyrethrin rinse, although shampooing with the gamma isomer of hexachlorocyclohexane is also effective. Nits may be removed with a fine comb dipped in vinegar.

Body lice are most easily treated by a good bath and a change in clothing. Antibiotics may be prescribed for the secondary bacterial infection.

PTHIRUS (OR *PHTHIRUS*) *PUBIS* (PUBIC LOUSE)

This organism (Figs. 19.23, 19.24) is shorter and more compact than the *Pediculus humanus* var. *corporis* or *capitis* and prefers only short hair, usually pubic hair.

• PATHOGENESIS •

The disease is transmitted easily by sexual intercourse. It may also be transferred by inanimate objects, since the louse may remain viable for several hours without the presence of a host. Perhaps this is one of the few diseases that in fact may be caught from a toilet seat.

• CLINICAL FEATURES •

Pruritus is the usual clinical feature. Careful examination discerns the nits on pubic hair and sometimes on other short hair—axillary hair, eyebrows, eyelashes (Fig. 19.25), and in males, body hair. In infestations of long standing, the saliva of the organism partially digests hemoglobin, leaving characteristic blue maculas (maculae ceruleae) in the inguinal areas.

• DIAGNOSIS AND TREATMENT •

Diagnosis is made by finding the organism or its eggs (Fig. 19.26). Other causes of itching localized to the genitalia include contact dermatitis, irritant dermatitis, candidiasis, and lichen simplex chronicus.

The preferred treatment is the synthetic pyrethrin compounds. In women, limited treatment of affected areas is sufficient. In men, treatment must include all involved body hair. Eyebrows and the nape of the neck may require treatment. All close contacts of both partners must be treated.

MYIASIS

Flies usually cause disease by biting, but myiasis is a disease form in which the larvae of a fly burrow into the flesh in order to obtain nutrients (Fig. 19.27). Animal hosts are most common, but humans are sometimes accidental hosts. In the United States, *Dermatobia hominis* (botfly) is the most common organism.

• PATHOGENESIS •

Dermatobia hominis requires the flesh of a warm-blooded mammal, usually a cow, to mature. The gravid fly lays its eggs on the underside of the mosquito Psorophora. In turn, as the mosquito attacks its host, the eggs hatch and the larvae burrow into the flesh of the host. The fly must go through four instars, or stages, before emerging from the animal host and dropping to the ground. As the fly grows through these stages, an inflammatory reaction develops.

Another form of this disease, cuterbrid myiasis, also occurs in North America. The fly lays eggs in soil, and humans are attacked while sitting or lying in the affected soil. A similar pattern of infestation occurs with the Tombu fly (*Cordylobia anthropophagia*) in Africa.

Maggots (fly larvae) may also be found in areas of necrotic tissue, such as a foot that has lost its arterial supply because of diabetic arterial disease (Fig. 19.28). This type of "passive housekeeping" involving maggots was used in the past for debridement of necrotic ulcers.

• CLINICAL FEATURES •

The accompanying inflammation caused by the maturing fly within the skin is called a warble. Since *Dermatobia hominis* is an air-breathing fly, an air tube is seen in the center of the warble. At this opening, single or multiple erythematous papules are noted (Fig. 19.29). The lesion most resembles a large abscess but is solid and nonfluctuant. The patient may complain of pain or itching and, sometimes, of movement under the skin. Larvae may invade vital structures such as the eye and sinuses.

• DIAGNOSIS AND TREATMENT •

The clinical features suggest the diagnosis. When there is doubt, the lesion can be opened surgically, revealing the organism.

Treatment involves incision of the lesions and removal of the larval forms or covering the opening with a layer of fat, such as petrolatum, to trap the migrating larvae. An untreated infestation ends with the expulsion of the fourth instar after about 4 weeks.

TUNGA PENETRANS

Tunga penetrans, the burrowing flea often called the "jigger," is found in both the eastern and western hemispheres. It is the smallest known flea, only 1 mm in length.

• PATHOGENESIS •

After mating, the female flea burrows into the keratin of the palms and soles and around nails to lay eggs. After the eggs have matured in (7 to 14 days), the cloacal (rear) end of the flea protrudes, and the eggs are released in another 7 to 10 days. The mother flea dies in the process and may be extruded with the maturing keratin or remain in situ.

• CLINICAL FEATURES •

In tungiasis, the keratin of the palms, soles, and periungual area contains black dots that, on first examination, may resemble warts. As the fleas enlarge, the swelling is characteristic (Fig. 19.30). The strands of released eggs indicate the diagnosis.

• DIAGNOSIS AND TREATMENT •

Opening the swollen areas with a scalpel blade produces the diagnostic findings of strings of eggs. Differential diagnosis includes warts, molluscum, and foreign bodies.

Surgical debridement of the affected areas is the best treatment. Foreign body granulomas from portions of retained flea may require further surgery or steroids. If secondary bacterial infection follows, antibiotics and local treatment are needed.

Unproven Insect Disease

The following disorders are included for completeness, although they are not proven to be related, in fact, to actual contact with insects.

ITCHY RED BUMP DISEASE

Red bumps resembling bites appear on the skin. Excoriation and secondary bacterial infection may occur.

• PATHOGENESIS •

Pathogenesis is unknown, but the disorder is thought to be due to unidentified insects.

• CLINICAL FEATURES •

Its sole clinical feature is the persistent recurrence of crops of bite-like lesions, often with excoriated surfaces.

• DIAGNOSIS AND TREATMENT •

The most important part of the workup is the search for other insects and mites that may be responsible, such as fleas, bedbugs, lice, scabies, cheylietella, bird mites, animal mites, and grain mites. Itching may be caused by foreign bodies, such as fiberglass, or internal disorders, such as dry skin or lymphomas, although these disorders usually lack the characteristic primary bite-like lesions. A careful history and detailed search for insects may be helpful. Examination of grooming material from pets may demonstrate unsuspected animal mites. Disappearance of the condition when the affected individual leaves home for a vacation is a strong clue that something at home may be responsible.

The best treatment is to identify and eliminate the offending insect. If this is impossible, blind treatment for scabies is warranted. Symptomatic treatment with lubricants, topical anesthetics, and antihistamines may be beneficial. Systemic steroids may be necessary in extreme cases.

DELUSIONS OF PARASITOSIS

This is thought to be a form of paranoid schizophrenia. Patients imagine the presence of insects on or in their bodies and often submit evidence, such as small bits of material on cellophane tape. Usually the material represents crusts and bits of fiber.

• PATHOGENESIS •

The cause is unknown, although organic brain syndrome, drug-induced toxicity, and vitamin deficiency have been implicated. In a few, the delusions may be brought on by a loss of vision and subsequent crawling sensation on the skin. Such patients are not truly delusional and are easily reassured.

• CLINICAL FEATURES •

There is usually evidence of severe self mutilation—deep excoriations or puncture wounds to "let out" the presumptive cause. The story is often very detailed and supported by a partner. Patients may resist aggressively any attempt to disprove their theory.

• DIAGNOSIS AND TREATMENT •

Most dermatologists will recognize the inconsistencies of the disease pattern. The sharp edges of excoriated skin, the presence of deep penetrating disease adjacent to normal skin, and the affect of the patient are often diagnostic. Any attempt to refer to a psychiatrist is usually refused vigorously. Differential diagnosis of "itchy red bump disease" must be considered in every case.

The best treatment would be psychiatric referral. However, most patients are unwilling and many psychiatrists refuse to accept these patients. The dermatologist, therefore, often must either discharge the patient or undertake treatment. Thioridazine at 25 to 75 mg per day helps some patients. Pimozide in doses of 2 to 8 mg per day has also proved beneficial (11, 12).

REFERENCES

1. Stafford CT, Hoffman DR, Rhoades RB. Allergy to imported fire ants. South Med J 1989;82:1520.
2. deShazo RD, et al. Dermal hypersensitivity reactions to imported fire ants. J Allergy Clin Immun 1984;74:841.
3. Melanby K. Man's reaction to mosquito bites. Nature 1946;158:554.
4. Gendron BP. *Loxosceles reclusa* envenomation. Am J Emerg Med 1990;8:51.
5. King LE, Rees RS. Dapsone treatment of a brown recluse bite. JAMA 1983;250:648.
6. Alexander JO. Arthropods and human skin. New York: Springer-Verlag, 1984:374.
7. Arlian LG, Estes SA, Vyszenski-Moher DL. Prevalence of *Sarcoptes scabei* in the homes and nursing homes of scabetic patients. J Am Acad Dermatol 1988;19:806.
8. Taplin D, et al. Permethrin 5% dermal cream: A new treatment for scabies. J Am Acad Dermatol 1989;20:134.
9. Friedman SJ. Lindane neurotoxic reaction in nonbullous congenital ichthyosiform erythroderma. Arch Dermatol 1987;123:1056.
10. Mellanby K. Epidemiology of scabies. In: Orkin MI, Mailbach HI, Parish

LC, Schwartzman RM, eds. Scabies and pediculosis. Philadelphia: JB
Lippincott, 1977.

11. Matas M, Robinson C. Diagnosis and treatment of monosymptomatic
hypochondriacal psychosis in chronic renal failure. Canadian J Psych
1988;33:748.

12. Ungvari G, Vladar K. Pimozide treatment for delusion of infection. Act
Nerv Super (Praha) 1986;28:103.

ANNOTATED BIBLIOGRAPHY

Alexander JO. Arthropods and human skin. New York: Springer-Verlag, 1984.
    The best single reference on arthropods for dermatologists.
Binford CH, Connor DH. Pathology of tropical and extraordinary diseases.
Washington, DC: Armed Forces Institute of Pathology, 1976.
    A classic reference containing descriptions of many of the diseases men-
tioned in this chapter, as well as many other infectious diseases. Although
this is a pathology text, there are many clinical pearls.
Elgart ML, ed. Insect bites and stings. Dermatol Clin 1990;8(2):219.
    A recent summary of many of these diseases.
Orkin MI, Mailbach HI, Parish LC, Schwartzman RM, eds. Scabies and pediculosis. Philadelphia: JB Lippincott, 1977.
    A wonderful reference to scabies and lice, including work by Mellanby.
    Treatment is somewhat dated.
Spach DH, et al. Tick-borne diseases in the United States. N Engl J Med
1993;329:936.
    An up-to-date review of tick-borne diseases.

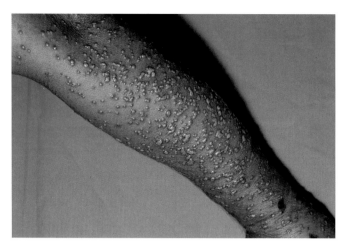

Figure 19.1.   Fire ant bites. Multiple pustules on arm. (Courtesy of Dr. Lee T. Nesbitt, Jr.)

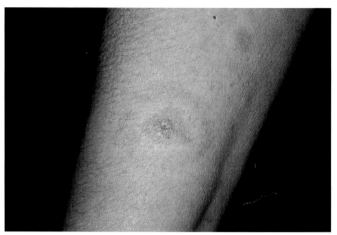

Figure 19.2.   Gnat bites. Cutaneous reaction with surrounding annular erythema. (Courtesy of Dr. Lee T. Nesbitt, Jr.)

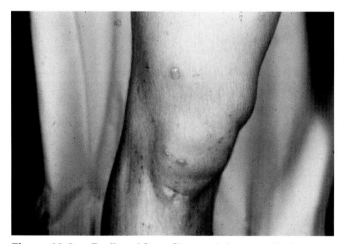

Figure 19.3.   Bedbug bites. Characteristic grouped lesions.

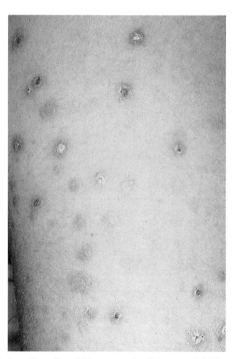

Figure 19.4.   Dog flea (*Ctenocephalides canis*) bites in a child.

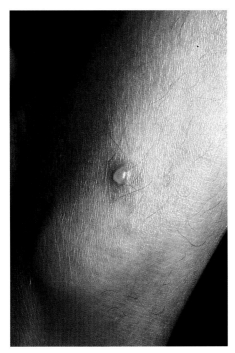

Figure 19.5.   Dog flea bites. Bullous reaction. (Courtesy of Dr. Lee T. Nesbitt Jr.)

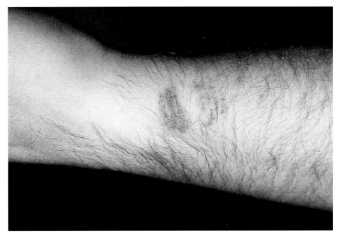

Figure 19.6.   *Megalopyge opercularis* sting. Local reaction. (Courtesy of Dr. Ted Rosen)

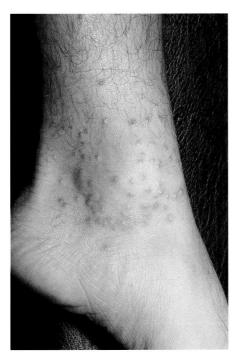

Figure 19.7.   Chigger bites. Around ankle: early stage. (Courtesy of Dr. Lee T. Nesbitt, Jr.)

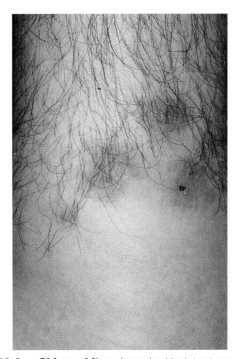

Figure 19.8.   Chigger bites. Around ankle: late stage.

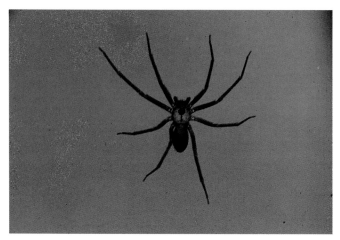

Figure 19.9.   Brown recluse spider, *Loxosceles reclusa.* Note the violin-like marking on the back of the thorax. (Courtesy of Dr. P.N. Morgan)

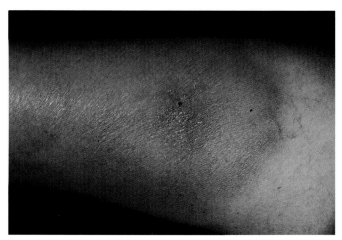

Figure 19.10.   Brown recluse spider. Necrotic brown recluse spider bite: early stage.

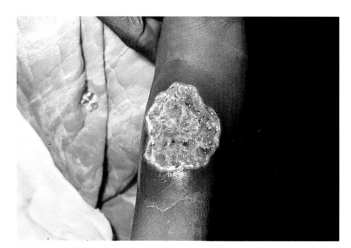

Figure 19.11.   Brown recluse spider. Necrotic brown recluse spider bite: late stage. (Courtesy of Dr. Lee T. Nesbitt, Jr.)

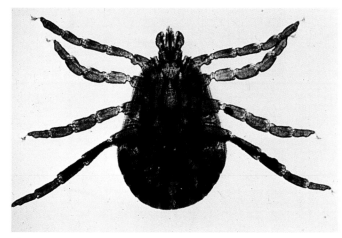

Figure 19.12.   *Dermacentor andersoni,* the wood tick. In hard ticks, mouth parts extend beyond a chitinous body.

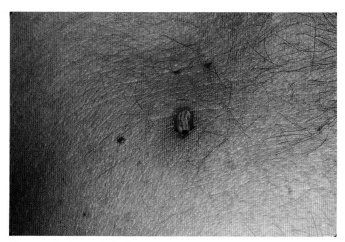

Figure 19.13.   Soft tick embedded in skin. The mouth parts, which protrude from the anterior portion of the body, are not visible.

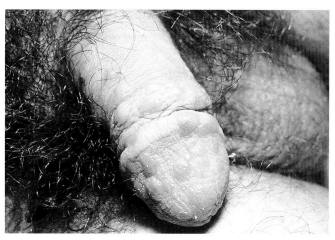

Figure 19.14.   Scabies. Papular lesions. (Courtesy of Dr. Lee T. Nesbitt, Jr.)

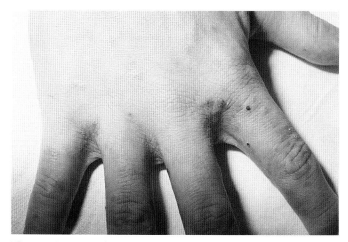

Figure 19.15.   Scabies. Pruritic papular lesions of the webbed spaces of the fingers (Courtesy of Dr. Lee T. Nesbitt, Jr.)

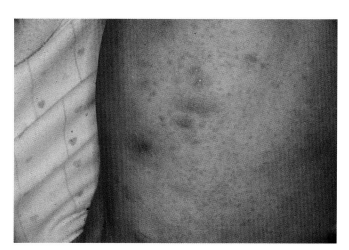

Figure 19.16.   Scabies. Erythematous papules on the trunk. Burrows not readily visible.

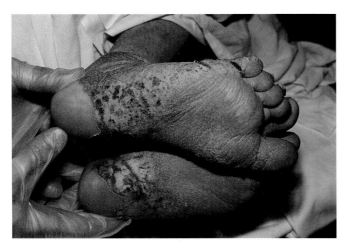

Figure 19.17.   Norwegian scabies. In an institutionalized patient with Down's syndrome. (Courtesy of Dr. Charles Sanders)

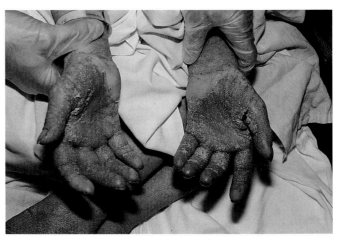

Figure 19.18.   Norwegian scabies. In an institutionalized patient with Down's syndrome. (Courtesy of Dr. Charles Sanders)

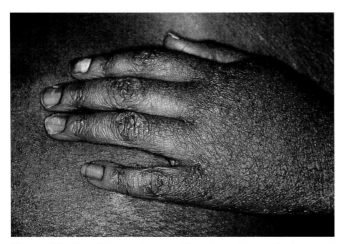

Figure 19.19.   Norwegian scabies. Itchy, dry eruption in a renal transplant patient. (From Elgart ML. Ant, bee, and wasp stings. Dermatol Clin 1990;8(2):253.)

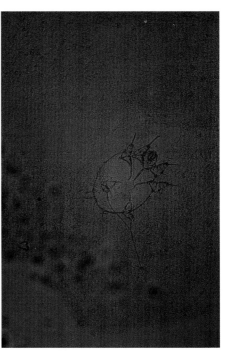

Figure 19.20.   Scabies nymph. Shows absence of the last pair of legs. (From Elgart ML. Ant, bee, and wasp stings. Dermatol Clin 1990;8(2):253.)

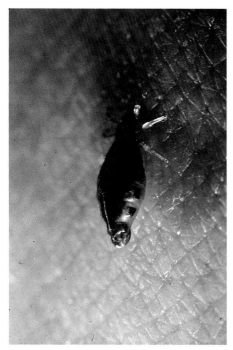

Figure 19.21. ***Pediculus humanus* var.** *corporis.* The body louse shown in the act of feeding. The head louse is similar but smaller. (From Elgart ML. Ant, bee, and wasp stings. Dermatol Clin 1990;8(2):219.)

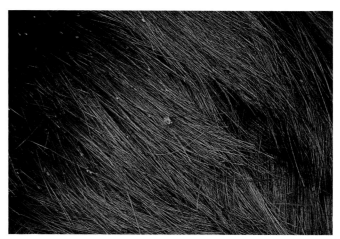

Figure 19.22.   Head lice. Head lice and nits on hair shafts. (Courtesy of Dr. Lee T. Nesbitt, Jr.)

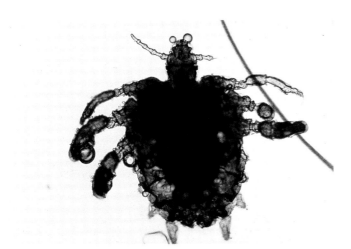

Figure 19.23.   Adult female pubic louse. (From Elgart ML. Ant, bee, and wasp stings. Dermatol Clin 1990;8(2):219.)

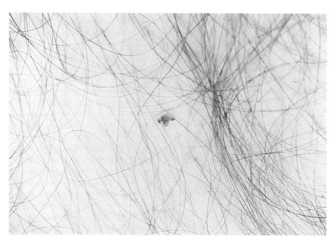

Figure 19.24.   Pubic louse. Pubic louse on the skin.

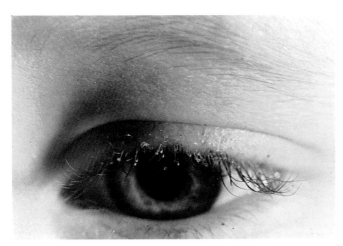

Figure 19.25.   Pediculosis. Nits on eyelashes. (Courtesy of Dr. Lee T. Nesbitt, Jr.)

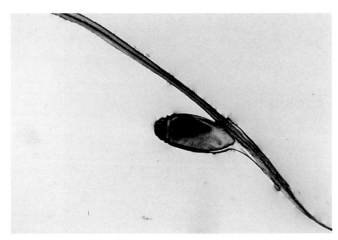

Figure 19.26.   Pubic louse nit. Operculum is intact and larva is probably alive. The nit of the head louse is similar. (From Elgart ML. Ant, bee, and wasp stings. Dermatol Clin 1990(2);8:219.)

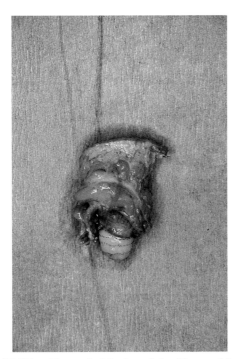

Figure 19.27.   *Dermatobia hominis.* Biopsy of the larva of *Dermatobia hominis* in the skin. (From Elgart ML. Ant, bee, and wasp stings. Dermatol Clin 1990;(2)8:237.)

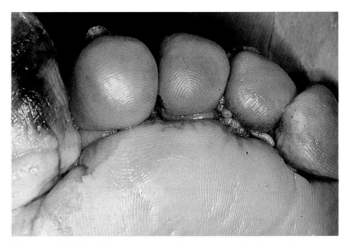

Figure 19.28.   *Musca domestica* maggots. Maggots from the common housefly attacking the necrotic foot of a diabetic patient. (From Elgart ML. Ant, bee, and wasp stings. Dermatol Clin 1990;(2)8:237.)

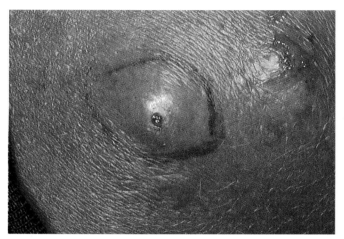

Figure 19.29. **Two *Dermatobia hominis* (botfly) warbles.**
Botfly warbles showing tiny spiracle at the apex of the papule. (From
Elgart ML. Ant, bee, and wasp stings. Dermatol Clin 1990;8(2):237.)

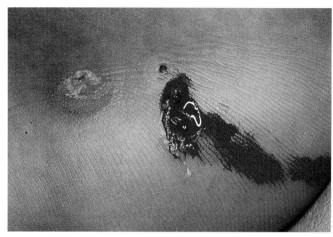

Figure 19.30. **Tungiasis.** Tungiasis in an American traveling in
Central America.

CHAPTER 20

Skin Infections in the Immunocompromised Host— NonHIV

RICHARD ALLEN JOHNSON, MARC AVRAM and EDWARD CHAN

During the past decade, the number of immunocompromised individuals has increased tremendously as a result of two major factors: the increasing use of immunosuppressive therapies for both malignancies and autoimmune disorders and the advent of human immunodeficiency (HIV) disease. The acquired immunocompromised state may be a consequence either of disease states (e.g., HIV, lymphoreticular malignancy, diabetes mellitus, collagen vascular disease, chronic inflammatory disorders), or therapies (e.g., long-term corticosteroid therapy, cytotoxic chemotherapy, cyclosporine, total bone marrow irradiation, antithymocyte and antilymphocyte globulins). These conditions accord a specific profile of immunologic deficits to the immunocompromised patient.

Splenectomized persons, for example, are at high risk for fulminant infections caused by *Streptococcus pneumoniae* (Figs. 20.1, 20.2), *Haemophilus influenzae*, and *Neisseria meningitidis*, the risk being higher in children than in adults. These individuals are also at increased risk for fulminant intraerythrocyte protozoal infections with *Babesia* and *Plasmodium malariae*.

The skin plays a vital role in the immunocompromised host. It is an important barrier to infection whose defenses may be easily breached, thus rendering these patients susceptible to both primary and opportunistic pathogens, most commonly bacteria (Figs. 20.3–20.5), environmental mycobacteria, fungi, viruses, and algae. Even pathogens with low invasive ability can cause primary cutaneous infections. Skin infections in and of themselves often produce morbidity and death and reportedly occur in 22% to 33% of severely immunocompromised patients. In addition, a defect in immunosurveillance in the skin may lead to premalignant, malignant, and inflammatory disorders.

Many patients have more than one type of immune system impairment, and specific defects in host immunity may present different profiles of cutaneous disease (Table 20.1). The immunocompromised host suffers not only from the typical skin

Table 20.1. Cutaneous Manifestations of Specific Defects in Host Immunity[a]

Defect in host immunity	Associated conditions	Common cutaneous manifestations
Cell-mediated immunity	Corticosteroid therapy, organ transplants, lymphoma	Infections (herpesviruses, *Mycobacteria*, *Nocardia*, *Cryptococcus neoformans*, *Histoplasma capsulatum*, *Coccidioides immitis*, *Toxoplasma gondii*); neoplasms (squamous cell carcinoma, Kaposi's sarcoma); drug reactions
Granulocyte number or function	Cytotoxic chemotherapy, myeloproliferative disorders	Infection, especially mucosal (*Staphylococcus aureus*, *Pseudomonas aeruginosa*, *Candida* species, *Aspergillus* species); mucormycosis; drug reactions
Humoral immunity	B-cell malignancies, acquired hypoglobulinemia	Infection (enteroviruses, *Neisseria meningitides*)
Complement	Acquired hypocomplementemia	Infection (*Neisseria* species)

[a]From Johnson RA, Dover JS. Cutaneous manifestations of human immunodeficiency virus disease. In: Fitzpatrick TB, et al. Dermatology in general medicine. 4th ed. New York: McGraw-Hill, 1993.

Table 20.2. Patterns of Cutaneous Disease in the NonHIV-infected Immunocompromised Host[a]

Pattern of cutaneous disease	Associated disorders
Cellulitis	Bacterial infection (Enterobacteriaceae, *Pseudomonas*, *Legionella micdadei*, anaerobes in patients with neutropenia); fungal infection (cryptococcosis, invasive candidiasis in patients with depressed cell-mediated immunity, disseminated *Aspergillus*, *Alternaria*). Inflammatory disorders such as erythema nodosum and pancreatic panniculitis.
Morbilliform	GM-CSF therapy, cutaneous eruption of lymphocyte recovery, neutrophilic eccrine hidradenitis, aspergillosis
Vesicular	Herpesvirus infections (herpes simplex virus 1 and 2, varicella-zoster virus), bullous impetigo, cryptococcosis, enterovirus, adverse cutaneous drug eruption
Follicular/pustular	Bacterial infection (Gram-positive cocci, *Pseudomonas*); fungal infection (*Candida*, *Coccidioides immitis*, *Trichophyton rubrum*); drug (oral, IV, or topical corticosteroid therapy {acneiform})
Abscess	Bacteria (*Staphylococcus aureus*, *Nocardia*); fungal (*Candida*, *C. immitis*); drug (IM pentamidine)
Verrucous/hyperkeratosis	Mycobacterial infection (tuberculosis verrucosa cutis); verruca vulgaris; crusted scabies
Hypertrichosis	Drug (cyclosporine A)
Wound infection	Bacterial infection (*Staphylococcus aureaus*, *Pseudomonas*); fungal infection (primary *Aspergillus* infection at inoculation site, mucormycosis)
Venous access device	Bacterial infection (*Staphylococcus aureus*, *Pseudomonas*)
Pruritus without rash	Drug (Tacrolimus, formerly FK506)

[a] From Brooks RG, et al. Am J Med 1985, 79:412.

diseases of the immunocompetent host, but also from atypical presentations and more difficult clinical courses (Table 20.2). Depending on host responses, infection can remain localized or extend into adjacent tissues, tissue planes, lymphatics, or blood vessels to produce life-threatening systemic infection. Conversely, infection may disseminate via blood to many organs, including the skin (Fig. 20.6), which can become a window to underlying internal disease. The prompt diagnosis of cutaneous disease in these patients, therefore, becomes both crucial and challenging.

The accessibility of mucocutaneous lesions makes lesional skin biopsy a highly valuable diagnostic test. In most cases, specimens should be processed for histological and microbiological examinations as outlined in Table 20.3. Infections of the cutaneous and subcutaneous tissue can be categorized variously by organism, underlying disease, mode of onset of illness, or pathophysiologic events (Table 20.1).

This chapter is a guide to the diagnosis and management of the major cutaneous diseases seen in the nonHIV-infected immunocompromised host.

Bacterial Infections

PSEUDOMONAS AERUGINOSA INFECTION

• PATHOGENESIS •

Pseudomonas aeruginosa sepsis in the immunocompromised host results in cutaneous lesions in 3% to 6% of cases. The organism is present in soil and water. It is a transient member of the normal skin flora on the external ear, axillae, and anogenital and periumbilical regions. In the normal host, the growth of *Pseudomonas* is inhibited by the resident Gram-positive organisms on the skin. In neutropenic patients, *Pseudomonas* gains access into deep cutaneous structures via adnexal structures, such as hair follicles. In patients with extensive thermal burns, it enters through devitalized skin, with resultant local infection and septicemia.

• CLINICAL FEATURES •

Ecthyma gangrenosum (Fig. 20.7) is the most common and distinct cutaneous pseudomonal infection occurring in the immunocompromised host. A septic vasculitis at the portal of entry results in a progressively enlarging necrotic plaque (Figs. 20.8, 20.9). Although most commonly found in the normally moist anogenital region and axillae (Figs. 20.10, 20.11), lesions may occur anywhere on the skin. Because of the vascular invasion associated with pseudomonal infection, bacteremia occurs early from the infected skin site. Petechial and ecchymotic eruptions may subsequently develop (Fig. 20.12).

• DIAGNOSIS AND DIFFERENTIAL DIAGNOSIS •

Bacteriological confirmation is made by direct culture and Gram's stains of biopsied lesions or from cultures of blood in patients with ecthyma gangrenosum. The differential diagnosis includes purpura fulminans, aspergillosis, atypical mycobacterial infections, and deep fungal infections.

• TREATMENT AND CLINICAL COURSE •

Appropriate antibiotics are mandatory, pending results of cultures in clinically suspicious lesions in an immunocompro-

Table 20.3. Processing of Lesional Skin Specimens in Immunocompromised Patients with Opportunistic Infections[a]

I. Laboratory identification of causative organisms from skin specimens (lesional skin biopsy, curettage, wound drainage)

A. Direct preparations for microscopic examination

1. Wet mount for fungal elements
   a. KOH
   b. Saline solution
   c. India ink

2. Stained smears
   a. Gram's stain
   b. Acid-fast stain

B. Dermatopathologic characteristics of infecting organisms

1. Actinomycetes: Delicate filaments <1 μm; with or without granules (*Nocardia, Actinomyces*)
2. Spherules: Thick-walled cells with endospores (*Coccidioides immitis*)
3. Zygomycetes: Aseptate hyphae; 10–15 μm (Mucoraceae: *Absidia, Mucor,* and *Rhizopus*)
4. Pseudohyphae: Hyphae with indentations at septa (*Candida*)
5. Yeasts
   a. Small: 1–3 μm (*Histoplasma capsulatum*)
   b. Medium: 2–5 μm (*Candida albicans*)
   c. Large
      i. 8–20 μm (*Blastomyces dermatitidis*)
      ii. 8–40 μm (*Paracoccidioides brasiliensis*)
      iii. 5–30 μm (*Cryptotoccus neoformans*)

II. Isolation of causative agents: Cultures of skin specimens

A. Aerobic and anaerobic bacteria

1. Thioglycollate broth
2. Sheep blood agar

B. Atypical mycobacteria (25°–37°C)

1. Löwenstein-Jensen medium
2. Middlebrook 7H10 agar

C. Fungal

1. Sabouraud's dextrose agar
2. Mycosal agar

D. Viral (holding media)

1. HSV
2. VZV
3. CMV

[a] KOH, potassium hydroxide; HSV, herpes simplex virus; VZV, varicella-zoster virus; CMV, cytomegalovirus

mised host. The prognosis of invasive *Pseudomonas* infection is best correlated with the severity of the underlying disease. Patients with severe prolonged neutropenia have a poor prognosis; however, availability of granulocyte-colony-stimulating factor (G-CSF) has improved their response to treatment.

NOCARDIOSIS

• PATHOGENESIS •

Nocardiosis is caused by the aerobic actinomycete *Nocardia asteroides*, which produces primary disease in the lungs with frequent subsequent hematogenous spread, most often to the brain. The skin is involved in 30% of disseminated nocardiosis. Primary cutaneous nocardiosis is rare.

• CLINICAL FEATURES •

Sinus tracts on the trunk arising from underlying deep abscesses are the most common skin finding. A sporotrichoid pattern (linear nodules following lymphatics) may occur as well.

• DIAGNOSIS AND DIFFERENTIAL DIAGNOSIS •

Lesional skin biopsy for Gram's stain and modified acid-fast stain demonstrates Gram-positive, partially acid-fast organisms. Cultures on Sabouraud's glucose agar at 37° C demonstrate the organism after 3 to 4 days. Atypical mycobacteria, sporotrichosis, other bacterial infections, and deep fungal infections may mimic the cutaneous lesions of nocardiosis.

• TREATMENT AND CLINICAL COURSE •

The prognosis without treatment is poor, primarily due to abscesses in the brain and lung. Incision and drainage are performed, and antibiotics, especially trimethoprim-sulfamethoxazole, are given. Minocycline, amikacin, erythromycin, and dapsone have been used as well.

Mycobacterial Infections

TUBERCULOSIS

Tuberculosis continues to be a major infectious disease in developing countries, where many persons have subclinical immunocompromise due to other infectious diseases or malnutrition. The incidence of tuberculosis has risen significantly in the United States, however, during the past decade. For a thorough description of disease features, see Chapters 21 and 11.

ATYPICAL MYCOBACTERIAL INFECTIONS

A variety of ubiquitous environmental mycobacterial species (a.k.a. atypical *Mycobacterium* or *Mycobacterium* other than tuberculosis or MOTT) cause invasive infection, usually in immunocompromised persons. Many environmental mycobacteria are capable of causing primary cutaneous infection, which may disseminate hematogenously via lymphatics or in the setting of compromised host defenses. Table 20.4 describes the clinical features and diagnosis of these lesions.

Treatment is discussed in Chapter 12.

Fungal Infections

Fungal infections in the immunocompromised host are classified by the depth of their tissue invasion, i.e., superficial or deep. Superficial fungal infections are caused by dermatophytes, which infect only keratinizing tissue such as skin, nails, and hair, and *Candida* species such as *C. albicans* (Fig. 20.13), which are discussed with regard to HIV disease in Chapter 21. *Candida* species are also capable of deep tissue invasion, as dis-

Table 20.4. Atypical Mycobacterial Infections

Mycobacterium	History	Physical Examination	Course
Group I *M. marinum*	More common in immunocompetent persons. Disseminated hematogenously in immunocompromised persons.	Verrucous nodule at inoculation site; ± nodular lymphangitis. Multiple disseminated ulceronodules in immunocompromised host.	Majority cured with antimicrobial treatment.
M. kansasii	Occurs in immunocompetent persons. Disseminates in immunocompromised host.	Scrofula-like lymphadenitis, sporotrichoid lesions. Tuberculosis-like pneumonia, osteomyelitis, tenosynovitis.	Poor prognosis if associated with advanced immuno-deficiency
Group III *M. haemophilum*	History of lymphoma, immunosuppressive therapy after renal transplant. HIV disease. Few cases in immunocompetent children. Mode of transmission poorly understood.	Ulcerating cutaneous nodules. Multiple lesions on extremities overlying joints; less common on face and trunk. Violaceous, fluctuant, 0.5–2.0 cm. Lesions enlarge and drain. Painful. Systemic infection. Lesions occur at site of lower skin temperature.	Prognosis poor because of advanced immunodeficiency and underlying disease.
Group IV *M. avium complex* (MAC)	Currently, the most commonly isolated species of *Mycobacterium* in clinical laboratories. Ubiquitous in environment.	Rarely associated with skin lesions. Cervical lymphadenitis and scrofuloderma. Reportedly causes granulomatous synovitis, osteomyelitis, meningitis, pericarditis.	Depends on severity of underlying immunodeficiency.
M. fortuitum-chelonae complex	Post-cardiac surgery; injury; post-infection. Neutropenia.	Soft-tissue infection; subcutaneous abscesses. Disseminated disease in immunocompromised host.	Majority of cases respond to treatment.

cussed below. *Trichosporon beigelii* not only causes infection of the hair shafts, white piedra, but also causes invasive infection, trichosporosis, in the immunocompromised host.

For a complete discussion of fungal infections see Chapters 14 and 15.

Superficial Mycoses

DERMATOPHYTOSIS

Dermatophytosis in the immunocompromised host, especially in solid organ transplant recipients, can be extensive with involvement of the trunk and extremities. Facial involvement, or tinea facialis, is often misdiagnosed as seborrheic dermatitis, atopic dermatitis, or lupus erythematosus. Extensive tinea corporis may be misdiagnosed as seborrheic dermatitis or psoriasis vulgaris.

PITYRIASIS VERSICOLOR

Pityriasis versicolor (tinea versicolor) is more prevalent under conditions of increased heat and humidity, as well as immunocompromise. The etiologic agent, *Pityrosporum ovale*, may also gain access to deeper structures via venous access devices, causing local infection as well as fungemia.

SUPERFICIAL CANDIDIASIS

A discussion of superficial candidiasis in the immunocompromised host appears in Chapter 20.

Deep Invasive Mycoses

SYSTEMIC INVASIVE CANDIDIASIS

• PATHOGENESIS •

The incidence of systemic invasive candidiasis (SIC) has increased during the past few decades. It is most commonly caused by *Candida albicans, C. tropicalis,* and less often, *C. krusei* and other species. The yeasts gain access to deeper structures by initially invading and colonizing the gastrointestinal tract, intravenous device access sites (Fig. 20.14), and intravenous drug injection sites. *Candida parapsilosis* and *Torulopsis glabrata* colonize intravenous device access sites, and, less often, disseminate to organs, such as the kidney or lung.

• CLINICAL FEATURES •

Cutaneous lesions occur in 10% to 15% of patients with SIC, presenting as small (5–10 mm) papules or nodules, at times hemorrhagic (Fig. 20.15). A newly described syndrome of hepatosplenic or chronic progressive candidiasis occurs in patients recovering from neutropenia who have been treated with broad-spectrum antibacterial agents, and often, with empirically administered amphotericin B.

• DIAGNOSIS AND DIFFERENTIAL DIAGNOSIS •

Diagnosis of SIC is made by isolation of *Candida* species on blood culture and/or sterile site culture or smear; antigen detection in urine or serum is still experimental. Greater than 80% of neutropenic patients with *C. albicans* or *C. tropicalis* fungemia are determined to have had SIC at autopsy.

• TREATMENT AND CLINICAL COURSE •

It is therefore recommended that fungemia patients be treated with amphotericin B, the response rate being 50% to 75%. Overall, the prognosis of SIC is poor because of difficulties in diagnosis and associated underlying granulocytopenia. Use of prophylactic intravenous miconazole in febrile granulocytopenic patients and granulocyte-macrophage-colony stimulating factor (GM-CSF) as well as better detection of *Candida* antigen may improve the prognosis.

TRICHOSPORONOSIS

• PATHOGENESIS •

Trichosporonosis is a systemic infection in the immunocompromised host with the fungus *Trichosporon beigelii*, the cause of a superficial hair shaft infection, white piedra. Factors predisposing to trichosporonosis include cytotoxic chemotherapy-induced granulocytopenia, corticosteroids, prosthetic valve surgery, hemochromatosis, and HIV disease.

• CLINICAL FEATURES •

Onset of acute infection is sudden, evolving over days, and is associated with skin lesions, fungemia, pulmonary infiltrates, renal involvement, and hypotension. Chronic trichosporonosis extends over several months and is characterized by progressive debilitation, persistent fever, hepatosplenomegaly, and elevated values in liver function tests.

• DIAGNOSIS AND DIFFERENTIAL DIAGNOSIS •

Diagnosis is made by demonstration of the fungus in lesional biopsy specimens, with confirmation by culture of the specimen or blood. Dermatopathology of lesional biopsy specimens show pseudohyphae, the presence of numerous rectangular arthroconidia, and a few blastoconidia. Trichosporonosis must be differentiated clinically and histologically from disseminated infection with species of *Candida, Aspergillus,* and members of the family Mucoraceae.

• TREATMENT AND CLINICAL COURSE •

To date, the prognosis of patients with disseminated *Trichosporon beigelii* has been very poor. The keystone of ther-

apy is early diagnosis followed by intravenous amphotericin B, and correction of underlying neutropenia. Hopefully, with increasing awareness of this emerging pathogen, more patients with trichosporonosis can be salvaged.

FUSARIUM SPECIES

• PATHOGENESIS •

Portals of entry include the paranasal sinuses, lungs, and skin. Neutropenia is the most common predisposing cause.

• CLINICAL FEATURES •

Fusarium species infection is associated with a high incidence of skin and subcutaneous lesions. Clinically, erythematous nodules with central necrosis are seen.

• DIAGNOSIS AND DIFFERENTIAL DIAGNOSIS •

Diagnosis is usually made easily by isolation of the organism on blood culture. *Fusarium* infection must be differentiated from *Aspergillus* infection.

• TREATMENT AND CLINICAL COURSE •

The optimal treatment of invasive *Fusarium* infections is amphotericin B, granulocyte transfusions, and in some individuals, granulocyte-macrophage-colony stimulating factor (GM-CSF). The prognosis is often poor and directly correlated with the severity and persistence of granulocytopenia.

ASPERGILLOSIS

• PATHOGENESIS •

Aspergillus species are saprophytes found in soil, decaying vegetation, and water. *Aspergillus fumigatus* and *A. flavus* are the two most common pathogens causing infections in immunocompromised hosts. Infection results from inhalation of spores or inoculation of spores through breaks in the integumentary barrier. Prolonged granulocytopenia is associated with the greatest risk for invasive aspergillosis; other risk groups include solid organ transplant recipients, patients on high-dose corticosteroid therapy, and persons with white blood cell functional defects.

• CLINICAL FEATURES •

Inhalation of *Aspergillus* spores is associated with a variety of bronchopulmonary infections, including allergic bronchopulmonary aspergillosis, aspergilloma, and invasive aspergillosis. The majority of cases of extrapulmonary aspergillosis occur via hematogenous dissemination from a primary pulmonary focus.

Primary cutaneous aspergillosis has occurred following the application of contaminated dressing to surgical wounds or venous access sites. The lesions begin as erythematous nodules that quickly ulcerate, forming a central eschar. This can lead to disseminated disease.

• DIAGNOSIS AND DIFFERENTIAL DIAGNOSIS •

Lesional biopsy specimens with "touch preparation" demonstrate narrow septated hyphae, branched at acute angles. Blood cultures are usually negative. *Aspergillus* invades blood vessels, causing infarction within the infected tissue. It must be differentiated from mucormycosis.

• TREATMENT AND CLINICAL COURSE •

Invasive aspergillosis is treated with high-dose intravenous amphotericin B alone or in combination with flucytosine. The prognosis is usually poor, depending on the rapidity of diagnosis and rate of recovery from granulocytopenia.

MUCORMYCOSIS

• PATHOGENESIS •

Mucormycosis is caused by genuses of the family *Mucoraceae* (i.e., *Absidia, Mucor,* and *Rhizopus*), which are found on fruits and vegetables. Mucormycosis is typically an airborne infection in immunocompromised patients. Clinical disease resembles aspergillosis in that both infections are characterized by invasion of large blood vessels with resultant infarctive lesions. Invasive mucormycosis is associated with ketoacidosis and defects in macrophage or neutrophil function and is seen mostly in the setting of uncontrolled diabetes mellitus, neutropenia, and high-dose corticosteroid therapy.

• CLINICAL FEATURES •

Several clinical patterns of mucormycosis are seen, including rhinocerebral and pulmonary infection and, less commonly, infection primarily involving the brain, kidneys, liver, heart, and gastrointestinal tract. Hematogenously disseminated infection may follow primary infection at any of these sites.

Cutaneous mucormycosis occurs primarily in extensive thermal burns, sites of minor trauma (Figs. 20.16, 20.17), or under contaminated dressings (e.g., Elastoplast), secondarily via extension from an underlying infection (i.e., rhinocerebral), or by hematogenous dissemination.

Cutaneous mucormycosis is characterized by a rapidly extending, necrotizing infection arising at breaks in the epidermis. Extension of infection from underlying periorbital or nasal infection presents as a rapidly spreading cellulitis in a severely toxic patient, associated with gangrene. Patients with early rhinocerebral infection complain of unilateral headache and nasal congestion early in their course. Within a few days, nasal and facial cellulitis extends to the sinuses and orbit, with involvement of cranial nerves and brain. Meningoencephalitis may result, with classic presentation of coma, proptosis, and ophthalmoplegia. In injecting drug users and patients with cancer, cerebral involvement may occur without nasal or facial infection as a result of hematogenous dissemination from a primary pulmonary focus.

• DIAGNOSIS AND DIFFERENTIAL DIAGNOSIS •

Diagnosis is most rapidly and predictably made by demonstrating the organism on a lesional skin biopsy specimen, which histopathologically shows large, broad, nonseptate hyphal forms in a "touch prep," and wide and nonseptate hyphae branched at right angles. The infecting organism is best identified by isolation from infected tissue or blood, rather than pus or exudate. The differential diagnosis includes infections such as aspergillosis in the immunocompromised host, as well as other types of cellulitis, Wegener's granulomatosis, or lethal midline granuloma.

• TREATMENT AND CLINICAL COURSE •

In spite of aggressive therapy, morbidity and mortality are high. Treatment should be directed at correcting underlying conditions. High-dose intravenous amphotericin B and surgical debridement of necrotic tissue are recommended.

MISCELLANEOUS DEEP MYCOSES

A group of deep mycoses—blastomycosis, coccidioidomycosis, cryptococcosis, and histoplasmosis (Figs. 20.18, 20.19)—have a similar epidemiology and pathogenesis. Spores exist in the environment in certain geographic regions and are inhaled into the lungs, where asymptomatic primary pulmonary infection occurs. Infection in the immunocompetent host is usually localized by an intact immune system; however, viable spores persist at the pulmonary focus for decades. In patients with immune compromise, spores can escape confinement and begin to grow, resulting in local pulmonary infection that may disseminate hematogenously to many organ systems. The clinical characteristics of the deep mycoses are outlined in Table 20.5. More information can be found in Chapter 15.

Viral Infections

HERPES GROUP VIRUSES

Human herpes viruses—i.e., herpes simplex virus (HSV) type 1 and type 2, varicella-zoster virus (VZV), cytomegalovirus (CMV), Epstein-Barr virus (EBV), and human herpesvirus-6 (HHV-6)—commonly exist in a latent state of infection in most adults and in many children. With the immunocompromised state, primary herpes virus infection is less common than reactivation of latent virus, which is associated with a broad clinical spectrum of disease.

Herpes Simplex Virus

• PATHOGENESIS AND CLINICAL FEATURES •

Immunocompromised individuals are most likely to experience eczema herpeticum, chronic herpetic ulcers, and disseminated HSV infection. Eczema herpeticum occurs in patients with mild immunocompromise, such as those with atopic dermatitis, extensive thermal burns, cutaneous T-cell lymphoma, or Sézary syndrome. Eczema herpeticum is characterized by multiple erosive lesions in involved skin. The area involved may be relatively minor or widespread and must be differenti-

Table 20.5. Characteristics of Blastomycosis, Coccidioidomycosis, Cryptococcosis, and Histoplasmosis[a]

Findings	Blastomycosis	Coccidioidomycosis	Cryptococcosis	Histoplasmosis
Organism	*Blastomyces dermatitidis*	*Coccidioides immitis*	*Cryptococcus neoformans*	*Histoplasma capsulatum, H. capsulatum* var. *duboisii*
Geographic distribution	U.S. (south-central and midwestern); Canada (central provinces); Africa	Western hemisphere; desert climate; Central and South America	Worldwide	Western hemisphere in river valleys of MS and OH; Africa (*H. capsulatum* var. *duboisii*)
Immuno-compromised state	Transplant recipient (solid organ or BMT); drugs (immunosuppressive, cytotoxic); HIV disease	T-cell dysfunction; transplant recipent (solid organ or BMT); drugs (immunosuppressive, cytotoxic); HIV disease	Transplant recipient (solid organ or BMT); drugs (immunosuppressive, cytotoxic); HIV disease	Transplant recipient (solid organ or BMT); drugs (immunosuppressive, cytotoxic); HIV disease
Clinical findings of skin	Verrucous or ulcerative lesions	Papules, plaques on face; abscess	Papules/nodules; cellulitis	Oropharyngeal ulcers; papules
Other involvement	Lungs, bone	Lungs, meninges	Lungs, meninges	Lungs, liver, spleen, lymph nodes
Histology	Budding yeast with wide base; granulomas and microabscesses	Spherules and endospores; granulomas	Encapsulated yeast cells; minimal cell response	Multiple small yeast within macrophages; granulomas

[a] BMT, bone marrow transplant

ated from systemic dissemination of HSV (Fig. 20.20).

With moderate cell-mediated immune deficiency, herpetic outbreaks may be extensive, deep, and accompanied by much tissue necrosis; progressive eruption of new vesicles may occur around older ulcerative lesions (Fig. 20.21).

Reactivation of HSV occurs in 70% to 80% of HSV-seropositive bone marrow transplant recipients who receive high-dose chemotherapy and total body irradiation. The infection appears a median of 18 days after treatment or 8 days following the transplant. Prior to effective antiviral therapy, 10% of these patients died of disseminated HSV infection.

Chronic herpetic ulcers develop most commonly at sites of herpes labialis or herpes genitalis, but with more persistence of the infection and more enlargement of the involved mucocutaneous site (Figs. 20.22, 20.23). Chronic epithelial breaks combined with chronic neutropenia facilitate invasive infection by a variety of bacteria and fungi.

• DIAGNOSIS AND DIFFERENTIAL DIAGNOSIS •

Diagnosis of HSV infections is most practical by isolation of the virus in culture, detection of HSV antigen in smears from lesional samples, or by identification in HSV-specific histologic stains of lesional skin biopsy specimens. In the majority of patients, HSV infection must be differentiated from VZV infections. Since there is a high likelihood of reactivation of latent HSV infection, seropositive patients are treated with prophylactic acyclovir before bone marrow transplants.

• TREATMENT AND CLINICAL COURSE •

Please see Chapters 17 and 21.

Varicella-zoster virus

• PATHOGENESIS •

The incidence of varicella-zoster in the immunocompromised host is very high, occurring, for example, in 25% of children with acute lymphocytic leukemia. While visceral dissemination is rare in the normal host, it occurs in 8% of untreated immunocompromised hosts with zoster. The severity of varicella-zoster virus (VZV) infection varies depending on the degree of immunocompromise. In the normal host, new lesions continue to form for a mean of 4 days after onset and half are healed by 8 days. In immunocompromised children, new lesions are reported to form for longer than 5 days; patients not treated with antiviral agents have a 28% incidence of pneumonitis and a 7% mortality rate. The untreated immunocompromised adult with herpes zoster sheds VZV for a longer period than the normal host (7.0 versus 5.3 days) and is much more likely to experience cutaneous dissemination.

• CLINICAL FEATURES •

Varicella-zoster virus infections in the immunocompromised host are often much more extensive than in the healthy host, with more cutaneous involvement and more severe systemic symptoms. In patients with varicella, lesions may be large, necrotic, and hemorrhagic (Figs. 20.24, 20.25). Neutropenic patients with varicella are more likely to experience secondary infection of cutaneous lesions. Zoster may be severe with a confluence of vesicopustules involving the entire dermatome or contiguous dermatomes. Hematogenous dissemination of VZV to the skin occurs in approximately 15% of healthy individuals with zoster and more frequently in the immunocompromised host (Figs 20.26, 20.27). VZV may also be disseminated to liver, lung, brain, and other organs, resulting in organ failure and death. The pain of both acute zoster and post-zoster neuralgia is likely to be more severe in the immunocompromised patient.

• DIAGNOSIS AND DIFFERENTIAL DIAGNOSIS •

Diagnosis of VZV infection is best confirmed by laboratory testing, mainly to differentiate it from HSV infections, which are treated with a lower dose of acyclovir. VZV infections are most readily diagnosed by detection of VZV antigen in a smear from fluid at the base of the lesion. Isolation of VZV from lesions is unreliable.

• TREATMENT AND CLINICAL COURSE •

Immunocompromised persons who have not had varicella should be immunized with the Oka vaccine. Nonimmunized persons exposed to VZV should be treated with varicella-zoster immune globulin as well as with acyclovir, which is most predictably effective when administered intravenously. With established zoster, patients should be treated with acyclovir as early in the course as possible; however, the effect of early antiviral therapy on post-zoster neuralgia is still unclear. Foscarnet, ganciclovir, and vidarabine are effective against acyclovir-resistant VZV strains.

Varicella-zoster virus is further discussed in Chapters 16, 17, and 21.

Cytomegalovirus

• PATHOGENESIS •

Cytomegalovirus (CMV) is the most common opportunistic pathogen in transplant patients, causing overt disease in approximately 1 of 3 renal transplant recipients. This incidence is lower in immunocompromised patients with malignancies, presumably because transplant recipients are at risk for both reactivation of latent CMV infection by immunosuppressive therapies and new infection transmitted via the transplanted organ or blood products. In contrast to the usually asymptomatic CMV infection in the "normal" host, infection in the immunocompromised host is often symptomatic and sometimes fatal. In one series of renal transplant patients, symptoms developed in 91% of those with primary CMV infection and in 35% of those with reactivated infection.

• CLINICAL FEATURES •

The most common sites of involvement of CMV infection are the lungs and the gastrointestinal tract. Cutaneous lesions directly attributable to CMV infection are extremely rare. Only 25 such cases have been reported, and their 6-month mortality rate was 85% because of serious concomitant systemic CMV infection (1, 2). In contrast to HSV and VZV infections, lesions associated with cutaneous CMV infection are not distinctive. A

wide variety have been reported, including ulcerations of the oral, anorectal, and perianal epithelium; erythematous macules and papules; petechiae associated with vasculitis; and bullous lesions.

• DIAGNOSIS AND DIFFERENTIAL DIAGNOSIS •

The cytopathic changes associated with CMV-induced lesions are homogeneous intranuclear inclusions with a clear halo in endothelial cells of dermal blood vessels. These changes, however, do not necessarily indicate that CMV is the etiologic agent of the lesion (3).

• TREATMENT AND CLINICAL COURSE •

Intravenous ganciclovir is the first-line antiviral agent used to treat systemic CMV infections. Ganciclovir-resistant CMV strains often emerge after prolonged therapy, necessitating the use of intravenous foscarnet. The course and prognosis depend on the severity of the underlying immunocompromised state. Bone marrow transplant recipients with CMV infection associated with fever, viremia, and wasting tend to do well with intravenous ganciclovir; those with CMV pneumonia have a poor prognosis.

See Chapters 17 and 21 for more information on CMV infections.

Human Papillomavirus

Human papillomavirus (HPV) infections can be more extensive than those of CMV or HSV. They respond poorly to conventional therapy in solid organ transplant recipients (Fig. 20.28) and in patients with autoimmune diseases (such as systemic lupus erythematosus) on long-term immunosuppressive therapy. Since opportunistic neoplasms occur more often in this patient population, verruca vulgaris must be distinguished from actinic keratosis and both in situ and invasive squamous cell carcinoma. Mucosal HPV types (HPV16, HPV18, HPV31) have been detected in squamous cell carcinoma in patients undergoing long-term suppression of cellular immunity.

HPV is further discussed in Chapters 17 and 21.

MOLLUSCUM CONTAGIOSUM

The prevalence of molluscum contagiosum is strikingly increased in HIV disease but not in other immunocompromised states. See Chapters 8, 17, and 21 for further discussion.

Cutaneous Neoplasia

KAPOSI'S SARCOMA

Kaposi's sarcoma (KS), a neoplasia of the vascular endothelium, is often associated with immunocompromised states. Classic Kaposi's sarcoma occurs in older males, often of Mediterranean heritage with no obvious immunodeficiency other than senescence and is also associated with other lymphoreticular malignances, including Hodgkin's lymphoma, nonHodgkin's lymphoma, leukemia, multiple myeloma, cutaneous T-cell lymphoma, Sézary syndrome, hairy cell leukemia, and angioimmunoblastic lymphadenopathy. In the past, Kaposi's sarcoma was diagnosed in 0.4% of renal transplant recipients receiving prednisone and azathioprine; the addition of cyclosporine A to the immunosuppressive regimen has resulted in a 2- to 4-fold increase in KS and an earlier occurrence (mean of 20 months compared with 60 months with prednisone/azathioprine alone). A genetic diathesis for KS is supported by the observation that KS occurs in 2.5% of iatrogenically immunosuppressed persons in Tel Aviv (4).

• PATHOGENESIS •

The etiology and nature of proliferating cells and factors that perpetuate and spread KS are not fully understood. Recent epidemiological evidence suggests that an infectious agent, possibly a retrovirus other than HIV, plays a role in the pathogenesis of HIV-induced Kaposi's sarcoma.

• CLINICAL FEATURES •

Lesions may arise in nearly any organ system; cutaneous lesions are common on the lower legs. In that Kaposi's sarcoma is associated with a proliferation of new blood vessels, lesions are angiomatous, with red-to-violaceous nodules and greenish-yellow halos resulting from the breakdown of red blood cells and biliverdin formation. Early lesions may be mistaken for an ecchymosis. In time, with the appearance of new lesions and enlargement of old lesions, large nodules and plaques may form. A second type of cutaneous lesion is edema, which can arise around large cutaneous lesions or as a result of proximal occlusion of lymphatic vessels. While edema is usually associated with obvious cutaneous lesions, it may present as an isolated finding on an extremity or the face. The gastrointestinal tract is commonly involved, especially with asymptomatic lesions of the palate. Lesions anywhere from the esophagus to the anus can become eroded and give rise to hemorrhage of varying degrees.

• DIAGNOSIS AND DIFFERENTIAL DIAGNOSIS •

The diagnosis is made when a lesional skin biopsy specimen shows early angiomatous and later sarcomatous patterns. The differential diagnosis of cutaneous KS includes vascular lesions such as pyogenic granuloma, prurigo nodularis, dermatofibroma, stasis dermatitis, pseudolymphoma, pigmented basal cell carcinoma, amelanotic melanoma, bacillary angiomatosis, and angiosarcoma.

• TREATMENT AND CLINICAL COURSE •

Kaposi's sarcoma-related iatrogenic immunosuppression should be treated by tapering or reducing immunosuppressants. About a quarter of Kaposi's sarcoma cases resolve following this adjustment. If additional therapy is indicated because of systemic involvement, many combinations of systemic chemotherapeutic agents can be used, with or without radiotherapy.

More information on Kaposi's sarcoma can be found in Chapter 21.

Nonmelanoma Skin Cancer (Basal Cell Carcinoma and Squamous Cell Carcinoma)

Patients treated with immunosuppressive therapy are at a significantly increased risk of developing cutaneous malignant neoplasms. Risk is estimated at 4-to-20 times that of nonimmunocompromised persons (5), the duration of immunosuppression being directly related to the magnitude of risk. The two major etiologic factors in nonmelanoma skin cancer in immunocompromised individuals are cumulative ultraviolet radiation (particularly UVB) exposure prior to the onset of immunosuppression and injection with oncogenic human papillomavirus strains. The ratio of squamous cell carcinoma to basal cell carcinoma is 2.3:1 compared with 0.2:1 in the general population. Nonmelanoma skin cancers in the immunocompromised host tend to be more aggressive and more likely to present with multiple primary lesions.

Adverse Cutaneous Drug Reactions Associated With Drugs Causing Immunosuppression

Please see Table 20.6.

Table 20.6. Adverse Cutaneous Drug Reactions Associated with Immunosuppressive Drugs

Bleomycin	Common: Alopecia, glossitis and oral ulcer. Flagellate hyperpigmentation is common, occurring at sites of mild "trauma," such as scratching, resulting in linear postinflammatory hyperpigmentation. Uncommon: Systemic sclerosis-like skin changes and Raynaud's phenomenon.
Busulfan	Cutaneous reactions to busulfan are rare. Diffuse pigmentation, urticaria, and erythema multiforme have been reported.
Corticosteroids	Common: Striae distensae, purpura, hypertrichosis, cutaneous atrophy, and a monomorphic acneiform eruption on the chest and back.
Cyclosporine A	Common: Hypertrichosis on the face, upper back, and upper arms; gingival hyperplasia. Uncommon: Acne, folliculitis.
(Tacrolimus FK506)	Many of the same side effects as cyclosporine A. Also alopecia and pruritus.
Antithymocyte globulin	Common: Serum sickness occurs 5–21 days after administration; characterized by fever, urticaria, angioedema, joint swelling, lymphadenopathy, and nephritis.

Miscellaneous Reactions Occurring in the Immunocompromised Host

Please see Table 20.7.

Table 20.7. Miscellaneous Reactions Occurring in the Immunocompromised Host

Graft-versus-host disease (GVHD)	Occurs in 50%–70% of patients following bone marrow transplantation; also following transfusion of nonirradiated blood and after maternofetal transfer of lymphoid cells. Onset 10–21 days after transplantation of immunocompetent lymphoid cells. Cutaneous GVHD is characterized by a morbilliform eruption on the hands, feet, forehead, and postauricular regions, which may become generalized. Uncommonly, cutaneous inflammation is severe with bullous, ulcerative, or toxic epidermal necrolysis lesions developing. Liver and GI involvement is manifested by increased bilirubin and alkaline phosphatase and diarrhea. Chronic GVHD occurs months after bone marrow transplant and may be manifested by violaceous lichenoid papules, systemic sclerotic changes, bullae formation, and hyperpigmentation.
Cutaneous eruptions of lymphocyte recovery	Occurs in patients with leukemia who undergo aggressive chemotherapy resulting in marrow suppression. Occurs in conjunction with recovery of lymphocytes after a chemotherapeutic-induced nadir in lymphocytes. Characterized by a morbilliform rash, similar to that which occurs with an adverse cutaneous drug eruption, viral exanthem, and acute GVHD. Histologically, resembles findings of acute GVHD or drug hypersensitivity reaction. Resolves in several days.
Eruption associated with recombinant human GM-CSF	Macular and papular generalized eruption and/or immediate localized angioedematous reaction at the site of injection. Same differential diagnosis as for cutaneous eruptions of lymphocyte recovery.
Sweet's syndrome	Characterized by painful, plaque-forming inflammatory papules and associated with fever, arthralgia, and peripheral luekocytosis. Associated with acute myeloid leukemia, transient myeloid proliferation, and various malignant tumors.
Neutrophilic eccrine hidradenitis	Characterized by dusky plaques. Usually associated with chemotherapy, especially with cytarabine, for new-onset lymphoma or leukemia. Must be differentiated from Sweet's syndrome.

REFERENCES

1. Lee LY. Cytomegalovirus infection involving the skin in immunocompromised hosts. Am J Clin Pathol 1989;92:96.
2. Toome BK, et al. Diagnosis of cutaneous cytomegalovirus infection: A review and report of a case. J Am Acad Dermatol 1991;24:857.
3. Drew WL. Diagnosis of cytomegalovirus infection. Rev Infect Dis 1988;10:S468.
4. Shmueli D, et al. The incidence of Kaposi's sarcoma in renal transplant patients and its relation to immunosuppression. Transplant Proc 1989;21:3209.
5. Bavinck JNB, et al. Relation between skin cancer and HLA antigens in renal-transplant recipients. N Engl J Med 1991;325:843.

ANNOTATED BIBLIOGRAPHY

Ackerman CD, Jegasothy BV. Cutaneous manifestations of the immunosuppressed host. In: Fitzpatrick TB, et al, eds. Dermatology in general medicine. 4th ed. New York: McGraw-Hill, 1993: 1519–1530.

A concise up-to-date summary with an excellent reference source.

Anaissie E. Opportunistic mycoses in the immunocompromised host: Experience at a cancer center and review. Clin Infect Dis 1992;14(suppl 1):S43.

Discussion of the clinical aspects of aspergillosis, invasive candidiasis, and emerging pathogens such as *Fusarium* sp., *Curvularia* sp., *Alternaria* sp., and *Trichosporon beigelii*.

Bencini PL, et al. Cutaneous manifestations in renal transplant recipients. Nephron 1983;34:79.

Authors call for close dermatological surveillance in transplant recipients. Skin lesions occurred in 100 of 105 renal transplant patients: 55% iatrogenic, 74% infectious, 12% precancerous or cancerous, and 4% miscellaneous.

Brooks RG, et al. Infectious complications in heart-lung transplant recipients. Am J Med 1985;79:412.

A study of infectious complications in 14 heart-lung transplant patients demonstrates their importance in morbidity and mortality. Most patients had bacterial pulmonary infections, half occurring the first two weeks after transplant.

Goldstein GD, Gollub S, Gill B. Cutaneous complications of heart transplantation. J Heart Transplant 1986;5(2):143.

A description of the most common cutaneous findings associated with heart transplantation: hypertrichosis, herpes simplex, warts, tinea, and steroid acne.

Morrison VA, Haake RI, Weisdorf DJ. The spectrum of non-Candida fungal infections following bone marrow transplantation. Medicine 1993;72:78.

The most common non-*Candida* fungal infections during the first 180 days after bone marrow transplantation were caused by *Aspergillus*, *Fusarium*, and *Alternaria*.

O'Hanley P, Easaw I, Rugo H, Easaw S. Infectious disease management of adult leukemic patients undergoing chemotherapy: 1982–1986 experience at Stanford University Hospital. Am J Med 1989;87:605.

Report of the incidence and profile of infections occurring during 226 induction and/or consolidation/maintenance chemotherapy courses for acute myelogenous leukemia and acute lymphoblastic leukemia.

Rowe JM, et al. Recommended guidelines for the management of autologous and allogenic bone marrow transplantation. A report from the Eastern Cooperative Oncology Group (ECOG). Ann Intern Med 1994;120:143.

Guidelines for the treatment of graft-versus-host disease, infections (PCP, fungal, CMV) and hepatic venoocclusive disease. Discussions on the use of hematopoietic growth factors, reconstitution of hematopoiesis after transplantation, and use of intravenous immunoglobulins.

Saral R. *Candida* and *Aspergillus* infections in immunocompromised patients: An overview. Rev Infect Dis 1991;13:487.

Diagnosis and empiric treatment of *Candida* and *Aspergillus*, the most common fungal pathogens causing disseminated infection in the immunocompromised host.

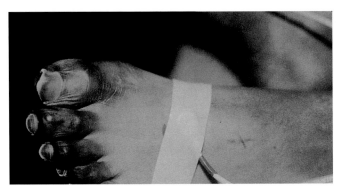

Figure 20.1.   Pneumococcal bacteremia with septic shock. In a patient splenectomized years earlier for idiopathic thrombocytopenia purpura. Gangrenous toes secondary to prolonged hypotension and tissue ischemia. (Courtesy of Dr. Charles V. Sanders)

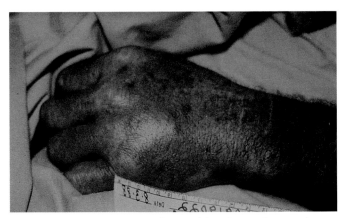

Figure 20.2.   Purpuric lesions with edema. Same patient as Figure 20.1 showing lesions of the dorsal hand and arm. (Courtesy of Dr. Charles V. Sanders)

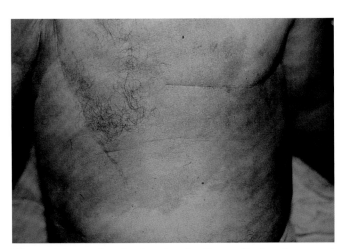

Figure 20.3.   Erysipelas due to Group A streptococcal infection. Erythema with sharp margins on the chest and abdomen following surgery for carcinoma of the breast. (Courtesy of Dr. Charles V. Sanders)

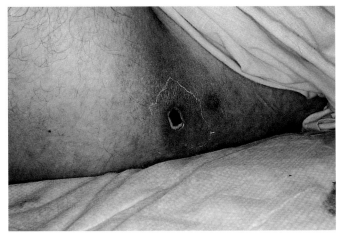

Figure 20.4.   *Aeromonas* septicemia. In a patient with acute leukemia showing a small cutaneous infarct on the hip which resolved with antibiotics. (Courtesy of Dr. Charles V. Sanders)

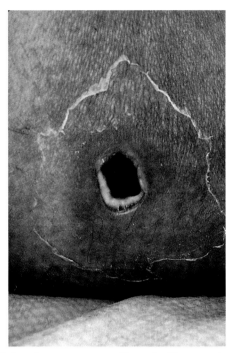

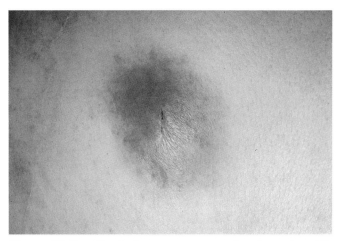

Figure 20.5. ***Aeromonas* septicemia.** Close-up view of patient in Figure 20.4. Necrotic ulcer with surrounding erythema and desquamation. (Courtesy of Dr. Charles V. Sanders)

Figure 20.6. ***Staphylococcus aureus* bacteremia with cutaneous nodules.** Large inflammatory nodule resulted from staphylococcal sepsis and seeding of the skin.

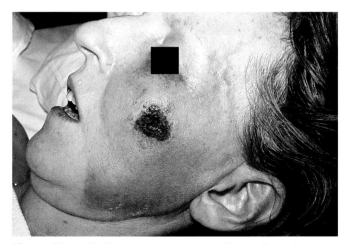

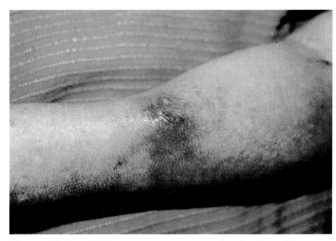

Figure 20.7. **Ecthyma gangrenosum due to *Pseudomonas aeruginosa.*** Lesion with surrounding erythema in a patient with Hodgkin's disease. (Courtesy of Dr. Charles V. Sanders)

Figure 20.8. **Ecthyma gangrenosum due to *Pseudomonas aeruginosa.*** Cellulitis with central infarction in a patient with Felty's syndrome (rheumatoid arthritis, neutropenia, and splenomegaly). (Courtesy of Dr. Charles V. Sanders)

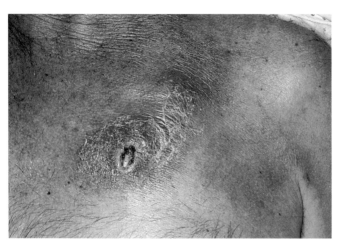

Figure 20.9.   Ecthyma gangrenosum due to *Pseudomonas aeruginosa*. Cellulitis at a Hickman catheter site in a patient with acute leukemia and neutropenia. (Courtesy of Dr. Charles V. Sanders)

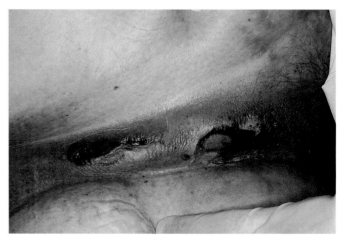

Figure   20.10.   Ecthyma   gangrenosum   due   to *Pseudomonas aeruginosa*. Early cellulitis with central necrosis in the inguinal region of a patient with acute leukemia. (Courtesy of Dr. Charles V. Sanders)

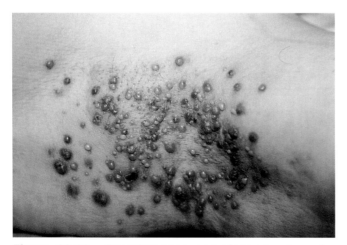

Figure 20.11.   *Pseudomonas aeruginosa* bacteremia. Polymorphous pustular eruption with surrounding erythema in the axilla of a patient with acute leukemia. (Courtesy of Dr. Charles V. Sanders)

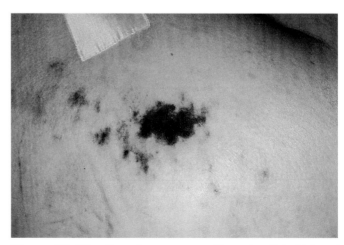

Figure 20.12.   *Pseudomonas* septicemia. Petechial and ecchymotic eruption on the upper thigh in a patient with acute leukemia. (Courtesy of Dr. Charles V. Sanders)

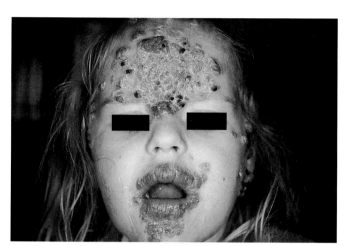

Figure 20.13.   Chronic mucocutaneous candidiasis. In a child with a specific immune defect to *Candida albicans*. Erythematous and crusted granulomatous lesions of the forehead and perioral area.

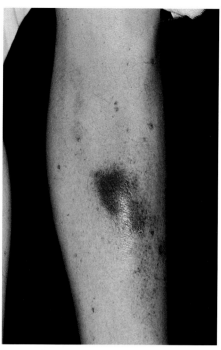

Figure 20.14.   Disseminated *Candida tropicalis* infection. Hemorrhagic nodule of hematogenous dissemination on the arm in a 73-year-old man with acute myelogenous leukemia with thrombocytopenia.

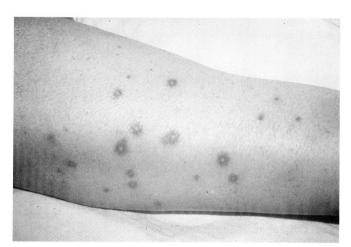

Figure 20.15.   Disseminated candidiasis. Pustular lesions on erythematous bases over the right forearm in a patient with acute leukemia.

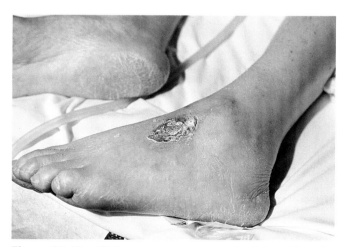

Figure 20.16.   Cutaneous mucormycosis. A 6-cm ulceration at an IV site on the dorsum of the foot in a patient with diabetic ketoacidosis.

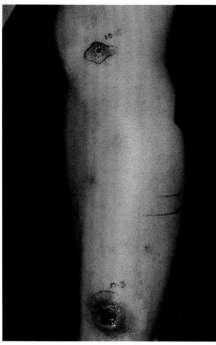

Figure 20.17.   Cutaneous mucormycosis. Two large, crusted, ulcerated nodules on the leg in a patient with acute myelogenous leukemia, arising at the site of insect bites.

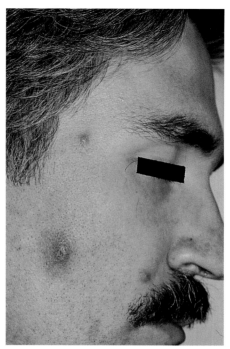

Figure 20.18.   Disseminated histoplasmosis. Pustular lesions on erythematous bases of the face. (Courtesy of Dr. Alan Stamm)

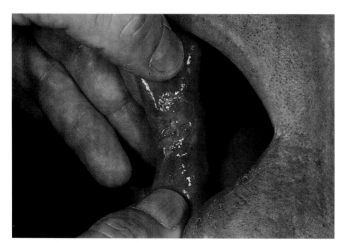

Figure 20.19.   Disseminated histoplasmosis. Ulcerative lesion on the oral mucosa. (Courtesy of Dr. Lee T. Nesbitt, Jr.)

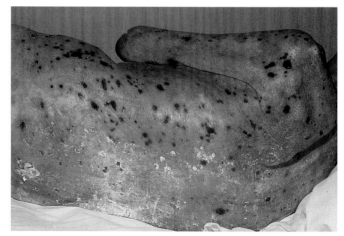

Figure 20.20.   Disseminated herpes simplex. Generalized eruption of hemorrhagic crusted lesions in a thrombocytopenic patient undergoing cancer chemotherapy. (Courtesy of Dr. Klaus Wolff)

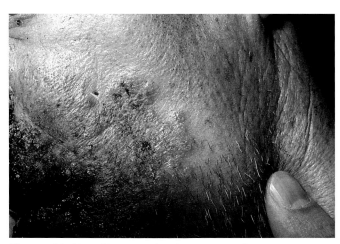

Figure 20.21.   Herpes simplex, extensive and severe. Persistent vesiculation and hemorrhagic crusts on the lips and cheeks of a patient with leukemia. (Courtesy of Dr. Lee T. Nesbitt, Jr.)

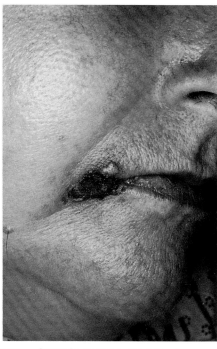

Figure 20.22.   Chronic herpes simplex. Large, crusted ulcer on the cheek of a patient with leukemia. (Courtesy of Dr. Charles V. Sanders)

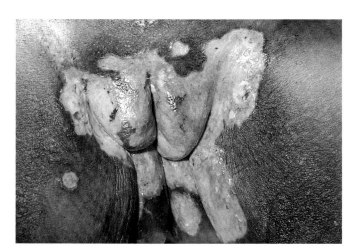

Figure 20.23.   Chronic herpes simplex. Extensive ulceration on the genitalia and surrounding area in a patient with leukemia undergoing chemotherapy. (Courtesy of Dr. Lee T. Nesbitt, Jr.)

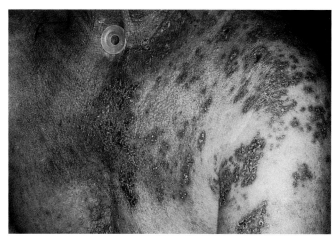

Figure 20.24.   Herpes zoster. Grouped vesicopustules on erythematous bases in a multidermatomal pattern on the shoulder. Patient had squamous cell carcinoma of the vocal cord. (Courtesy of Dr. Charles V. Sanders)

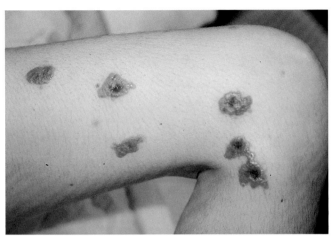

Figure 20.25.   Herpes zoster. Large vesicobullous lesions of the leg in a patient with malignancy. (Courtesy of Dr. Charles V. Sanders)

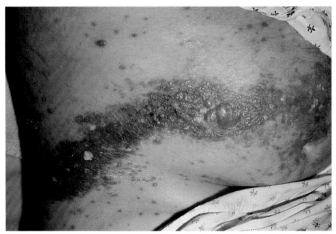

Figure 20.26.   Disseminated herpes zoster. Zosteriform eruption on the flank with hundreds of disseminated vesicopustules in a patient with lymphoma. (Courtesy of Dr. Charles V. Sanders)

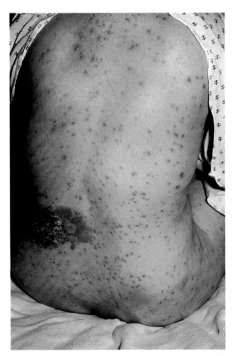

Figure 20.27.   Disseminated herpes zoster. Showing dermatomal lesion on the back and disseminated vesicopustules on the trunk. Same patient as in Figure 20.26. (Courtesy of Dr. Charles V. Sanders)

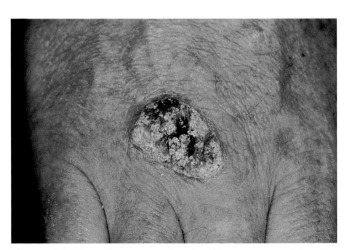

Figure 20.28.   Verruca vulgaris. Huge wart, recalcitrant to cryosurgery and electrosurgery, on the hand of a renal transplant patient. The wart resolved after the transplanted kidney failed and immunotherapy was discontinued.

CHAPTER **21**

Infections in the Immunocompromised Host— HIV and AIDS

RICHARD ALLEN JOHNSON and ROBERT H. RUBIN

HIV Disease Overview

CUTANEOUS AND MUCOUS MEMBRANE INVOLVEMENT

Cutaneous and mucous membrane involvement in HIV infection and its endstage disease, AIDS, is important for at least four reasons:

1. These lesions may be the first manifestation of the progression from the asymptomatic carrier state to overt disease;

2. The lesions may contribute considerably to the morbidity and mortality of HIV-infected patients;

3. Mucocutaneous sites may serve as the portal of entry for infection that will subsequently disseminate into life-threatening systemic infection;

4. Mucocutaneous sites, being highly visible, may serve as the first warning that disseminated infection or malignancy is present.

In the HIV-infected patient, the morphology of a lesion is primarily determined not by the nature of the invading microbe, but by the nature of the inflammatory response to this microbe. Because this inflammatory response may be greatly altered, the appearance of the lesion is also altered. There are three important corollaries to this central precept:

1. Since the extent of the inflammatory response to microbial invasion is constantly changing in the course of HIV infection (from essentially normal to essentially absent), the appearance of lesions caused by the identical organism may be very different at different points in time;

2. The broader range of infections to which this population is susceptible (Table 21.1), combined with the decreased inflammatory response, creates an effect that broadens the differential diagnosis, compared with the normal host;

3. The net result is an increased need to biopsy even seemingly innocuous lesions for histological and microbiological assessment (Table 21.2).

Table 21.3 presents the differential diagnostic considerations in the HIV-infected patient with a mucocutaneous abnormality.

Table 21.1 Conditions Included in the 1993 AIDS Surveillance Case Definition for Adolescents and Adults[a]

Candidiasis of bronchi, trachea, or lungs
Candidiasis, esophageal
Cervical cancer, invasive
Coccidioidomycosis, disseminated or extrapulmonary
Cryptococcosis, extrapulmonary
Cryptosporidiosis, chronic intestinal (> 1 mo)
Cytomegalovirus (CMV) disease (other than liver, spleen, or nodes)
CMV retinitis (with loss of vision)
Encephalopathy, HIV-related
Herpes simplex virus (HSV): chronic ulcer(s) (> 1 month's duration), or pneumonitis, or esophagitis
Histoplasmosis, disseminated or extrapulmonary
Isosporiasis, chronic intestinal (> 1 month's duration)
Kaposi's sarcoma (KS)
Lymphoma, Burkitt's
Lymphoma, immunoblastic
Lymphoma, primary, of brain
Mycobacterium avium complex or *M. kansasii*, disseminated or extra-pulmonary
M. tuberculosis, any site (pulmonary or extrapulmonary)
Mycobacterium, other species or unidentified, disseminated or extra-pulmonary
Pneumocystis carinii pneumonia (PCP)
Pneumonia, recurrent
Progressive multifocal leukoencephalopathy (PML)
Salmonella septicemia, recurrent
Toxoplasmosis of brain
Wasting syndrome due to HIV

[a] From Castro KG, et al. 1993 revised classification system for HIV infection and expanded surveillance case definition for AIDS among adolescents and adults. MMWR 41(RR-17), 1992.

PATHOGENESIS OF HIV INFECTION

HIV infection (both HIV-1, the retrovirus responsible for virtually all cases of AIDS outside of Africa, and HIV-2, a related retrovirus isolated from West Africans and their direct contacts) is transmitted among humans in one of three ways: *a)* through sexual contact with an infected individual (heterosexual or homosexual), *b)* through the inoculation with blood from an infected individual (including organ transplantation), and

Table 21.2. Definitive Diagnostic Methods for Diseases Indicative of AIDS[a]

Disease	Diagnostic Methods
Cryptosporidiosis Isosporiasis Kaposi's sarcoma (KS) Lymphoma *Pneumocystis carinii* pneumonia (PCP) Progressive multifocal leukoencephalopathy (PML) Toxoplasmosis Cervical cancer	Microscopy (histology or cytology)
Candidiasis	Gross inspection by endoscopy or autopsy or by microscopy (histology or cytology) on a specimen obtained directly from the tissues affected (including scrapings from the mucosal surface, not from a culture)
Coccidioidomycosis Cryptococcosis Cytomegalovirus (CMV) Herpes simplex virus (HSV) Histoplasmosis	Microscopy (histology or cytology), culture, or detection of antigen in a specimen obtained directly from the tissue affected or a fluid from those tissues
Tuberculosis Other mycobacterioses Salmonellosis	Culture
HIV encephalopathy (dementia)	Clinical findings of disabling cognitive or motor dysfunction interfering with occupation or activities of daily living, progressing over weeks to months, in the absence of a concurrent illness or condition other than HIV infection that could explain the findings. Methods to rule out such concurrent illness and conditions must include cerebrospinal fluid examination and either brain imaging (CT or MRI) or autopsy.
HIV wasting syndrome	Findings of profound involuntary weight loss of > 10% of baseline body weight plus either chronic diarrhea (at least 2 loose stools per day for > 30 days), or chronic weakness and documented fever (for > 30 days, intermittent or constant) in the absence of a concurrent illness or condition other than HIV infection that could explain the findings (e.g., cancer, tuberculosis, cryptosporidiosis, or other specific enteritis).
Pneumonia, recurrent	Recurrent (more than 1 episode in a 1-year period), acute (new X-ray evidence not present earlier) pneumonia diagnosed by both: a) culture (or other organism-specific diagnostic method) obtained from a clinically reliable specimen of a pathogen that typically causes pneumonia (other than *Pneumocystis carinii* or *Mycobacterium tuberculosis*), and b) radiologic evidence of pneumonia; cases that do not have laboratory confirmation of a causative organism for one of the episodes of pneumonia will be considered to be presumptively diagnosed.

[a] From Castro KG, et al. 1993 revised classification system for HIV infection and expanded surveillance case definition for AIDS among adolescents and adults. MMWR 41(RR-17), 1992.

Table 21.3. Differential Diagnosis by Type of Cutaneous Lesions Occurring in HIV Disease[a]

Papules, nodules

Any location — Botryomycosis, staphylococcal; Mycobacterial, environmental; Verruca vulgaris, verruca plana; Bacillary angiomatosis; Scabies, scabetic nodules; Disseminated deep mycotic infection; Cryptococcosis; Histoplasmosis; Coccidioidomycosis; Kaposi's sarcoma; Basal cell carcinoma; Squamous cell carcinoma

Facial — Molluscum contagiosum; Verruca vulgaris, verruca plana; Disseminated deep mycotic infection; Kaposi's sarcoma; Basal cell carcinoma; Squamous cell carcinoma

Anogenital — Condylomata acuminata; Intraepithelial neoplasia; Molluscum contagiosum; Scabies, scabetic nodules; Kaposi's sarcoma; Squamous cell carcinoma arising in intraepithelial neoplasia

Crusted papules/nodules — Impetigo; Ecthyma; Mycobacterial, environmental; Ecthymatous varicella-zoster virus (VZV) infection (painful); Disseminated deep mycotic infection; Kaposi's sarcoma; Basal cell carcinoma; Herpes simplex virus (HSV), chronic ulcers

Vesicles, bullae, pustules

Solitary — Bullous impetigo; Ecthyma gangrenosum; Drug eruption

Multiple — Grouped: HSV infection, primary or recurrent; Zosteriform: herpes zoster, herpes simplex; Bullous impetigo; Ecthyma gangrenosum; Disseminated zoster; Disseminated herpes simplex; Infectious endocarditis; Pustular psoriasis; Reiter's syndrome/keratoderma blenorrhagica; Erythema multiforme; Toxic epidermal necrolysis

Acneiform — Acne vulgaris; Rosacea; Perioral dermatitis; Disseminated histoplasmosis; Eosinophilic folliculitis; Papular eruption of AIDS

Table 21.3. *Cont.*

Folliculitis	*Staphylococcus aureus* *Candida albicans* *Pityrosporum ovale* Papular eruption of AIDS
Psoriasiform (papulo-squamous)	Seborrheic dermatitis *Tinea versicolor* Dermatophytosis Psoriasis vulgaris Psoriasis, inverse pattern Reiter's syndrome Xerosis/icthyosis
Eczematous dermatitis	Atopic dermatitis Seborrheic dermatitis Scabies
Urticaria	Drug eruption Idiopathic
Erythema multiforme	Drug eruption HSV-associated
Morbilliform eruption	Acute HIV exanthem Infectious exanthem Drug eruption
Purpura ± palpable	Thrombocytopenic purpura Hypersensitivity vasculitis Extrapulmonary pneumocystosis Infectious endocarditis
Erosion(s), ulcer(s) Any size	HSV: primary, recurrent, chronic Cytomegalovirus (CMV) infection Ecthyma Nocardiosis Mycobacterial, environmental Deep mycotic infection Mycobacterial infection Fixed drug eruption
Anogenital	Fixed drug eruption, including foscarnet HSV ulcer, chronic CMV Bacterial infection: ecthyma gangrenosum Balanitis circinata (Reiter's syndrome)
Generalized pruritus ± skin changes	Atopic dermatitis Scabies HIV-associated eosinophilic folliculitis Papular eruption of HIV disease Adverse cutaneous drug reaction
Scars	Intravenous drug use Skin "popping"
Nail/paronychial changes	Dermatophytosis, proximal superficial Candida paronychia and onychomycosis *Staphylococcus aureus* whitlow Psoriasis: pits, onycholysis, subungual hyperkeratosis Beau's lines Zidovudine pigmentation Yellow nail syndrome

aFrom Johnson RA, Dover JS. Cutaneous manifestations of human immunodeficiency virus disease. In: Fitzpatrick TB et al., eds. Dermatology in general medicine. 4th ed. New York: McGraw-Hill, 1993.

c) through perinatal spread from an infected mother (either intrauterine or perinatal). Once HIV transmission occurs and other than a mononucleosis-like syndrome occurring in 10% to 20% of individuals 3 to 12 weeks after exposure, HIV infection remains asymptomatic, albeit transmissible, for an average of 5 to 9 years.

The immunopathological events that characterize HIV disease are primarily due to the interaction of HIV with cells that bear the CD4 surface molecule, this molecule being the high-affinity cell receptor for the virus. This means that the brunt of the events initiated by HIV infection will be borne by helper T-lymphocytes (which have the highest concentration of this molecule), certain populations of monocytes and macrophages, and certain neurons and glial cells, all of which bear the CD4 surface molecule. The hallmark of HIV infection is depletion of the CD4-positive (helper) T-lymphocyte population. Because of the central role of this cell population in virtually all immune processes, its depletion results in the crippling of a broad array of host defenses, making way for the repetitive occurrence of opportunistic infection and malignancy that characterizes clinical AIDS.

In addition to the primary effects on the helper T-cell population, HIV also affects cell populations that influence host defense. Monocytes and macrophages, for example, serve as reservoirs of infection and transport HIV to the central nervous system. HIV-induced defects in monocyte function probably play a role in the pathogenesis of such infections as *Pneumocystis carinii* pneumonia (PCP), and in the inappropriate elaboration of such cytokines as interleukin-1 and tumor necrosis factor, both of which probably contribute to fever and cachexia. B-lymphocytes show evidence of a severe dysregulation caused by polyclonal activation of these cells on exposure to the virus (as opposed to infection with the virus). This results in increased polyclonal hypergammaglobulinemia, circulating immune complexes, autoantibodies (and autoimmune clinical syndromes), atopic reactions, and a deficient antibody response to the polysaccharide capsules of such organisms as *Streptococcus pneumoniae* and *Hemophilus influenzae* type B. Thus, response to vaccines from these two organisms is poor and disseminated infection from them is more likely.

HIV-ASSOCIATED DISORDERS

The manifestations of HIV infection can be divided into four general categories: *a)* those that occur as a direct consequence of HIV infection, *b)* those caused by Kaposi's sarcoma, *c)* those related to opportunistic infections, and *d)* those that arise from the combined effects of immunosuppression and infection with certain oncogenic viruses. Mucocutaneous processes falling into these four categories may occur at three different points following HIV infection:

1. During the acute HIV mononucleosis syndrome (characterized by fevers, sweats, malaise, fatigability, headache, sore throat, diarrhea, generalized lymphadenopathy, and thrombocytopenia lasting 2 to 3 weeks and occurring 3 to 12 weeks postinfection), the following manifestations can be observed in as many as 75% of patients: a macular, erythematous truncal eruption that may be accompanied

by an exanthem; acute urticaria; and, less commonly, palatal and esophageal ulcers or oropharyngeal candidiasis.

2. During the prolonged version of this symptom complex, which usually occurs months to years later (AIDS-related complex or ARC), two major mucocutaneous problems are observed. The first is severe, often recurrent herpes simplex (HSV) infection with both HSV-1 (primarily affecting the orolabial region) and HSV-2 (primarily affecting the anogenital region); the second is mucocutaneous candidiasis predominantly affecting the pharynx and esophagus.

3. During full-blown AIDS (defined and described in Tables 21.4 and 21.5), the earlier mucocutaneous manifestations are joined by systemic and life-threatening processes.

Kaposi's Sarcoma

Kaposi's sarcoma (KS) is a hemangioma-like proliferation of endothelial-derived cells; the classic form of Kaposi's sarcoma was first reported in 1872 in men of Mediterranean or Eastern European ancestry. Variants of classic KS have been described in African males and in patients on long-term immunosuppressive therapy. In 1981, epidemic or HIV-associated KS became one of the first disorders identified in patients with AIDS with most cases subsequently present in homosexual or bisexual males. Early in the HIV epidemic, approximately 40% of homosexual or bisexual men with AIDS had KS, but the incidence has more recently fallen below 15%. In all other high-risk HIV groups, such as IV drug abusers, the prevalence of KS has remained at 1% to 3%.

• PATHOGENESIS •

Epidemiologic evidence suggests that KS is caused primarily by an infectious agent transmitted sexually. Various observations suggest that this infectious agent was present in the homosexual population at the time HIV was introduced, and that HIV plays a permissive role in both the development and accelerated course of KS in this patient population.

The increased incidence of HLA-DR5 in KS patients suggests that immunogenetic factors affect the occurrence of this condition. Male predominance is seen both in humans and in mice transfected with the transactivating gene of HIV.

• CLINICAL FEATURES •

The clinical course of KS in AIDS patients is usually aggressive, with frequent and widespread cutaneous and visceral lesions. Early lesions of HIV-associated KS present as slightly macular or barely papular discolorations of the skin. These dermal lesions lack any epidermal change and are pink in color with faint hues of tan, yellow, or green that give the appearance of a bruise (Fig. 21.1). Over time (weeks to years), early lesions may enlarge into nodules or frank tumors (Fig. 21.2) and darken to a violaceous color, often with a yellow-green halo. As lesions enlarge, epidermal changes may occur, with erosion or ulceration of the surface. Oral lesions are common and may be the first site involved, occurring typically on the hard palate as a violaceous stain.

Table 21.4. Revised Classification System for HIV Infection Based on CD4⁺ T-cell Count and Clinical Category[a]

CD4⁺ T-cell Categories	Category A Asymptomatic, acute (primary) HIV or persistent generalized Lymphadenopathy	Category B Symptomatic conditions not (A) or (C)	Category C AIDS-indicator conditions
(1) ≥ 500 µL	A1	B1	C1
(2) 200–499 µL	A2	B2	C2
(3) < 200 µL (AIDS-indicator T-cell count)	A3	B3	C3

Clinical Categories of HIV Infection—Definitions

Category A.
Category A consists of one or more of the conditions listed below in an adolescent or adult (> 13 years) with documented HIV infection. Conditions listed in Category B and C must not have occurred.

> Asymptomatic HIV infection
> Persistent generalized lymphadenopathy (PGL)
> Acute (primary) HIV infection with accompanying illness or history of acute HIV infection

Category B.
Category B consists of symptomatic conditions in an HIV-infected adolescent or adult that are not included among conditions listed in clinical Category C and that meet at least one of the following criteria: a) the conditions are attributed to HIV infection or are indicative of a defect in cell-mediated immunity, or b) the conditions are considered by physicians to have a clinical course or to require management that is complicated by HIV infection. Examples of conditions in clinical Category B include, but are not limited to:

> Bacillary angiomatosis
> Candidiasis, oropharyngeal
> Candidiasis, vulvovaginal; persistent, frequent, or poorly responsive to therapy
> Cervical dysplasia (moderate or severe)/cervical carcinoma in situ
> Constitutional symptoms, such as fever (38.5°C) or diarrhea lasting > 1 month
> Hairy leukoplakia
> Herpes zoster, involving at least two distinct episodes or more than one dermatome
> Idiopathic thrombocytopenic purpura
> Listeriosis
> Pelvic inflammatory disease, particularly if complicated by tubo-ovarian abscess
> Peripheral neuropathy

Note: For classification purposes, Category B conditions take precedence over those in Category A. For example, someone previously treated for oral or persistent vaginal candidiasis (and who has not developed a Category C disease but who is now asymptomatic) should be classified in clinical Category B.

Category C.
Category C includes the clinical conditions listed in the AIDS surveillance case definition (Table 21.1). For classification purposes, once a Category C condition has occurred, the person will remain in Category C.

---

[a] From Castro KG, et al. 1993 revised classification system for HIV infection and expanded surveillance case definition for AIDS among adolescents and adults. MMWR 41(RR-17), 1992.

Table 21.5. Presumptive Diagnosis of Diseases Indicative of AIDS

Disease	Diagnostic Findings
Candidiasis of esophagus	*a)* Recent onset of retrosternal pain on swallowing and *b)* oral candidiasis diagnosed by the gross appearance of white patches or plaques on an erythematous base or by the microscopic appearance of fungal mycelial filaments from a noncultured specimen scraped from the oral mucosa.
Cytomegalovirus (CMV) retinitis	Characteristic appearance on serial ophthalmoscopic examinations (e.g., discrete patches of retinal whitening with distinct borders, spreading in a centrifugal manner along the paths of blood vessels, progressing over several months, and frequently associated with retinal vasculitis, hemorrhage, and necrosis). Resolution of active disease leaves retinal scarring and atrophy with retinal pigment epithelial mottling.
Mycobacteriosis	Microscopy of a specimen from stool or normally sterile body fluids or tissue from a site other than lungs, skin, or cervical or hilar lymph nodes that shows acid-fast bacilli or a species not identified by culture.
Kaposi's sarcoma (KS)	Characteristic gross appearance of an erythematous or violaceous plaque-like lesion on skin or mucous membrane. (Note: Presumptive diagnosis of KS should not be made by clinicians who have seen few cases of it.)
Pneumocystis carinii pneumonia (PCP)	*a)* History of dyspnea on exertion or nonproductive cough of recent onset (within the past 3 months), and *b)* chest x-ray evidence of diffuse bilateral interstitial infiltrates or evidence by gallium scan of diffuse bilateral pulmonary disease, and *c)* arterial blood gas analysis showing an arterial pO_2 of <70 mm Hg or a low respiratory diffusing capacity (<80% of predicted values) or an increase in the alveolar-arterial oxygen tension gradient, and *d)* no evidence of bacterial pneumonia.
Pneumonia, recurrent	Recurrent (more than one episode in a 1-year period), acute (new symptoms, signs, or x-ray evidence not present earlier) pneumonia diagnosed on clinical or radiologic grounds by the patient's physician.
Toxoplasmosis of brain	*a)* Recent onset of a focal neurologic abnormality consistent with intracranial disease or a reduced level of consciousness, and *b)* evidence on brain imaging (by CT or MRI) of a lesion having a mass effect or the radiographic appearance of which is enhanced by injection of contrast medium, and *c)* serum antibody to toxoplasmosis or successful response to therapy for toxoplasmosis.
Tuberculosis, pulmonary	When bacteriologic confirmation is not available, other reports may be considered to be verified cases of pulmonary tuberculosis if the criteria of the Division of Tuberculosis Elimination are used.

[a]From Castro KG, et al. 1993 revised classification system for HIV infection and expanded surveillance case definition for AIDS among adolescents and adults. MMWR 41(RR-17), 1992.

HIV-associated KS can occur anywhere on the skin but has a predilection for certain sites. On the head and neck, lesions commonly develop on the tip of the nose, cheeks, eyelids, and ears. Occasionally, KS lesions may form on the bulbar conjunctiva, appearing as a subconjunctival hemorrhage. Facial edema is common, due to lymphatic obstruction by the KS lesions, and is sometimes extreme. Edema of the extremities may also occur, even when visible lesions are scanty or absent.

Truncal KS lesions often are multiple and may have a pityriasis rosea-like pattern of oval lesions along the normal skin lines of the trunk. In a study of 173 patients with epidemic KS, the distribution of lesions was as follows: trunk, 52% (Fig. 21.3); legs, 45% (Fig. 21.4); arms, 38%; face, 33%; and oral cavity, 40% (Fig. 21.5) (1). Köbnerization of KS lesions has been reported at sites of venipuncture, BCG (Bacille bilié de Calmette-Guérin) injection, abscess formation, and contusion (2).

• DIAGNOSIS AND DIFFERENTIAL DIAGNOSIS •

Although the diagnosis of KS can usually be suspected clinically, it should usually be confirmed histologically with a lesion biopsy. The differential diagnosis depends on the stage of disease encountered. An early, macular (patch stage) lesion can be mistaken for a bruise, hemangioma, dermatofibroma, insect bite, or benign nevus. More advanced, nodular, or plaque KS lesions must be differentiated from psoriasis, lichen planus, secondary syphilis, insect bites, benign nevi, skin tumors including melanoma, bacillary angiomatosis and metastatic visceral malignancies. Once the individual KS plaques or tumors have coalesced, the major differential diagnosis is lymphoma.

• TREATMENT AND CLINICAL COURSE •

The course of HIV-associated KS is highly variable. Although this condition is associated with significant morbidity, few patients die from complications directly related to it. Some individuals will develop only a few lesions over the 2 to 5 years following diagnosis, or their lesions may spontaneously regress. If opportunistic infections do not intervene, these patients remain in relatively good health. In most patients, however, established KS lesions tend to enlarge and darken, at times coalescing while new lesions appear. Occasionally, internal organs may be involved in the absence of any visible mucocutaneous involvement. At autopsy, most patients with KS will be found to have lesions in the gastrointestinal tract, lymph nodes, liver, lung, spleen, and/or kidneys. There also appears to be an increased incidence of second malignancies.

Treatment for AIDS-associated KS is determined by the stage of the disease:

1. Localized KS: Treatment is considered when lesions are cosmetically disfiguring, large or bulky, ulcerative and bleeding, painful, rapidly growing, or edematous. Such lesions can be treated with local radiation therapy. Other local treatments include cryotherapy, surgical excision, and intralesional injection of vinblastine, bleomycin, or alpha interferon.

2. Indolent disseminated cutaneous KS: This entity is best treated with systemic immunotherapy or chemotherapy. Systemic alpha inter-

feron (36 million units/day) is most effective in patients with CD4-lymphocyte counts >400/mm who have few systemic symptoms and no opportunistic infections. Because of its slow onset of action, systemic alpha interferon is inappropriate therapy for rapidly growing KS. In these patients and in nonresponders, aggressive chemotherapy may be employed.

3. Aggressive disseminated KS: The beneficial treatment is systemic chemotherapy with vincristine and bleomycin, usually in combination with adriamycin. Over three-fourths of patients respond, but therapy at this stage is often complicated by opportunistic infections.

Although each of these therapeutic approaches is effective, none improves patient survival. Corticosteroids are best avoided, as they appear to accelerate the clinical progression of KS if given for prolonged periods.

Important Mucocutaneous Infections

VIRAL INFECTIONS

Herpes Group Viruses (Herpes Simplex Virus, Cytomegalovirus, Varicella-Zoster Virus, Epstein-Barr Virus, and Human Herpesvirus-6).

The herpes group viruses share three characteristics that make them highly effective pathogens in the HIV-infected patient: latency (with reactivation due to immunosuppression); cell association (rendering humoral immunity inefficient and cell-mediated immunity paramount in their control); and oncogenicity (all are potentially oncogenic, the clearest demonstration being EBV-related lymphoproliferative disease). The mucocutaneous tissues of the HIV-infected individual are most affected by herpes simplex, varicella-zoster, and, to a lesser extent, Epstein-Barr virus.

Herpes Simplex Virus (HSV) Infection. Reactivation HSV infection, both types 1 and 2, has a major impact on the HIV patient, typically causing recurrent disease whose severity is a marker for the degree of advancement of the HIV infection. During the asymptomatic phase of HIV infection, the clinical manifestations of HSV infection are no different from those occurring in normal orolabial lesions (usually due to HSV 1) or anogenital lesions (usually due to HSV 2), triggered by such factors as fever, stress, other viral infections, or exposure to intense ultraviolet light. However, with progression of immunodeficiency, one sees more recurrences (even after effective therapy), delayed healing, and chronic ulcers, occasionally due to treatment-resistant strains of HSV.

Symptomatically, recurrent herpetic infection is characterized by a tingling sensation at the site, usually prior to lesion development. Grouped vesicopustules on erythematous bases appear and rupture, leaving superficial erosions and ulcers that are associated with varying degrees of discomfort. Regional lymphadenopathy may be present. Healing by reepithelialization will occur within 7 to 14 days in patients with mild-to-moderate immunodeficiency. In patients with advanced immunodeficiency, recurrent lesions may fail to heal and may

continue to enlarge, forming large, chronic ulcers (Figs. 21.6–21.11) with rolled margins. In the absence of other causes of immunocompromise, chronic herpetic ulcers present for more than a month are highly suggestive of AIDS. Such ulcers may develop on any mucocutaneous epithelium but are most common in the genital, anorectal, perioral, and digital sites. Untreated, these lesions may extend up to 20 cm in diameter.

The diagnosis of mucocutaneous herpetic infection can usually be made clinically and confirmed by the demonstration of multinucleated giant cells on lesional scraping. Multinucleated giant cells, however, also occur in the cutaneous lesions of varicella-zoster virus (VZV), but detection of viral antigens by immunofluorescence or ELISA (enzyme-linked immunoadsorbent assay) can now identify and differentiate these infections. Viral cultures of biopsied tissue will also yield the diagnosis. Differential diagnostic considerations include cytomegalovirus (CMV), perianal ulcers, ecthymatous VZV infection, ecthyma, syphilitic chancre, lues maligna, ecthyma gangrenosum, deep mycotic infection, ulcerated basal or squamous cell carcinoma, or foscarnet-induced genital ulcers.

The cornerstone of therapy of HSV infection in this patient population presently is acyclovir, although new herpes virus drugs will soon be available. For mild-to-moderate immunodeficiency, oral acyclovir 200 mg 5 times per day for 5–7 days is effective; as the HIV infection progresses, higher doses (800 mg 5 times daily) or intravenous therapy (5 to 10 mg/kg every 8 hours) for more prolonged periods becomes necessary. In the patient with advanced AIDS, prompt recurrences are the rule, and chronic acyclovir treatment is often necessary. An increasingly worrisome problem is the emergence of acyclovir-resistant infection, requiring the use of the far more toxic drug foscarnet (50mg/kg intravenously every 8 hours).

More information on HSV can be found in Chapter 17.

Varicella-Zoster Virus (VZV) Infection. Primary varicella infection in the advanced AIDS patient is a highly lethal process characterized by infection of the lungs, central nervous system, abdominal viscera, and mucocutaneous tissues, with common production of disseminated intravascular coagulation. HIV-infected persons who are seronegative for VZV and at risk for primary infection should receive zoster immune globulin on exposure to the virus and high-dose intravenous acyclovir (10 mg/kg every 8 hours) at the earliest signs of infection. This disastrous illness is a major concern, especially in HIV-infected children.

The more common problem is reactivation disease, where latent virus in the dorsal nerve root ganglia becomes reactivated due to HIV-induced immunosuppression. Typically, zoster occurs relatively early in HIV infection. The first manifestation of zoster is usually pain in the dermatome, followed by the appearance of the classic grouped vesicles on an erythematous base (Fig. 21.12). Multidermatomal involvement, either contiguous or noncontiguous, may occur. The majority of HIV-infected patients with zoster have an uneventful recovery, but lesions may persist for months or recur (Fig. 21.13) within the same dermatome. The dermatomal eruption in these patients is often hemorrhagic and/or necrotic. There may be hematogenously borne cutaneous dissemination. Persistent VZV lesions are often very painful and appear as crusted or hyperkeratotic plaques (Fig. 21.14), 1 to 2 cm in diameter, occasionally with marginal vesicles. These ecthymatous or chronic VZV infections are sparse and typically occur on the trunk or proximal extremities.

The diagnosis of VZV infection is usually made clinically, supported by the finding of giant and/or multinucleated cells on cytologic study of vesicle fluid. Alternatively, the diagnosis can be substantiated by biopsy or culture. The differential diagnosis of varicella includes disseminated HSV infection, cutaneous dissemination of zoster, eczema herpeticum, disseminated vaccinia, bullous impetigo, and various vesicular viral exanthems, such as *Enterovirus* infection. The prodromal pain of herpes zoster can mimic cardiac or pleural pain, an acute abdomen, or vertebral disc disease. The eruption must be distinguished from zosteriform HSV infection. Ecthymatous VZV lesions must be differentiated from impetigo, ecthyma, or deep mycotic infections.

The present cornerstone of treatment for VZV infection is acyclovir. As with HSV infection, acyclovir-resistant VZV has been reported. Famcyclovir and valacyclovir are highly effective drugs that are becoming available for VZV and other herpes viral infections.

VZV infection is further discussed in Chapter 17.

Epstein-Barr Virus (EBV) Infection. EBV infection facilitates three important clinical conditions in HIV-infected patients: oral hairy leukoplakia, classic Burkitt's lymphoma, and EBV-associated B-cell lymphoproliferative disease. Of these, oral hairy leukoplakia most affects mucocutaneous tissues.

Oral hairy leukoplakia (OHL) typically presents as hyperplastic, whitish, epithelial plaques on the lateral aspects of the tongue, frequently extending onto the contiguous dorsal or ventral surfaces. Usually, a single lesion or as many as three to six discrete plaques separated by normal-appearing mucosa are observed. Much less commonly, OHL occurs on the buccal mucosa opposing the tongue and on the soft palate. Although described as hairy, lesions are more likely to have a corrugated appearance, with nearly vertical, parallel white rows.

The characteristic clinical picture of OHL is a white lesion involving the lateral aspect of the tongue (Fig. 21.15), which cannot be rubbed off and which is unresponsive to antifungal therapy. Differential diagnostic considerations include hyperplastic oral candidiasis, condyloma acuminatum, geographic (migratory) glossitis, lichen planus, tobacco-assisted leukoplakia, mucous patches of secondary syphilis, squamous cell carcinoma, and traumatic hyperplasia.

OHL is asymptomatic, and waxes and wanes in severity from week to week. Treatment generally is not indicated, although acyclovir or foscarnet will induce a remission but only during their administration. The chief importance of OHL lies in its predictive nature: in HIV-infected individuals still lacking an AIDS diagnosis, 48% with OHL will develop overt AIDS within 16 months and 83% by 31 months.

Cytomegalovirus (CMV) Infection. CMV is the most common opportunistic viral pathogen to complicate HIV disease. The majority of high-risk individuals have asymptomatic CMV

infection acquired during childhood or as a sexually transmitted disease. Reactivation of CMV occurs in a wide variety of organs, including the eye, liver, adrenal glands, lung, brain, or gastrointestinal tract. One of the most common and devastating CMV manifestations occurs in the retina of one or both eyes, showing progressive retinal inflammation with hemorrhages and exudates and causing progressive visual impairment and blindness. Lung infection with CMV results in a pneumonitis that must be differentiated from PCP. Infection of the intestinal mucosa is associated with disabling diarrhea. Symptomatic cutaneous infection, however, is rare. Even when skin biopsy specimens reveal pathologic or culture evidence of CMV, the lesion is usually caused by some other pathogen.

Human Papillomavirus

Human papillomavirus (HPV) commonly infects both keratinized and nonkeratinized skin and mucous membranes. Common clinical presentations of HPV infections include those of keratinized skin—verruca vulgaris, verruca plantaris, and verruca plana—and infections of nonkeratinized skin and of mucous membranes—condylomata acuminata and intraepithelial neoplasia. The incidence and severity of HPV infections is increased in HIV-infected persons in direct proportion to the degree of immunocompromise.

• PATHOGENESIS •

The prevalence of HPV infection of nonkeratinized and mucous epithelium in HIV-infected homosexual men is high. Similarly, HIV-infected women have rates of HPV-induced cervical dysplasia 5 to 10 times higher than nonHIV-infected women.

• CLINICAL FEATURES •

Verrucae usually present asymptomatically in HIV-infected persons, the most common complaint being a cosmetic one (Fig. 21.16). Some, however, can become large (Fig. 21.17) and painful, especially warts on the plantar aspect of the foot. Some HIV-infected patients have unusually widespread or recalcitrant verrucae.

Condylomata acuminata are usually asymptomatic, although voluminous lesions may be painful and bleed. Condylomata appear as well demarcated papules or plaques arising anywhere on the anogenital (Fig. 21.18), vaginal, cervical, rectal, or oropharyngeal (Fig. 21.19) epithelium. Lesions may be numerous and become confluent. In situ or invasive squamous cell carcinoma must always be suspected in warty lesions of unusual appearance within a cluster of condylomata; biopsies should be obtained.

• DIAGNOSIS AND DIFFERENTIAL DIAGNOSIS •

The diagnosis of HPV infection is usually made on a clinical basis. The whitish appearance of micropapules or macules after the application of 5% acetic acid to the anogenital epithelium can be helpful in defining the extent of HPV infection. The diagnosis of intraepithelial neoplasia and invasive squamous cell carcinoma can only be made histologically, so typical lesions must be biopsied.

The differential diagnosis of common warts usually includes molluscum contagiosum and various benign and malignant epidermal neoplasms. The differential diagnosis of condylomata acuminata includes various benign and malignant mucocutaneous neoplasms, condylomata lata of secondary syphilis, and molluscum contagiosum.

• TREATMENT AND CLINICAL COURSE •

Treatment of HPV infection in HIV-infected patients varies with the stage of HIV disease. In the HIV-seropositive person with little or no demonstrable immunodeficiency, lesions should be managed as in the normal host. In patients with advanced immunodeficiency, complete eradication of benign HPV-induced lesions is usually not possible, and aggressive treatment such as laser surgery is not indicated. Cytologic smears and/or lesional biopsies should be obtained to monitor the evolution from cytologic atypia to intraepithelial neoplasia or invasive squamous cell carcinoma.

More information on HPV can be found in Chapter 8.

Molluscum Contagiosum

Molluscum contagiosum (MC) is a common epidermal poxvirus infection causing multiple papular and nodular lesions. In the normal host, mollusca tend to resolve spontaneously in 6 to 12 months; in the HIV-infected individual with immunodeficiency, mollusca usually fail to resolve even with treatment. Approximately 10% of AIDS patients have MC.

• PATHOGENESIS •

The poxvirus causing MC is transmitted by autoinoculation, close interpersonal contact, sexual contact, or fomites. In the normal host, the bases of mollusca demonstrate an inflammatory response to the epidermal viral infection, after which lesions regress and heal without scarring. This immune response to MC is not observed in the HIV-infected host, and lesions persist.

• CLINICAL FEATURES •

Mollusca are usually not associated with pruritus, pain, or tenderness unless there is bacterial superinfection. They usually occur as multiple lesions and are typically grouped in one bodily region, i.e., the face (Fig. 21.20), axilla, or groin. Individual mollusca are skin-colored, dome-shaped papules of 2–4 mm that commonly have a central umbilication (Fig. 21.21). In patients with moderate-to-advanced immunodeficiency, hundreds of facial lesions may occur. Multiple MC can also develop into a confluent mass in the beard area (Fig. 21.22) as the result of shaving, or be clustered on the margins of the eyelids.

• DIAGNOSIS AND DIFFERENTIAL DIAGNOSIS •

The diagnosis is usually suspected clinically and confirmed by cytological or histological examination. Differential diagno-

sis of MC in HIV-infected patients includes verruca vulgaris, keratoacanthoma, and hematogenous dissemination of systemic fungal infections, especially disseminated cryptococcosis.

• TREATMENT AND CLINICAL COURSE •

MC is usually treated with liquid nitrogen destruction. Both curettage and electrodestruction are probably best avoided in HIV-infected patients. Some patients can apply topical keratolytic or peeling agents with partial response. In HIV-infected patients, however, lesions usually recur and spread despite diligent treatment, although if zidovudine therapy improves immune function, MC lesions may regress.

BACTERIAL INFECTIONS

***Staphylococcus aureus* Infection**

Staphylococcus aureus is the single most common bacterial cause of cutaneous and systemic infection in HIV-infected patients. Both the incidence of staphylococcal infections, and the range of clinical syndromes, is far greater in this population than in normal hosts.

• PATHOGENESIS •

The usual reservoir for staphylococcal infection is the nose. Once the nasal passages are firmly colonized, the organism spreads predictably both to normal skin and to skin whose integrity has been breached by catheters, drainage tubes, or primary skin disease. *S. aureus* may also be locally invasive in the nose, causing nasal abscess.

• CLINICAL FEATURES •

A wide range of *S. aureus* infections occurs in HIV-infected individuals: impetigo (Fig. 21.23); bullous impetigo; ecthyma; folliculitis, especially of the beard, buttocks, and extremities; furuncles (Fig. 21.24) and carbuncles (Fig. 21.25); cellulitis; secondary infection of skin damaged by scabies, eczematous dermatitis, herpetic ulcerations, Kaposi's sarcoma, molluscum contagiosum (Fig. 21.26), or vascular access lines (Fig. 21.27) and drainage tubes.

Staphylococcus aureus botryomycosis occurs with the extension of staphylococcal folliculitis into the perifollicular skin, producing a draining pustular lesion. A typical plaque-like staphylococcal folliculitis has been described in AIDS. Clinically, these lesions appear as violaceous plaques up to 10 cm in diameter, at times with superficial pustules and crusts, occurring in the groin, axillae, or scalp.

Adult-onset chronic pruritic eczematous dermatitis has been reported in HIV-infected individuals with no history of atopy. *Staphylococcus aureus* can be cultured from the nares and skin and can be associated with peripheral eosinophilia and very high serum IgE antibody titers. Eczema and pruritus may resolve with antistaphylococcal antibiotic therapy.

• DIAGNOSIS AND DIFFERENTIAL DIAGNOSIS •

The differential diagnosis of the various types of *S. aureus* infections differs widely according to the morphology of the lesions and whether the infection is a primary pyoderma or a secondarily infected dermatosis. The diagnosis of *S. aureus* botryomycosis can be aided by skin biopsy, which reveals colonies of basophilic-staining coccal bacterial forms surrounded by eosinophilic amorphous material with a radiating appearance. Staphylococcal botryomycosis must be distinguished from a deep fungal infection of the skin.

• TREATMENT AND CLINICAL COURSE •

The cornerstone of treatment is anti-staphylococcal antibiotic therapy with such drugs as nafcillin, dicloxacilin, cefazolin, oxacillin, or vancomycin in penicillin-allergic patients. Intranasal administration of mupiricin ointment may deter the spread of the organism from the nose.

Bacillary Angiomatosis

Bacillary (epithelioid) angiomatosis (BA) is an infection of HIV-infected persons that produces vascular tumor-like growths of the skin.

• PATHOGENESIS •

The cause of BA is a Gram-negative organism similar to the cat-scratch disease bacillus, which can be identified with a Warthin-Starry stain of lesional biopsy specimens. Indeed, contact with cats can sometimes be documented, with lesions at the scratch site appearing in 1 to 4 weeks. By polymerase chain reaction, the etiologic agents have been demonstrated to be the *Rochalimaea* species, *R. quintana* and *R. henselae*, rickettsia-like microbes. Impaired cell-mediated immunity clearly plays a role in the pathogenesis of this process, as this entity only occurs in patients with significant immunocompromise and tends to spread to visceral organs in patients with advanced AIDS.

• CLINICAL FEATURES •

The lesions of BA are papular or nodular, dome-shaped, and hemangioma-like (Fig. 21.28), ranging in size from a few millimeters to 3 cm and, at times, becoming pedunculated. They are usually violaceous to bright-red but may be skin-colored. Usually situated in the dermis, these lesions may also occur deeper in the subcutaneous tissue in which case they are firm, nontender, and nonblanching. They may occur at any site, but palms, soles, and the oral cavity are usually spared. Bronchial lesions have been reported. Lesions may be solitary or number in the hundreds.

Some patients may have systemic spread to the bone, marrow, liver, and spleen. Peliosis hepatitis (cystic, blood-filled spaces in the liver) has also been noted. Histologically, organisms may be visualized within the myxoid stroma of these lesions.

• DIAGNOSIS AND DIFFERENTIAL DIAGNOSIS •

Diagnosis of BA is made by demonstrating the rod-like organism in biopsy material stained with the Warthin-Starry or a similar silver stain. The histological appearance of this lesion is that of endothelium-lined vascular spaces in the dermis with a variable amount of edema and inflammatory infiltrate. The endothelial cells are typically large and cuboidal, with prominent nuclei. Culture of the organism from tissue has been reported but is not routinely done. Differential diagnosis includes Kaposi's sarcoma, pyogenic granuloma, epithelioid (histiocytoid) angioma, cherry angioma, sclerosing hemangioma, verruga peruana lesions of bartonellosis, and disseminated cryptococcosis.

• TREATMENT AND CLINICAL COURSE •

The course of bacillary angiomatosis is variable and can include spontaneous regression of lesions. Particularly in patients with extensive or systemic disease, treatment with broad-spectrum antibiotics, such as erythromycin (250 to 500 mg 4 times per day) or doxycycline (100 mg twice daily), can be effective. (See Chapter 10 for more information).

Syphilis

Syphilis is an important problem in HIV-infected patients for at least four reasons:

1. Persons at high risk for HIV acquisition are also at high risk for syphilis;

2. Genital ulcer disease facilitates the transmission and acquisition of HIV;

3. Immunologic defects may block the appearance of the usual antibody response to *Treponema pallidum*, so that false-negative serologic tests for syphilis can be observed in the face of active and even progressive infection;

4. Manifestations of the disease may be altered, response to therapy decreased, and duration of the stages of syphilis greatly telescoped, all due to the host's immunocompromised state.

• PATHOGENESIS •

Shortly after *T. pallidum* penetrates the intact mucous membrane or abraded skin, it spreads via lymphatics and the systemic circulation. The degree of immunocompromise greatly influences development and healing of the infection. Severe immunocompromise is likely to be associated with a larger organism burden, systemic spread, rapid development of "late stage" disease, and failure of conventional antimicrobial therapy, particularly with bacteriostatic drugs, such as doxycycline or erythromycin.

• CLINICAL FEATURES •

The clinical presentation of primary syphilis in the HIV-infected individual may be identical to that in the normal host: a single painless papule appearing 3 to 90 days after inoculation that erodes and becomes indurated. However, the HIV-infected patient may have multiple chancres, larger ulcers, and painful infection with *Staphylococcus aureus* or other bacteria. Instead of healing in 3 to 6 weeks, ulcers may persist much longer.

HIV patients may demonstrate the same clinical manifestations of secondary syphilis as the normal host. Also possible are lues maligna (Figs. 21.29, 21.30), an uncommon form of secondary syphilis characterized by pleomorphic skin lesions—pustules, plaques, nodules, and ulcers, with a necrotizing vasculitis. The most notable aspect of secondary and tertiary syphilis in the HIV-infected individual, however, is the rapid progression of disease, such that normally late sequelae may be observed less than 6 months after primary infection, even in the face of normally adequate therapy.

The late cutaneous manifestations of syphilis are gummas, granulomatous-like lesions that produce superficial nodules and deeper lesions that may break down and ulcerate. Areas of trauma are likely to be involved.

In general, HIV-infected persons with syphilis have atypical skin eruptions, more systemic symptoms, simultaneous multiorgan involvement, and greater development of neurosyphilis and uveitis. Because of the severe course of the disease and the unreliability of traditional diagnostic and therapeutic approaches, an aggressive biopsy and treatment program are essential.

• DIAGNOSIS AND DIFFERENTIAL DIAGNOSIS •

In nonHIV-infected persons, diagnosis is usually confirmed by serologic testing. However, since false-positive and false-negative results are common in HIV-infected patients, serology must be supplemented by biopsies of suspicious lesions. If possible, fluid from early lesions should be examined by dark-field microscopy. In addition, specific immunofluorescent or immunoperoxidase staining of pathologic specimens can assist in the definitive diagnosis.

The differential diagnosis of cutaneous syphilitic lesions is broad, influenced by the stage of infection. Primary lesions of syphilis must be distinguished from herpes simplex infection, chancroid, and bacterial infections. Under appropriate epidemiologic conditions, such entities as donovanosis, lymphogranuloma venereum, mycobacterial infection, and tularemia must also be considered. The differential diagnosis of secondary syphilis includes drug eruption, pityriasis rosea, infectious exanthems, tinea corporis, tinea versicolor, scabies, "id" reaction, condylomata acuminata, guttate psoriasis, and lichen planus. The differential diagnosis of cutaneous tertiary syphilis includes lymphoma, tuberculosis, sarcoidosis, and deep fungal infections.

• TREATMENT AND CLINICAL COURSE •

- Primary and secondary syphilis and early latent syphilis of less than 1 years' duration:
    Benzathine penicillin G, 2.4 million units IM, in 1 dose. Some experts advise repeating the dose in 1 week.
    Alternative regimen for penicillin-allergic (nonpregnant) patients:
    Doxycycline, 100 mg orally b.i.d. for 2 weeks; or

    Tetracycline, 500 mg orally q.i.d. for 2 weeks; or
    Erythromycin, 500 mg orally q.i.d. for 2 weeks; or
    Ceftriaxone, 250 mg IM once a day for 10 days.
- Late latent syphilis of more than 1 years' duration, gummas, and cardiovascular syphilis:
    Benzathine penicillin G, 7.2 million units total, administered as 3 doses of 2.4 million units IM, given 1 week apart for 3 consecutive weeks.
    Alternative regimen for penicillin-allergic (nonpregnant) patients:
    Doxycycline, 100 mg orally b.i.d. for 4 weeks, or
    Tetracycline, 500 mg orally q.i.d. for 4 weeks.
- Neurosyphilis:
    Aqueous crystalline penicillin G, 2–4 million units every 4 hours IV (total of 12–24 million units per day), for 10–14 days.
    Alternative regimen (for compliant outpatients):
    Procaine penicillin, 2 to 4 million units IM daily and
    Probenecid, 500 mg orally q.i.d., both for 10–14 days.
- Syphilis in HIV-infected patients:

    Penicillin regimens should be used whenever possible for all stages of syphilis in HIV-infected patients. Some authorities advise CSF examination and/or treatment with a regimen appropriate for neurosyphilis for all patients coinfected with syphilis and HIV, regardless of the clinical stage of syphilis. Patients should be followed clinically and with quantitative nontreponemal serologic tests (VDRL, RPR) at 1, 2, 3, 6, 9, and 12 months after treatment. Patients with early syphilis whose titers increase or fail to decrease 4-fold within 6 months should undergo CSF examination and be treated again. In such patients, CSF abnormalities could be due to HIV-related infection, neurosyphilis, or both.

Pneumococcal Infections

HIV-positive patients have an increased susceptibility to pneumococcal infections. Pneumococcal disease in HIV patients may have unusual manifestations, such as soft tissue abscesses, multiple brain abscesses, and purpura fulminans (Fig. 21.31) (3).

Tuberculosis and Other Mycobacterioses

Tuberculosis is a common opportunistic infection in HIV disease. Of particular concern is the emergence of strains of *M. tuberculosis* resistant to multiple antituberculous drugs. As with tuberculosis in the immunocompetent patient, cutaneous involvement is uncommon; however, transmission to health care workers has been reported from cutaneous lesions in HIV-infected patients.

Several nontuberculous *Mycobacteria* have been reported to cause cutaneous lesions, usually via hematogenous dissemination to the skin. *Mycobacterium avium-intracellulare* complex (MAC), a common opportunistic pathogen, rarely causes specific cutaneous lesions, although as with CMV infections MAC can be cultured from skin biopsy specimens as a manifestation of widespread infection.

FUNGAL INFECTIONS

Mucosal Candidiasis

Oropharyngeal and esophageal candidiasis were recognized early as important manifestations of HIV-initiated clinical disease. Mucosal candidiasis occurs nearly universally in patients with advanced HIV-induced immunodeficiency. Candidiasis of moist, keratinized cutaneous sites, such as the anogenital region, however, occurs uncommonly, and systemic infection with visceral seeding is rare, even in patients with advanced HIV infection.

• PATHOGENESIS •

The occurrence of mucosal candidal infection is directly related to the severity of HIV cell-mediated immune dysfunction. The diagnosis of thrush in the absence of predisposing local or systemic causes (previous antibiotic therapy, oral contraceptive use, pregnancy, steroid administration), should always raise the possibility of HIV infection.

• CLINICAL FEATURES •

Although often asymptomatic, the presence of white curd-like colonies of *Candida* in the mouth is a constant reminder of HIV disease to the patient. When symptoms are present, they often include a soreness or burning sensation in the mouth, sensitivity to spicy foods, and/or altered sense of taste. Symptomatic esophageal candidiasis is less common than oropharyngeal infection, but may produce symptoms of retrosternal burning and odynophagia. Female patients with HIV infection are increasingly subject to vulvovaginal candidiasis associated with vulvar pruritus, dysuria, dyspareunia, and vaginal discharge.

On physical examination and esophagoscopy, oropharyngeal and esophageal candidiasis usually demonstrate a pseudomembranous pattern (thrush) (Fig. 21.32) and, less often, a chronic hyperplastic and/or atrophic pattern (Figs. 21.33, 21.34). Pseudomembranous candidiasis is characterized by white-to-creamy curd-like plaques on any surface of the oral mucosa, the white areas being colonies of *Candida*. The "curds" are easily removed with dry gauze (in contrast to lesions of oral hairy leukoplakia, which are relatively fixed to the underlying mucosa) with some bleeding of the mucosa. Atrophic candidiasis is often overlooked on examination of the mouth and is often the initial presentation of oropharyngeal candidiasis; it appears as patches of erythema, usually in the vault of the mouth on the hard and/or soft palate. On the dorsal surface of the tongue, atrophic candidiasis causes areas of depapillation, resulting in a smooth red mucosa. Some sites show areas of pseudomembranous involvement, while others manifest the atrophic pattern. Chronic hyperplastic candidiasis presents as both red and white patches at any site in the oropharynx. In patients with dentures, pseudomembranous and/or atrophic candidiasis is typically seen under the occluded mucosa.

Candidal angular cheilitis occurs at the corners of the mouth (Fig. 21.35) and is more common in edentulous patients; it may occur in conjunction with oropharyngeal or esophageal disease or as the only manifestation of candidal infection.

Chronic candidal vulvovaginitis is a common opportunistic infection in HIV-infected women with moderate-to-advanced immunodeficiency. Children with HIV infection commonly experience candidiasis in the diaper area, intertrigo in the axillae and neck folds, and chronic candidal paronychia with nail dystrophy.

• DIAGNOSIS AND DIFFERENTIAL DIAGNOSIS •

The diagnosis of mucocutaneous candidal infection is based on clinical manifestations of infection plus the demonstration of pseudohyphae on a potassium hydroxide preparation. Since *Candida* is a commensal organism in the oral cavity, its isolation on culture in the absence of a clinically overt abnormality is not very meaningful. At times, lesional biopsy is required for the diagnosis of hyperplastic candidiasis.

The differential diagnosis of oropharyngeal candidiasis includes oral hairy leukoplakia, migratory glossitis (geographic tongue), lichen planus, bite line irritation, and smoker's leukoplakia.

• TREATMENT AND CLINICAL COURSE •

Two different strategies are available for controlling mucosal candidal infections: topical therapy with nystatin or clotrimazole troches, administered 4–5 times per day, or systemic therapy with once-a-day ketoconazole or fluconazole. Although topical therapy can be effective, particularly when HIV-induced immunocompromise is minimal, systemic therapy gives a better initial clinical response and a higher rate of eradication of the organism. Fluconazole is the more reliable of the two systemic drugs, probably because its absorption is not dependent on gastric acidity. Typically, as AIDS advances, patients develop recurrent episodes of mucosal candidiasis. These can sometimes be prevented by maintaining the patient on long-term fluconazole therapy.

Systemic Mycoses Disseminated to the Skin

The first important clues to the presence of a systemic mycotic infection may be the presence of cutaneous manifestations from dissemination. The most important examples of this phenomenon are disseminated *Cryptococcus neoformans* infection, which occurs in approximately 10% of AIDS patients, and infection due to *Histoplasma capsulatum* (Fig. 21.36) or *Coccidioides immitis,* which occur primarily in geographically restricted areas. *Sporothrix schenckii* occurs worldwide, and can uncommonly show cutaneous infection due to dissemination from a pulmonary focus of sporotrichosis rather than the usual primary inoculation disease seen in immunocompetent persons.

• PATHOGENESIS •

As in tuberculosis, primary infection from these organisms usually occurs in the lungs following inhalation. The initial response by polymorphonuclear leukocytes limits the extent of primary infection, but the cell-mediated immune response limits the subsequent breakdown of sites of dormant infection and the impact of postprimary systemic dissemination. Thus, AIDS patients are at risk for three patterns of infection:

1. Progressive, primary infection with systemic spread due to a failure of the normal cell-mediated immune response;

2. Reactivation of dormant sites of infection, with systemic dissemination of the organisms;

3. Reinfection through loss of the protective immunity of past exposure, producing a disease pattern resembling progressive primary infection.

• CLINICAL FEATURES •

About 10% of patients with disseminated mycotic infections develop skin or mucosal disease, often as the first recognizable manifestation of the infection. These skin lesions are usually asymptomatic, except for their appearance. Thus, the patient's presenting symptoms are determined primarily by other sites of involvement. Oral and/or esophageal ulcerations due to *Histoplasma capsulatum* may, however, be painful.

Skin lesions due to systemic fungal infection in the HIV-infected individual most commonly occur on the face in the form of multiple molluscum contagiosum-like lesions, papules, or nodules; lesions can also be seen on the trunk and extremities. These lesions may become ulcerated. Other reported cutaneous findings include erythematous macules; necrotic or keratin-plugged papules and nodules; pustules or acneiform lesions; vegetative plaques; and panniculitis. Oral mucosal lesions occurring in disseminated disease include nodules, vegetations, and ulcerations on the lips, soft palate, oropharynx, epiglottis, and/or nasal vestibule. Mucosal lesions occur most commonly with histoplasmosis, occasionally in cryptococcosis, but, essentially, not in coccidioidomycosis. Hepatosplenomegaly and/or lymphadenopathy occur commonly in patients with disseminated histoplasmosis. Patients with disseminated sporotrichosis have widespread crusted nodules on the skin. Meningitis, arthritis, and endophthalmitis have also been reported.

• DIAGNOSIS AND DIFFERENTIAL DIAGNOSIS •

Diagnosis in this clinical situation is by skin biopsy for culture and pathological examination. Because of the need for early diagnosis and recognition of disseminated infection in an immunocompromised host, any unexplained skin lesion in the patient with HIV infection should be biopsied.

The differential diagnosis of patients with skin lesions possibly due to systemic fungal infection includes molluscum contagiosum, verruca vulgaris, verruca plana, disseminated herpetic or varicella infection, bacillary angiomatosis, and furunculosis.

• TREATMENT AND CLINICAL COURSE •

The diagnosis of cutaneous infection with *Cryptococcus neoformans*, *Coccidioides immitis*, or *Histoplasma capsulatum* is evidence of disseminated infection. Primary infection of the skin from these organisms is rare, only occurring in unusual circumstances, such as direct inoculation in a laboratory. The traditional therapy for these infections has been a prolonged course of intravenous amphotericin. Recent experience suggests that lifelong therapy with drugs such as fluconazole is necessary to prevent relapse in these patients.

Dermatophytosis

Infection by dermatophytes in HIV-infected persons may occur on keratinized surfaces—skin (Fig. 21.37), nails (Figs. 21.38, 21.39), and hair. Because of the impaired cell-mediated immunity in these patients, extensive infection poorly responsive to traditional topical therapies is not uncommon. Such infections are important for three reasons: *a*) morbidity and disfigurement can be extensive; *b*) breakdown in the skin integrity can provide a portal of entry for other pathogens, particularly *Staphylococcus aureus*; and *c*) these infections can mimic other dermatologic conditions, such as tinea facialis mimicking the more common seborrheic dermatitis. Prolonged courses of oral antifungal agents have been an effective treatment.

Pityrosporum ovale

Pityrosporum ovale normally resides in regions of the skin with active sebaceous activity, such as the scalp, face, upper back, and central chest. It is implicated in the pathogenesis of seborrheic dermatitis, a condition extremely common in HIV infected patients. Seborrheic dermatitis often responds to topical antifungal agents, such as ketoconazole cream or shampoo. *Pityrosporum ovale* also may cause a folliculitis on the trunk in the immunocompromised host as well as nonimmunocompromised persons under certain situations.

PROTOZOAN INFECTION

Pneumocystis carinii (PC) is the most common pulmonary opportunistic pathogen in the developed world, resulting in *Pneumocystis carinii* pneumonia (PCP). Prophylaxis of PCP in HIV disease has resulted in a marked reduction in its prevalence. In patients treated solely with aerosolized pentamidine, only the lung receives the benefit; therefore, patients are susceptible to disseminated PC infection. Cutaneous manifestations in this situation are nodules in or around the external auditory canals and acral infarctive lesions secondary to arteriolar occlusion.

Important Noninfectious Forms of Mucocutaneous Disease

ADVERSE DRUG REACTIONS PRODUCING CUTANEOUS ABNORMALITIES

HIV-infected persons have an inordinately high incidence of cutaneous eruptions in reaction to a variety of drugs, especially antibiotics. The most common offending agents are sulfonamides and amoxicillin-clavulanate. Multiple drug reactions are also more common.

The greatest clinical problem is with trimethoprim-sulfamethoxazole (TMP-SMZ). Over half of patients with *Pneumocystis carinii* pneumonia treated with TMP-SMZ develop a widespread macular or papular erythematous eruption and fever 8 to 10 days after starting therapy, almost 10 times higher than that of the general population. Parenteral pentamidine, an alternative to TMP-SMZ, also can cause severe adverse reactions in up to 20% of AIDS patients. Even aerosolized pentamidine may cause a widespread erythematous, maculopapular eruption. Fansidar (sulfadoxine-pyrimethamine), another alternative drug, has been reported to cause erythema multiforme and fatal toxic epidermal necrolysis.

The most common cutaneous reaction to zidovudine (AZT) is hyperpigmentation of the nails. Blue to brown-black nail discoloration can occur in over 40% of zidovudine-treated individuals, particularly in those of African ancestry. Dyschromia usually develops 4 to 8 weeks after initiating treatment but may occur up to 1 year later. Longitudinal streaks are most common, but diffuse pigmentation and transverse bands may occur, especially on the thumbnail. Hyperpigmentation of mucous membranes and skin also occurs, although mucosal pigmentation is usually only seen in those of African descent. Diffuse hyperpigmentation mimicking primary adrenal insufficiency has also been reported in patients treated with zidovudine. Although infrequent, severe exanthematous eruptions warranting drug withdrawal occur in the first 8 to 12 days of therapy in about 1% of patients receiving zidovudine. Successful desensitization has been accomplished in such circumstances.

Foscarnet (trisodium phosphonoformate) induces localized, painful, penile ulceration in almost 30% of patients beginning high-dose induction therapy for CMV retinitis. The ulcers clear spontaneously in one-half of those affected, whether patients receive treatment or not.

Systemic treatment with methotrexate for psoriasis and corticosteroids for vasculitis or lymphoma has been associated with the sudden appearance and rapid proliferation of Kaposi's sarcoma.

CUTANEOUS CONDITIONS OF UNCLEAR ETIOLOGY

Seborrheic dermatitis (Fig. 21.40) occurs to varying degrees in nearly all persons with HIV disease. Its anatomic distribution is typical, but it tends to be more hyperkeratotic than in nonHIV-infected individuals.

Psoriasis vulgaris (Fig. 21.41) occurs in 1% to 2% of HIV-infected patients and psoriatic arthritis in 2% to 10% of those with skin involvement. Psoriasis may develop spontaneously after HIV seroconversion in a person who has never before had clinical disease, or mild, preexisting psoriasis may suddenly exacerbate once AIDS develops. Eosinophilic folliculitis is relatively common in advanced HIV disease, characterized clinically by pruritic follicular papules and associated with eosinophilia in lesions and the blood.

Perspective

About 100 million persons are expected to be infected with HIV by the turn of the century. As these numbers grow, and as patients live longer, more mucocutaneous disorders associated with HIV disease will be reported. For example, dual infection of HIV with human T-cell lymphotropic virus I or leprosy may produce a different set of cutaneous disorders or atypical disease

courses. Also, with the rise in both tuberculosis and HIV disease, more cutaneous tuberculous infections will likely be seen.

REFERENCES

1. Myskowski PL, et al. AIDS-associated Kaposi's sarcoma: Variables associated with survival. J Am Acad Dermatol 1988;18:1299.
2. Janier M, Morel P, Civatte J. The Köbner phenomenon in AIDS-related Kaposi's sarcoma. J Am Acad Dermatol 1990;22:125.
3. Barradas MCR, et al. Unusual manifestations of pneumococcal infection in human immunodeficiency virus-infected individuals: The past revisited. Clin Infect Dis 1992;14:192.

ANNOTATED BIBLIOGRAPHY

Alessi E, et al. Oral hairy leukoplakia. J Am Acad Dermatol 1990;22:79.
   Report of 59 cases of hairy leukoplakia with description of the clinical findings, dermatopathology, and course.
Berger TG, Greene I. Bacterial, viral, fungal, and parasitic infections in HIV disease and AIDS. Dermatol Clin 1991;9:465.
   Comprehensive review of the infectious complications of HIV disease manifesting in the skin and mucous membranes.
Cockerell CJ. Human immunodeficiency virus infection and the skin. A crucial interface. Arch Intern Med 1991;151:1295.
   Review of the cutaneous findings in HIV disease with excellent clinical photographs.
Cockerell CJ. Noninfectious inflammatory skin diseases in HIV-infected individuals. Dermatol Clin 1991;9:531.
   Extensive review of the numerous noninfectious cutaneous disorders occurring in HIV disease.
Coopman SA, Johnson RA, Platt R, Stern RS. Cutaneous disease and drug reactions in HIV infection. N Engl J Med 1993;328:1670.
   In a large Boston HMO, the medical records of 684 HIV-infected members were reviewed to determine the frequency of dermatologic disorders. Diagnoses of skin conditions increased according to the stage of disease. The authors concluded that cutaneous diseases, including drug reactions, are extremely common in HIV infection and that their incidence increases as immune function deteriorates.
Dover JS, Johnson RA. Cutaneous manifestations of human immunodeficiency virus infection. (parts I, II) Arch Dermatol 1991;127(10):1383,1549.
   Comprehensive review of the mucocutaneous manifestations of HIV disease.
Friedman-Kien AE, et al. Herpes zoster: A possible early clinical sign for development of acquired immunodeficiency syndrome in high-risk individuals. J Am Acad Dermatol 1986;14:1023.
   A retrospective review of 300 cases of HIV-associated Kaposi's sarcoma reports that 8% had prior zoster, a rate that is seven-fold greater than historical controls of the same age.
Friedman-Kien AE, Saltzman BR. Clinical manifestations of classical, endemic African and epidemic AIDS-associated Kaposi's sarcoma. J Am Acad Dermatol 1990;22:1237.
   Discussion of the various forms of Kaposi's sarcoma, with excellent color illustrations.
Gaines H. Primary HIV infection. Clinical and diagnostic aspects. Scand J Infect Dis 1989;(suppl 61).
   A very comprehensive review of the clinical findings and diagnosis of symptomatic primary HIV infection.
Gottlieb MS, et al. Pneumocystis carinii pneumonia and mucosal candidiasis in previously healthy homosexual men. Evidence of a new acquired cellular immunodeficiency. N Engl J Med 1981;305:1425.
   Initial case report of AIDS in four homosexual men with mucosal candidiasis and Pneumocystis carinii pneumonia.
Greenspan D, Greenspan JS. Oral manifestations of HIV infection. Dermatol Clin 1991;9:517.
   Review of candidiasis, hairy leukoplakia, condyloma, ulcers, and necrotizing gingivitis in HIV disease.
Johnson RA, Dover JS. Cutaneous manifestations of human immunodeficiency

virus disease. In: Fitzpatrick TB, et al, eds. Dermatology in general medicine. New York: McGraw-Hill, 1994: 2637–2689.

Comprehensive current review article with excellent color photographs of the oral and cutaneous manifestations of HIV disease.

Krigel RL, Friedman-Kien AE. Epidemic Kaposi's sarcoma. Semin Oncol 1990;17:350.

Excellent current review of HIV-associated Kaposi's sarcoma.

Musher DM. Syphilis, neurosyphilis, penicillin, and AIDS. J Infect Dis 1991;163:1201.

Comprehensive review of the clinical aspects of neurosyphilis in the HIV-infected patient with discussion of treatment and follow-up.

Schwartz JJ, Dias BM, Safai B. HIV-related malignancies. Dermatol Clin 1991;9:503.

Discussion of Kaposi's sarcoma, nonHodgkin's B-cell lymphoma, primary central nervous system lymphoma, T-cell lymphoma, and anorectal carcinoma occurring in HIV disease.

Siegal FP, et al. Severe acquired immunodeficiency in male homosexuals, manifested by chronic perianal ulcerative herpes simplex lesions. N Engl J Med 1981;305:1439.

A report of the first cases of AIDS at the beginning of the epidemic. Four homosexual men with chronic herpetic ulcers and a previously unrecognized acquired immunodeficiency are described.

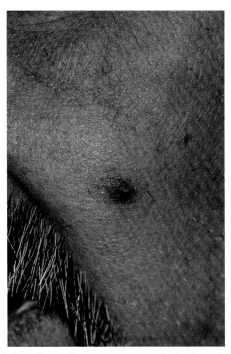

Figure 21.1.   Kaposi's sarcoma, early lesion. Solitary violaceous nodule on the cheek.

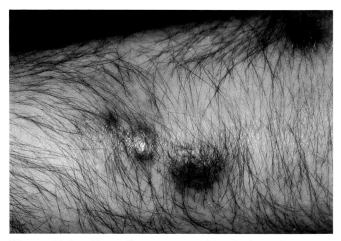

Figure 21.2.   Kaposi's sarcoma, older lesions. Three large tuberous lesions on the forearm, surrounded by a wide greenish halo, which occurs because of extravasation of blood from these vascular lesions and subsequent breakdown to hemosiderin.

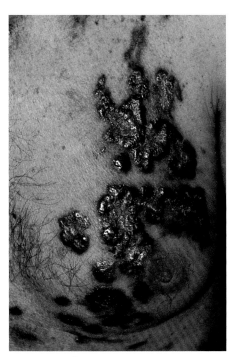

Figure 21.3.   Kaposi's sarcoma, older tuberous lesions. Very large lesions, present for more than 2 years, are becoming confluent. Note edema of the skin overlying the breast.

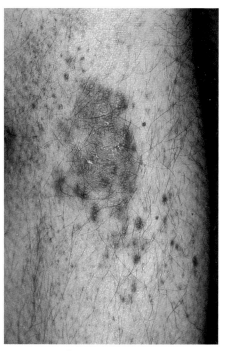

Figure 21.4.   Kaposi's sarcoma appearing in a follicular pattern. Central plaque formed by the confluence of small lesions surrounded by small, early papules on the thigh.

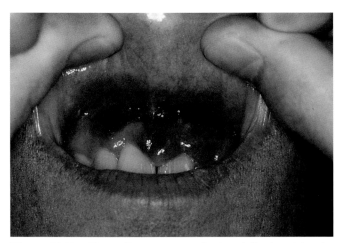

Figure 21.5.   Kaposi's sarcoma, gingiva. Infiltration of the gingival tissue. Disfiguring nodular KS lesions are also present on the adjoining area of the hard palate.

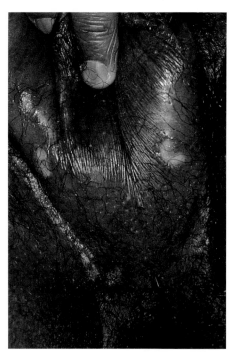

Figure 21.6.   Chronic herpes simplex. Well-circumscribed ulcerations, present for 8 weeks, on the scrotum and inguinal folds. This was the initial presentation of this 33-year-old Haitian male and, in the absence of other causes of immunocompromise, an AIDS-defining condition.

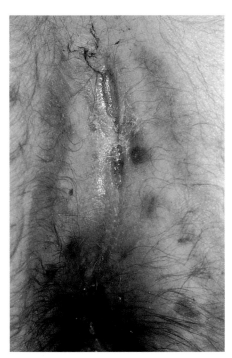

Figure 21.7.   Chronic herpes simplex. Linear herpetic ulcer in the intergluteal cleft. Numerous violaceous nodules of KS and an inverse pattern psoriasis are also seen on the buttocks.

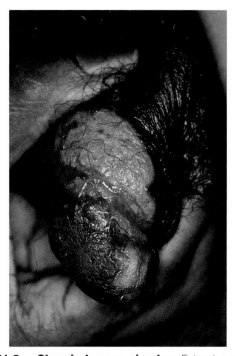

Figure 21.8.   Chronic herpes simplex. Extensive ulcerations on the shaft of the penis, which resolved on oral acyclovir.

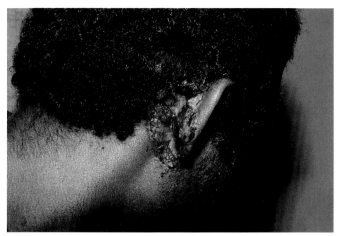

Figure 21.9.   Chronic herpes simplex. Chronic herpes simplex of the posterior ear and neck. (Courtesy of Dr. Lee T. Nesbitt, Jr.)

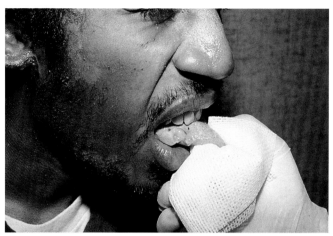

Figure 21.10.   Chronic herpes simplex. Chronic herpes simplex of the tongue in the patient shown in Figure 21.9. (Courtesy of Dr. Lee T. Nesbitt, Jr.)

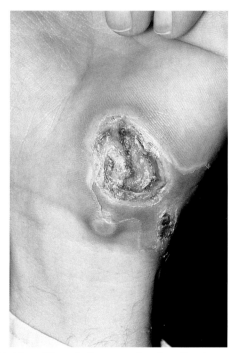

Figure 21.11.   Chronic herpes simplex. Persistent ulcer of the wrist with surrounding vesicular lesion. (Courtesy of Dr. Lee T. Nesbitt, Jr.)

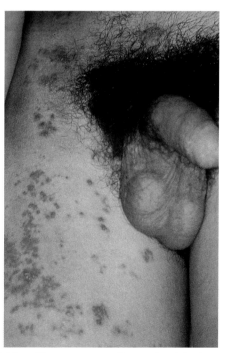

Figure 21.12.   Herpes zoster. Grouped vesicles in a dermatomal pattern on the thigh of an 18-year-old hemophiliac infected with HIV 7 years previously.

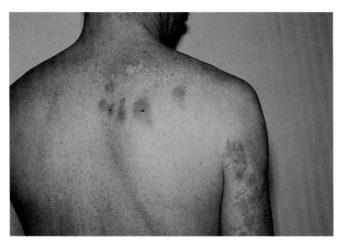

Figure 21.13.   Recurrent herpes zoster. Erythema and grouped vesicles, with scars from a previous outbreak. (Courtesy of Dr. Lee T. Nesbitt, Jr.)

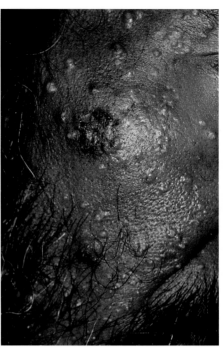

Figure 21.14.   Ecthymatous varicella-zoster virus infection. Painful, thickly crusted ulcerations on the cheek. Patient had 9 similar lesions at other sites, which cleared on IV-administered ganciclovir for CMV retinitis. Numerous mollusca contagiosa are also seen.

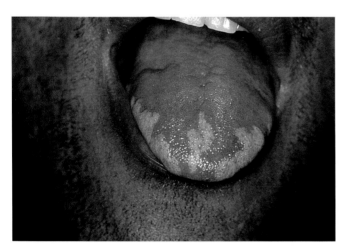

Figure 21.15.   Hairy leukoplakia. Well-demarcated white plaques on the lateral aspects of the tongue. Lesions cleared with oral acyclovir.

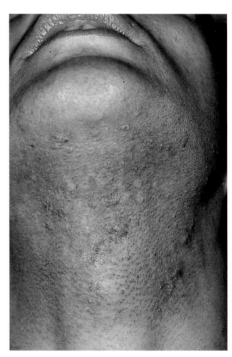

Figure 21.16.   Verruca plana. Hundreds of brown papules in the beard area, a major cosmetic stigma to the patient.

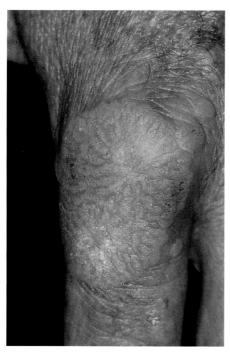

Figure 21.17.   Verruca vulgaris. A wart, 3 cm in diameter, on the dorsum of the metacarpophalangeal joint with other smaller warts.

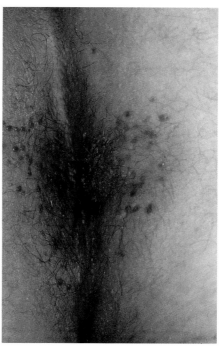

Figure 21.18.   Condylomata acuminata and intraepithelial neoplasia. Numerous brown soft papules on the perianal skin, which proved to be intraepithelial neoplasia on lesional biopsy.

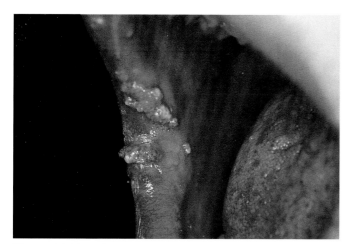

Figure 21.19.   Condylomata acuminata. Soft pink papules on the lips and oral mucosa in a 20-year-old woman who also had genital warts.

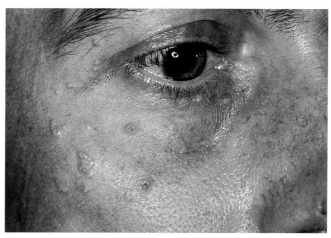

Figure 21.20.   Mollusca contagiosa. Numerous skin-colored papules on the face, resembling dermal nevi. Such a profusion of facial lesions is rare except in HIV disease.

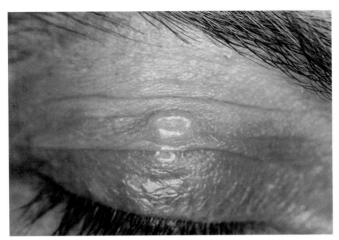

Figure 21.21.   Mollusca contagiosa. Close-up view of mollusca occurring on the eyelids, exhibiting a giant molluscum with the typical central umbilication.

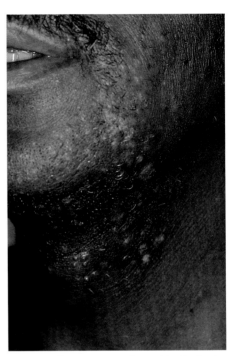

Figure 21.22.   Mollusca contagiosa. Hundreds of mollusca present in the beard area that were spread by shaving. Lesions must be distinguished from flat warts, which also occur as multiple papules in the beard area of HIV-infected men.

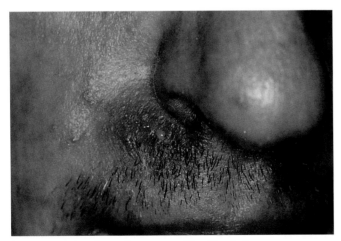

Figure 21.23.   Impetigo, caused by *Staphylococcus aureus*. Large crusted plaque on the upper lip and cheek.

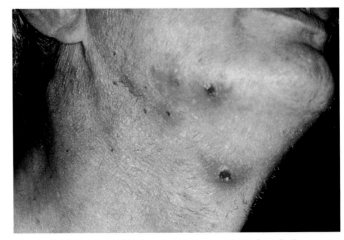

Figure 21.24.   Multiple furuncles caused by *Staphylococcus aureus*. Multiple abscesses on the neck in a patient who also had similar lesions on the scalp and buttocks. Chronic oral antibiotics were necessary to prevent recurrence.

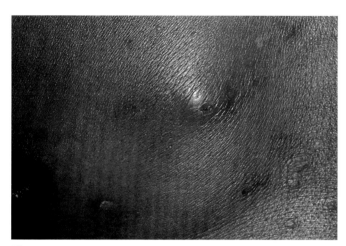

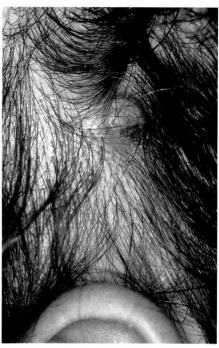

Figure 21.25. Abscess caused by *Staphylococcus aureus*. A large intact abscess, surrounded by cellulitis, on the pectoral area, accompanied by multiple abscesses on the back. Lesions arose over 2 to 3 days in sites of excoriation. Patient required chronic antibiotic suppressive therapy.

Figure 21.26. Giant molluscum contagiosum. A 1-cm solitary nodule with a halo of erythema on the scalp. Lesions were superinfected with *Staphylococcus aureus*.

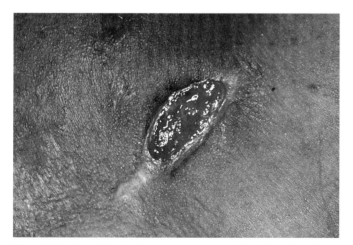

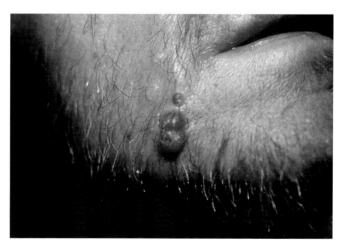

Figure 21.27. *Staphylococcus aureus* infection. Infection at the site of a central venous line, which had been in place for 1 month and which was removed during this infection.

Figure 21.28. Bacillary angiomatosis. Three hemangioma-like nodules on the cheek. Numerous skin-colored mollusca are also seen. (Courtesy of Dr. Neil S. Sadick)

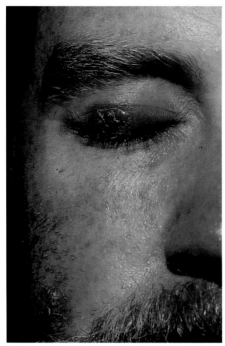

Figure 21.29.   Secondary syphilis. Edematous, erythematous lesion with central crusting of the upper eyelid. A crusted lesion is also present on the lower cheek. (Courtesy of Dr. Charles V. Sanders)

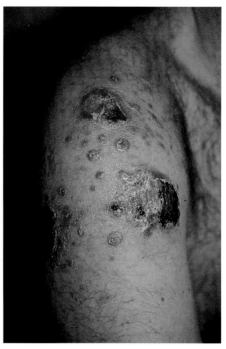

Figure 21.30.   Secondary syphilis. Vesiculopustular lesions with plaque formation. (Courtesy of Dr. Charles V. Sanders)

Figure 21.31.   Pneumococcal sepsis. Secondary to pneumonia in an HIV-positive patient, showing reticular pattern of purpura on the abdomen and flank. (Courtesy of Dr. Charles V. Sanders)

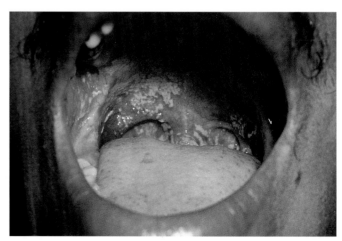

Figure 21.32.   Oral candidiasis, pseudomembranous (thrush). White curd-like candidal colonies on an erythematous, atrophic mucosa seen on the soft palate. (Courtesy of Dr. Charles V. Sanders)

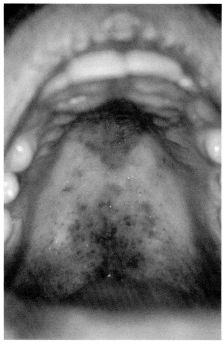

Figure 21.33.   Oral candidiasis, atrophic. Confluent erythematous patches on the palate.

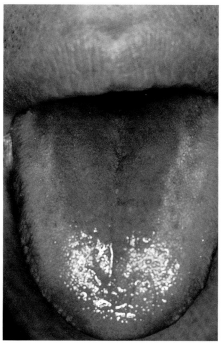

Figure 21.34.   Oral candidiasis, atrophic and hyperplastic. The median part of the tongue is red and atrophic, and the lateral aspects are hyperplastic.

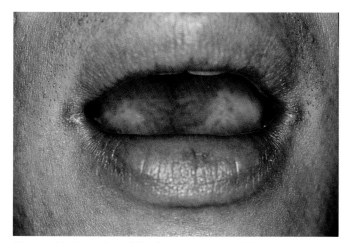

Figure 21.35.   Candidiasis, angular cheilitis. Same patient as Figure 21.34. The erythema at the corners of the mouth represents candidal intertrigo.

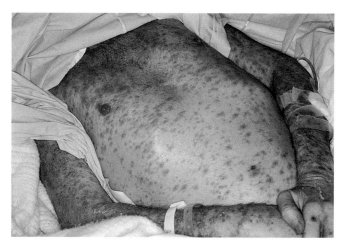

Figure 21.36.   Disseminated histoplasmosis in a patient with AIDS. Generalized maculopapular eruption and vesiculopustules resemble varicella-zoster. (Courtesy of Dr. Charles V. Sanders)

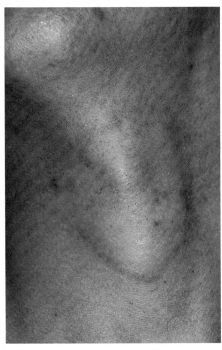

Figure 21.37.   Dermatophytosis: tinea corporis. A large annular lesion on the anterior neck that spread rapidly from tinea pedis.

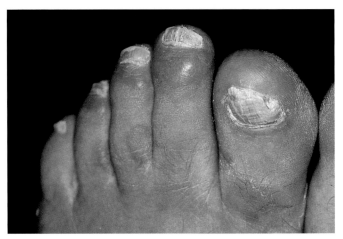

Figure 21.38.   Dermatophytosis: tinea pedis, tinea unguium. Erythema and scaling on the skin of the feet, with thickened and dystrophic toenails. An incidental finding is the KS, manifested as a violaceous color and enlargement of the distal toes.

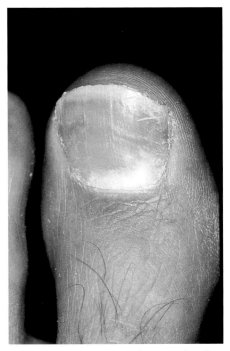

Figure 21.39.   Dermatophytosis: proximal superficial tinea unguium. This rare variant of dermatophytic infection of the nails is relatively common in HIV disease.

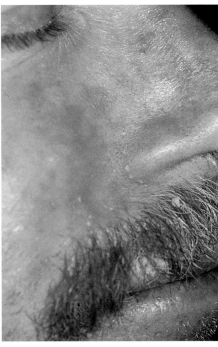

Figure 21.40.   Seborrheic dermatitis. Erythema and scaling at the nasolabial region and upper lip within the mustache.

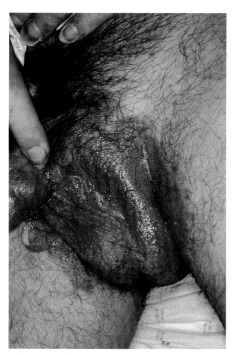

Figure 21.41.   Psoriasis vulgaris. Erythematous, partially eroded, and scaling plaques in the groin region. Generalized involvement
occurred within 1 week.

CHAPTER 22

Approach to the Diagnosis of the Patient with Fever and Rash

CHARLES V. SANDERS

The skin provides a large, easily accessible window to the diagnosis of many illnesses, including those due to infectious microorganisms. The clinical syndrome of fever and skin rash represents a challenging and often urgent diagnostic problem that may alarm both patient and physician. If not diagnosed promptly, many infectious diseases can spur irrevocable changes that may result in death, despite treatment with large doses of appropriate antimicrobials (e.g., acute meningococcemia and Rocky Mountain spotted fever). A skin rash may be the initial clue to the diagnosis of a febrile illness caused by a broad spectrum of infectious agents—bacteria, viruses, spirochetes, and rickettsiae. These agents can produce a wide variety of skin lesions (Table 22.1), some of which are nonspecific while others, such as erythema migrans, are pathognomonic of the disease, as is the case in Lyme disease. In addition, one agent can produce many types of skin lesions, and many agents may produce similar skin lesions (Table 22.1).

An awareness of the various types of skin lesions associated with infectious agents will aid the physician in the diagnosis and treatment of illnesses caused by those agents. A careful history (Table 22.2), a complete physical exam (Tables 22.3, 22.4), and judicious use of ancillary laboratory tests (Table 22.5) are of paramount importance in the diagnosis of patients with fever and skin rash. Therapy may be presumptive or empiric (as for a patient with shock and purpuric skin lesions), specific (in the case of recognized bacterial infection such as Lyme disease), or supportive (as with most childhood viral exanthems).

Patients with erythema nodosum (Fig. 22.1) (Table 22.6), erythema multiforme (Fig. 22.2) (Table 22.7), and toxic epidermal necrolysis (Fig. 22.3) (Table 22.8) may present with fever and rash. Many infectious agents are associated with illnesses in which urticaria occurs (Fig. 22.4) (Table 22.9). A number of organisms may cause papular, nodular, or ulcerative skin lesions (Table 22.10).

When the physician is confronted with a patient with fever and skin rash, several questions must be answered during the initial assessment:
- Can the patient (or someone with the patient) offer a history?
- Is isolation required (as in the case of a patient with acute meningococcemia)?
- Should the patient be admitted to the intensive care unit (a patient with toxic shock syndrome)?
- Is rapid resuscitation relevant (a hemodynamically unstable patient)?

The tables in this chapter provide a concise and easily referenced overview of the range of infectious agents and drug-related conditions associated with skin manifestations. Additionally, they suggest initial clinical approaches to patients who present with concomitant fever and rash. Much of the material outlined here is handled in greater detail elsewhere in the text.

ANNOTATED BIBLIOGRAPHY

Kingston ME, Mackey D. Skin clues in the diagnosis of life threatening infections. Rev Infect Dis 1986;8:1.

An excellent review of skin lesions seen in several systemic infections. These authors note that skin lesions, an important clue in the diagnosis of septicemia, result from five main processes:
1. Disseminated intravascular coagulation;
2. Direct vascular invasion and occlusion caused by bacteria or fungi;
3. Immune complex formation and vasculitis;
4. Emboli associated with infective endocarditis;
5. Vascular effects due to toxins.

Weber DJ, et al. The acutely ill patient with fever and rash. In: Mandell GL, Douglas RG, Jr, Bennett JE, eds. Principles and practice of infectious diseases. New York: Churchill Livingstone, 1990:479–489.

An excellent review that discusses the diagnosis and differential diagnosis of the acutely ill patient with fever and rash.

Table 22.1. Fever and Rash: Differential Diagnosis Based on Appearance of Rash

Macules, papules, nodules or plaques	Vesicles, bullae, or pustules	Purpuric macules, purpuric papules, or purpuric vesicles	Widespread erythema with or without edema followed by desquamation
Bacterial[a] *Bacillus anthracis* *Borrelia burgdorferi* (Lyme Disease) *Borrelia* sp. (relapsing fever) *Brucella* sp. (brucellosis)[c] Cat-scratch bacillus (*Afipia felis, Rochalimaea henselae* [will be renamed *Bartonella*]) *Chlamydia psittaci* (psittacosis) *Corynebacterium haemolyticum* *Ehrlichia canis* *Erypsipelothrix rhusiopathiae* (erysipeloid) *Francisella tularensis* (tularemia) *Listeria monocytogenes* *Leptospira* sp (leptospirosis)[c] *Mycoplasma pneumoniae* *Neisseria gonorrhoeae* (gonorrhea)[c] *Neisseria meningitidis* (meningococcemia)[c] *Pseudomonas aeruginosa* *Rickettsia akari* (rickettsialpox) *Rickettsia prowazekii* (epidemic/louse-borne typhus) *Rochalimaea quintana* (trench fever) *Rickettsia rickettsii* (RMSF-early lesions)[c,d] *Rickettsia tsutsugamushi* (scrub typhus) *Rickettsia typhi* (endemic/murine typhus) *Salmonella typhi* (typhoid fever)[c] *Spirillum minor* (rat-bite fever) *Staphylococcus aureus* (toxic shock syndrome TSS,[c] staphylococcal scalded skin syndrome [SSSS]) *Streptobacillus moniliformis* (rat-bite fever)[a] Streptococcus Group A (erysipelas, scarlet fever, erythema marginatum, toxic shock-like syndrome) *Treponema pallidum* (secondary syphilis)[c] *Vibrio vulnificus*[c]	*Bacillus anthracis* *Ehrlichia canis* *Listeria monocytogenes* *Mycoplasma pneumoniae* *Neisseria gonorrhoeae* *Neisseria meningitidis* *Pseudomonas aeruginosa* *Rickettsia akari* *Rickettsia rickettsii* *Staphylococcus aureus* (TSS, SSSS) Streptococcus Group A *Treponema pallidum* (secondary syphilis) *Vibrio vulnificus*	Bacteremia[b] *Borrelia* sp. *Clostridium* sp. Infective endocarditis (many organisms) *Haemophilus influenzae* type B *Neisseria gonorrhoeae* (disseminated gonococcal infection)[d] *Neisseria meningitidis* (acute or chronic meningococcemia)[d] *Pseudomonas aeruginosa* *Rickettsia prowazekii* *Rickettsia rickettsii*[d] *Spirillum minor* *Staphylococcus aureus* (bacteremia) *Streptobacillus moniliformis* Streptococcus Group A (toxic shock-like syndrome, scarlet fever) *Streptococcus pneumoniae* (asplenic patient) *Vibrio vulnificus* *Yersinia pestis*	Streptococcus Group A (scarlet fever) *Staphylococcus aureus* (TSS, SSSS)
Fungal *Candida* sp. *Coccidioides immitis* *Cryptococcus neoformans* *Histoplasma capsulatum* Other disseminated deep fungal infections in immunocompromised patients	*Histoplasma capsulatum*		

Table 22.1. *Cont*

Macules, papules, nodules or plaques	Vesicles, bullae, or pustules	Purpuric macules, purpuric papules, or purpuric vesicles	Widespread erythema with or without edema followed by desquamation
Viral			
Adenovirus	Colorado tick fever	Adenovirus (rare)	Kawasaki syndrome (presumed viral)
Arborvirus	Coxsackie A5, 9, 10, 16, B2, 7	Atypical measles	
Atypical measles	Echoviruses	Colorado tick fever	
Colorado tick fever	Eczema herpeticum[e]	Congenital cytomegalovirus	
Coxsackieviruses A and B	Herpes simples (disseminated)[e]	Coxsackie A and B (rare, types A9, B2-5)	
Cytomegalovirus, primary infection	Varicella (chickenpox)[e]	Dengue fever	
Dengue virus	Varicella-zoster (disseminated)[e]	Epstein-Barr virus (rare)	
Epstein-Barr virus, primary infection		Echoviruses (rare, types 3, 4, 9)	
Echoviruses		Rubella	
Hepatitis B (urticaria)[c]		Varicella-zoster virus	
Human herpesvirus 6 (exanthem subitum)		Viral hemorrhagic fevers (many)	
Human immunodeficiency virus (HIV-1)		Yellow fever	
Kawasaki syndrome, presumed viral			
ORF			
Parvovirus B19 (erythema infectiosum, fifth disease)			
Rubella (German measles)[c,d]			
Rubeola (measles)[c]			
Varicella (chickenpox)			
Varicella-zoster (disseminated)			
Protozoal			
Toxoplasma gondii (toxoplasmosis)		*Plasmodium falciparum* (blackwater fever)	
Trichinella spiralis (trichinosis)		*Trichinella spiralis*	
		Toxoplasma gondii	
Noninfectious			
Erythema multiformed	Erythema multiforme bullosum	"Allergic" vasculitis[a,d]	Erythroderma
Systemic lupus erythematosus	Toxic epidermal necrolysis	Cholesterol embolization	Graft-versus-host reaction
Dermatomyositis	Dermatitis from plants	Disseminated intravascular coagulation (purpura fulminans)[b]	Toxic epidermal necrolysis
Gianotti-Crosti syndrome	Drug hypersensitivities	Fat embolism	von Zumbusch pustular psoriasis
Pityriasis rosea (fever rare)		Henoch-Schönlein purpura	Stevens-Johnson syndrome
Sarcoidosis		Immune thrombocytopenia purpura	Drug hypersensitivities
"Serum sickeness"[d]		Wegener's granulomatosis	
Acute febrile neutrophilic dermatosis (Sweet's syndrome)		Drug hypersensitivities	
Juvenile rheumatoid arthritis (Still's disease)			
Inflammatory bowel disease			
Drug hypersensitivities			

Modified from Fitzpatrick TB, et al. Color atlas & synopsis of clinical dermatology—Common and serious diseases. New York: McGraw-Hill, 1992.
[a] specific therapy available
[b] often present as infarcts
[c] reportable disease
[d] may have arthralgia or musculoskeletal pain
[e] umbilicated papule or vesicle a characteristic of these exanthems

Table 22.2. Fever and Rash: History

1. Age of patient?

2. Season of year?

3. Geographic setting?

4. Travel history?

5. Occupational exposures?

6. Recent medications (prescription and nonprescription)?

7. Immunizations?

8. Exposure to sexually transmitted disease?

9. Risk factors for HIV (homosexual orientation, intravenous drug abuse, unprotected casual sex)?

10. Immunologic status:
    Malignancy?
    Cancer chemotherapy?
    Corticosteroids?
    Asplenia?

11. Valvular heart disease?

12. Exposure to febrile or ill individuals in recent past?

13. Exposure to wild or rural habitats and wild animals?

14. Pets?

15. Prior illnesses, including a history of drug and/or antibiotic allergies?

16. Type of prodrome?

17. When did rash start?

18. Duration of rash?

19. Where did it start?

20. Progression: Slow? Rapid?

21. Has the rash changed since onset (evolution)?

22. How has the rash spread?

23. Previous treatment of rash?

Table 22.3. Fever and Rash: Physical Examination

1.	Vital signs	Temperature?
		Pulse?
		Respiration?
		Blood pressure?
2.	General appearance	Alert?
		Acutely ill?
		Chronically ill?
		Toxic?

3. Adenopathy? Location?

4. Conjunctival, mucosal, or genital lesions?

5. Hepatosplenomegaly?

6. Arthritis?

7. Nuchal rigidity or neurological dysfunction?

8.	Features of rash	Type? (See Table 22.1)
		Discrete or uniform?
		Desquamation?
		Configuration of individual lesion:
		Annular? Iris?
		Arrangement of lesion:
		Zosteriform? Linear?
		Distribution pattern:
		Exposed areas? Centripetal or centrifugal?

Table 22.4. Differential Diagnosis of Fever and Rash With Accompanying Signs

Arthritis or arthralgia	Desquamation	Lymphadenopathy	Meningitis

Acute meningococcemia
Disseminated gonococcal
  infection
Erythema marginatum (acute
  rheumatic fever)
Hepatitis B virus, prodromal
  phase
Lyme disease
Parvovirus B19
Rocky Mountain spotted fever
Roseola (especially in adults)
Rubella
Allergic purpura
Reiter's syndrome
Serum sickness
Still's disease
Systemic lupus erythematosus
	Corynebacterium
	  haemolyticum infection
	Kawasaki syndrome
	Measles
	Rocky Mountain spotted fever
	Scarlet fever
	Staphylococcal scalded skin
	  syndrome (SSSS)
	Stevens-Johnson syndrome
	Toxic shock syndrome
	Drug hypersensitivity
	Graft-versus-host reaction
	Toxic epidermal necrolysis
	von Zumbusch pustular
	  psoriasis
		Cervical
		  Kawasaki syndrome
		  Rubella
		  Scarlet fever
		
		Generalized
		  Infectious mononucleosis
		  Secondary syphilis
		  Serum sickness
		  Sarcoidosis
		  Systemic lupus
		    erythematosus
		  Toxoplasmosis
		
		Hilar
		  Atypical measles
		  Sarcoidosis
		
		Local
		  Cat-scratch disease
		  Tularemia
			Acute meningococcemia
			Cryptococcosis
			
			Enterovirus (Coxsackieviruses,
			  echoviruses)
			Leptospirosis
			Lyme disease
			Rocky Mountain spotted fever
			Secondary syphilis

Table 22.4. *Cont.*

Mucosal membrane lesions (enanthems)	Palm-sole involvement	Pulmonary infiltrate	Rash predominantly on extremities	Ulcerative or vesicular stomatitis
Herpes simplex Infectious mononucleosis (palatal petechiae) Measles (Koplick's spots) Varicella-zoster Atypical measles (strawberry tongue) Kawasaki disease (strawberry tongue) Scarlet fever (strawberry tongue) Toxic shock syndrome (strawberry tongue)	Acute meningococcemia Atypical measles (rubeola) Dengue Hand-foot-mouth disease (Coxsackieviruses) Measles Rocky Mountain spotted fever Secondary syphilis *Staphylococcus aureus* endocarditis Drug rash Erythema multiforme Kawasaki syndrome	Atypical measles (rubeola) Coccidioidomycosis Cryptococcosis Histoplasmosis *Mycoplasma pneumoniae* infection North American blastomycosis Rocky Mountain spotted fever Varicella-zoster Fat embolism Psittacosis Sarcoidosis	Brucellosis Disseminated gonococcal infection Ecthyma gangrenosum Erythema nodosum Sporotrichosis (fever rare) Allergic purpura	Hand-foot-mouth disease Herpes simplex Histoplasmosis Secondary syphilis Inflammatory bowel disease Systemic lupus erythematosus

Modified from Hurst, J W, ed. Medicine for the practicing physician. 3rd ed., Boston: Butterworth-Heinemann, 1992:274.

Table 22.5. Fever and Rash: Useful Diagnostic Tests

Test	Application
General: Complete blood count, urinalysis, chemistries	Nonspecific
Aspirate of skin lesion for Gram's stain and culture	Most helpful in pustular or petechial lesions. Positive in up to 50% of acute meningococcemia cases.
Biopsy	Fungal infections, granulomatous disease, vasculitis Immunofluorescence: Rocky Mountain spotted fever (RMSF), systemic lupus erythematosus (SLE)
Cultures of other sites Blood Throat/rectal swab Throat, rectum, urethra, cervix, joint	 All cases of bacteremia and some cases of fungemia Viral infections Disseminated gonococcal infection
Serologic tests	Streptococcal and rickettsial infections, spirochetal infections (syphilis, leptospirosis, Lyme disease), mycoplasma, fungal infections (cryptococcosis, coccidioidomycosis), viral infections (hepatitis B, Epstein-Barr virus, cytomegalovirus, measles, adenovirus, trichinosis, SLE)
Wright or Giemsa stain of vesicular fluid	Herpesvirus infections (multinucleated giant cells)

Modified from Stein JH, ed. Internal medicine. 4th ed., St. Louis: Mosby, 1994: 1854.

Table 22.6. Causes of Erythema Nodosum

Infectious	Noninfectious
Streptococcus pyogenes	Drug reactions
Mycobacterium tuberculosis	Oral contraceptives
Mycobacterium leprae	Antibiotics (especially
Atypical mycobacteria	sulfonamides)
Systemic fungal infections	Endocrine/hormonal conditions
Coccidioides immitis	Pregnancy
Histoplasma capsulatum	Thyroid disorders
North American blastomycosis	Idiopathic (40%)
Miscellaneous	Inflammatory and autoimmune
Cat-scratch disease	disorders
Chlamydia (lymphogranuloma	Crohn's disease
venerum, psittacosis)	Ulcerative colitis
Enteric pathogens *(Yersinia,*	Systemic lupus erythematosus
Campylobacter, Salmonella)	Malignancy
Parasites (e.g., amebiasis,	Leukemia
giardiasis)	Lymphoma
Rickettsiae	Sarcoidosis
Spirochetes (e.g., syphilis)	
Viruses (e.g., hepatitis B)	

Modified from Fox MD, Schwartz RA. Erythema nodosum. Am Fam Phys 1992; 46:821.

Table 22.7. Causes of Erythema Multiforme[a]

Infections	Herpes simplex 1 and 2
	Epstein-Barr virus
	Hemolytic streptococci
	Proteus sp.
	Salmonella sp.
	Staphylococcus sp.
	Mycobacterium tuberculosis
	Francisella tularensis
	Vibrio parahaemolyticus
	Yersinia sp
	Mycoplasma pneumoniae
	Histoplasma capsulatum
Drugs	Allopurinol
	Antituberculous agents
	Barbiturates
	Carbamazepine
	Phenytoin
	NSAIDs
	Sulfonamides
	Oral hypoglycemic agents
Physical Factors	Sunlight
	X-ray therapy
Endocrine Factors	Pregnancy
Contact Reactions	*Tadania ignis* (fire sponge)
Idiopathic	>50%

Modified from Fitzpatrick TB, et al. eds. Dermatology in general medicine. New York: McGraw-Hill, 1993.

Table 22.8. Causes of Toxic Epidermal Necrolysis (TEN)

Drugs	Sulfonamides[a] NSAIDs (esp. phenylbutazone)[a] Antibiotics (esp. tetracyclines and penicillin)[a] Anticonvulsants[a] Barbiturates[a] Allopurinol[a] Alka-seltzer® Amiodarone Antipyrine Brompheniramine Chlorpromazine Dapsone Ethambutol Fansidar Fenoprofen Gold Griseofulvin Ipecac Isoniazid Pentamidine Phenolphthalein Quinine Streptomycin Tolbutamide Trimethoprim
Vaccinations	BCG Diphtheria toxoid Measles Poliomyelitis Tetanus antitoxin
Infections	Measles virus Varicella-zoster virus Herpes simplex *Escherichia coli* (septicemia) Aspergillosis (pulmonary)
Neoplasia	Hodgkin's disease Nonhodgkin's lymphoma Leukemia
Miscellaneous	Graft-versus-host reaction Idiopathic

Modified from Rohrer TE, Ahmed AR. Toxic epidermal necrolysis. Int J Dermatol 1991; 30:457.
[a] Drugs most commonly associated with toxic epidermal necrolysis

Table 22.9. Infectious Agents Associated with Illnesses in Which Urticaria Occurs

Infectious Agent	Illness
Bedbugs, kissing bugs, ants, fleas, flies, and mosquitoes	Bites and stings
Coxiella burnetii	Q Fever
Coxsackieviruses A9, A16, B4, B5	Rash
Echinococcus sp	Echinococcosis
Echovirus	Rash
Epstein-Barr virus	Infectious mononucleosis
Entamoeba histolytica	Amebiasis
Enterobius vermicularis	Pinworm infestation
Giardia lambdia	Giardiasis
Hepatitis B virus	Hepatitis
Mumps virus	Mumps
Mycoplasma pneumoniae	*Pneumonia*
Necator americanus	Hookworm disease
Neisseria meningitidis	Meningococcemia
Mites	Mite bites
Plasmodium sp	Malaria
Pediculus humanus	Pediculosis
Sarcoptes scabiei	Scabies
Schistosoma sp	Schistosomiasis
Shigella sonnei	Shigellosis
Trichinella spiralis	Trichinosis
Trichobilharzia sp	Swimmer's itch; collector's itch
Trichomonas vaginalis	Vulvovaginitis
Trombicula irritans	Chigger bites
Wuchereria bancrofti	Filariasis
Yersinia enterocolitica	Yersiniosis

Modified from Feigin RD, Cherry JD, eds. Textbook of pediatric infectious diseases. 3rd ed., Vol. 1, Philadelphia; WB Saunders, 1992; 771.

Table 22.10. Infectious Agents Associated with Papular, Nodular, and Ulcerative Lesions

Agent	Papular	Nodular	Ulcerative	Illness
Atypical mycobacteria			X	Other skin lesions
Blastomyces dermatitidis		X	X	Blastomycosis
Bartonella bacilliformis		X		Bartonellosis
Calymmatobacterium granulomatis		X	X	Granuloma inguinale
Candida albicans		X		Systemic candidiasis
Cimex lectularius	X			Bedbug bites
Francisella tularensis			X	Tularemia
Fleas	X			Flea bites
Flies and mosquitoes	X			Fly and mosquito bites
Haemophilus ducreyi			X	Chancroid
Hepatitis B virus	X			Gianotti-Crosti syndrome
Leishmania braziliensis and *mexicana*	X		X	American cutaneous leishmaniasis
Leishmania tropica		X	X	Oriental sore
Loxosceles reclusus			X	Recluse spider bite
Molluscum contagiosum virus	X	X		Molluscum contagiosum
Mycobacterium leprae		X		Leprosy
Mycobacterium tuberculosis		X		Lupus vulgaris
Mycobacterium tuberculosis			X	Papulonecrotic tuberculids
Necator americanus	X			Hookworm disease
Onchocerca volvulus	X			Onchocerciasis
Orf virus		X		Ecthyma contagiosum
Mites	X			Mite bites
Paravaccinia virus		X		Milker's nodules
Pseudomonas aeruginosa			X	Ecthyma gangrenosa
Pseudomonas aeruginosa	X			Folliculitis
Sarcoptes scabiei	X			Scabies
Solenopsis saevissima	X	X		Fire ant bites
Schistosoma sp	X			Schistosomiasis
Sporothrix schenckii			X	Sporotrichosis
Ticks			X	Tick bites
Triatoma sanguisuga	X	X		Kissing bug bites
Treponema pallidum			X	Chancre
Treponema pertenue	X		X	Yaws
Trombicula irritans	X			Chigger bites
Trypanosoma sp		X		Trypanosomiasis
Wart virus	X	X		Warts

Modified from Feigin RD, Cherry JD, eds. Textbook of pediatric infectious diseases. 3rd ed. Vol. 1, Philadelphia: WB Saunders, 1992: 771.

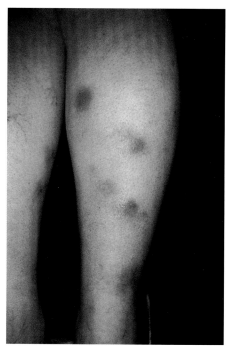

Figure 22.1.   Erythema nodosum. Erythematous-to-pigmented nodules of the legs. (Courtesy of Dr. Lee T. Nesbitt, Jr.)

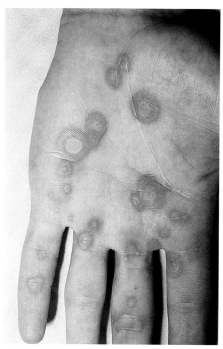

Figure 22.2.   Erythema multiforme. Target lesions of the palm with beginning central vesicle. (Courtesy of Dr. Lee T. Nesbitt, Jr.)

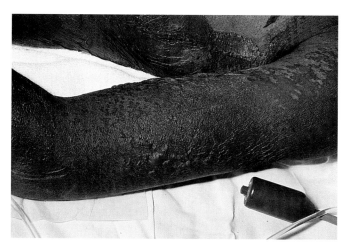

Figure 22.3.   Toxic epidermal necrolysis. Large, confluent, vesicular and necrotic areas of the arm and trunk showing peeling away of skin with underlying erythema. (Courtesy of Dr. Lee T. Nesbitt, Jr.)

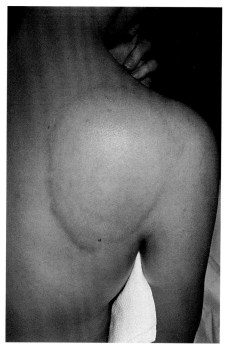

Figure 22.4.   Giant urticaria. Very large, erythematous annular lesion of the shoulder with central clearing. Patient had several large lesions of this type simulating erythema migrans. (Courtesy of Dr. Lee T. Nesbitt, Jr.)

INDEX

Page numbers followed by *t* and *f* indicate tables and figures, respectively.
Page numbers followed by *b* indicate citations in the Annotated Bibliography.

characteristics of, 181
culture, 256 *t*
infection, 12 *f*, 201. *See also* Herpes zoster;
    Varicella
    disseminated, 298 *t*
    in HIV-infected (AIDS) patient, 276–277,
        287 *f*–288 *f*
    in immunocompromised host, 259–261, 269
        f–270 *f*
Variola, 204–205
Vascular damage
    bacteria-induced, 39
    immune-mediated, 39
Vasculitis, 19 *t*
    cutaneous, differential diagnosis of, 43
    differential diagnosis of, 40
    herpesvirus, histopathology of, 26 *f*
    of rickettsioses, 120
    and thrombosis, 19 *t*
Venom. *See also* Hymenoptera venom
    caterpillar, 239
    fire ant, 237
    spider, 240
Verruca plana, in HIV-infected (AIDS) patient,
        288 *f*
Verruca vulgaris, 14 *t*, 211 *f*–212 *f*. *See also*
        Wart(s), common
    diagnosis of, 133 *t*
    in HIV-infected (AIDS) patient, 288 *f*
    in immunocompromised host, 260, 270 *f*
Vesicle(s), 3, 9 *f*
    differential diagnosis based on, 297 *t*–298 *t*
    of disseminated gonococcal infection, 42
    in enteroviral infections, 186, 186 *t*
    in HIV-infected (AIDS) patient, differential
        diagnosis of, 272 *t*
    in *Pseudomonas aeruginosa* bacteremia, 43
    purpuric, differential diagnosis based on,
        297 *t*–298 *t*
Vesicular reaction, 16, 16 *t*, 24 *f*
Vesiculopustules, differential diagnosis of, 181,
        181 *t*
Vespidae, 236
Vibrio, infections, 50–51
    clinical course of, 51
    clinical features of, 50–51, 57 *f*
    diagnosis of, 51
    differential diagnosis of, 51
    histology of, 50–51
    pathogenesis of, 50
    treatment of, 51
Vibrio alginolyticus, infections, 50
Vibrio damsela, infections, 50

Vibrio parahaemolyticus, infections, 50
Vibrio vulnificus, 19 *t*–20 *t*, 70 *b*, 297 *t*
    infections, 50–51
        clinical course of, 51
        clinical features of, 50–51, 57 *f*
        diagnosis of, 51
        differential diagnosis of, 51
        pathogenesis of, 50
        treatment of, 51
    morphology, in histological sections, 21 *t*
    necrotizing fasciitis caused by, 65
    necrotizing infection, 68
Vidarabine, for varicella-zoster virus, in immuno-
        compromised host, 261
Vincristine, for Kaposi's sarcoma, in HIV-infect-
        ed (AIDS) patient, 276
Viral encephalitis, transmission, 236 *t*
Viral exanthems, 16, 17 *t*, 181–199, 194 *b*
Viral infection(s), 194 *b*, 200–213. *See also spe-
        cific virus*
    in HIV-infected (AIDS) patient, 276–278
    in immunocompromised host, 254 *t*–255 *t*,
        259–261
    insect vectors, 236 *t*–237 *t*
    rash of, differential diagnosis based on, 298 *t*
Virus
    culture, 256 *t*
    morphology, in histological sections, 21 *t*
Visceral larva migrans, 223
von Zumbusch pustular psoriasis, differential
        diagnosis of, 298 *t*
Vulvovaginitis, candidal
    clinical features of, 160
    in HIV-infected (AIDS) patient, 281
VZV. *See* Varicella-zoster virus

Walking dandruff, 242
Wangiella dermatitidis, 17 *t*
Warble(s), botfly, 243, 253 *f*
Wart(s), 20 *b*. *See also* Human papillomavirus;
        Verruca vulgaris
    clinical features of, 203, 211 *f*–212 *f*
    common, 203, 211 *f*–212 *f*
    cutaneous manifestations of, 304 *t*
    diagnosis of, 203
    differential diagnosis of, 203
    filiform, 203
    flat, 203
    genital, 100–101, 111 *f*, 203. *See also*
        Condylomata acuminata
        malignant transformation, 100, 111 *f*, 203,
            206 *b*

in immunocompromised host, 203
periungual, 211 *f*
plantar, 203
treatment of, 203
Wasp(s), stings, 236–237
Wegener's granulomatosis, differential diagnosis
        of, 298 *t*
Weil-Felix reaction, in rickettsioses, 121–122
Weil's disease, 83, 89 *f*
Western equine encephalitis, transmission, 237 *t*
Wheal(s), 3
Wiskott-Aldrich syndrome, herpes infection in,
        201
Wuchereria bancrofti, 221, 232 *f*

Xenopsylla cheopis, disease transmission by,
        122–123, 236 *t*, 239

Yaws, cutaneous manifestations of, 304 *t*
Yeast(s), dermatopathologic characteristics of,
        256 *t*
Yellow fever, 205–206
    differential diagnosis of, 298 *t*
    transmission, 237 *t*, 238
Yersinia enterocolitica, 51
    bacteremia, cutaneous manifestations, 43
Yersinia pestis, 78–79, 297 *t*
    bacteremia, cutaneous manifestations, 43
    infection. *See* Plague

Zidovudine (Azidothymidine; AZT; ZDV)
    adverse effects of, in HIV-infected (AIDS)
        patient, 283
    for Epstein-Barr virus infection, 204
Zoonoses. *See also* Anthrax; Brucellosis; Cat-
        scratch disease; Chagas disease;
        Erysipeloid; Glanders; Leptospirosis;
        Listeriosis; Melioidosis; *Pasteurella
        multocida* infection; Plague; Rat-bite
        fever; Tularemia
    skin signs of, 76–90
Zosteriform eruptions, in enteroviral infections,
        186, 186 *t*
Zosteriform grouping, 4–5, 13 *f*
Zoster immune globulin, for HIV-infected
        (AIDS) patient, 276
Zygomycetes, 19 *t*–20 *t*
    dermatopathologic characteristics of, 256 *t*
    morphology, in histological sections, 22 *t*
Zygomycosis, 19 *t*